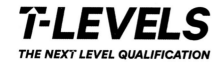

CW01024501

HEALTH T LEVEL: SUPPORTING THE ADULT NURSING TEAM

OCCUPATIONAL SPECIALISM

Alison Burton

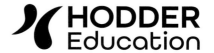

This resource has been endorsed by national awarding organisation, NCFE. This means that NCFE has reviewed them and agreed that they meet the necessary endorsement criteria.

Whilst NCFE has exercised reasonable care and skill in endorsing this resource, we make no representation, express or implied, with regard to the continued accuracy of the information contained in this resource. NCFE does not accept any legal responsibility or liability for any errors or omissions from the resource or the consequences thereof.

'T-LEVELS' is a registered trade mark of the Department for Education.

'T Level' is a registered trade mark of the Institute for Apprenticeships and Technical Education. The T Level Technical Qualification is a qualification approved and managed by the Institute for Apprenticeships and Technical Education.

Although every effort has been made to ensure that website addresses are correct at time of going to press, Hodder Education cannot be held responsible for the content of any website mentioned in this book. It is sometimes possible to find a relocated web page by typing in the address of the home page for a website in the URL window of your browser.

Hachette UK's policy is to use papers that are natural, renewable and recyclable products and made from wood grown in well-managed forests and other controlled sources. The logging and manufacturing processes are expected to conform to the environmental regulations of the country of origin.

To order, please visit www.hoddereducation.com or contact Customer Service at education@hachette.co.uk / +44 (0)1235 827827.

ISBN: 978 1 0360 0568 9

© Alison Burton 2024

First published in 2024 by
Hodder Education
An Hachette UK Company
Carmelite House
50 Victoria Embankment
London EC4Y 0DZ

www.hoddereducation.com

Impression number 10 9 8 7 6 5 4 3 2 1

Year   2028 2027 2026 2025 2024

All rights reserved. Apart from any use permitted under UK copyright law, no part of this publication may be reproduced or transmitted in any form or by any means, electronic or mechanical, including photocopying and recording, or held within any information storage and retrieval system, without permission in writing from the publisher or under licence from the Copyright Licensing Agency Limited. Further details of such licences (for reprographic reproduction) may be obtained from the Copyright Licensing Agency Limited, www.cla.co.uk

Cover photo © Drazen - stock.adobe.com

Illustrations by Barking Dog Art, Integra Software Services Pvt. Ltd and Aptara, Inc.

Typeset in India by Aptara, Inc.

Printed and bound in Great Britain by Bell and Bain Ltd, Glasgow

A catalogue record for this title is available from the British Library.

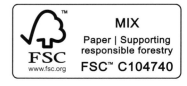

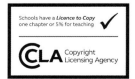

Contents

Supporting Healthcare

Supporting the Adult Nursing Team

Assessment

Answers can be found online at: https://www.hoddereducation.com/answers-and-extras

Acknowledgements

I shall start by thanking the best husband ever, Dave, for the endless cups of tea and support whilst writing – I am blessed. My gratitude goes to my children and my dad who inspire me to be the best I can be. Thanks also to Tola for embarking on the T-Level Health journey with me – the dream team; I learned a lot. And finally, thank you to my publishing team, I am grateful for their guidance and hard work.

About the author

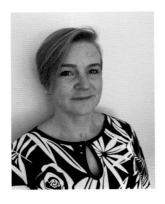

Raised in Leicestershire, the daughter of a farmer who did his best as a single parent, Alison Burton was not the easiest teenager. From a very early start, Alison lacked safety and security, leading to a mistrust of adults. This was then restored by a primary school teacher, Mrs. Chisholm. A secondary school teacher dedicated her lunchtimes to support Alison with improving behaviour and was a significant influence, allowing her to successfully gain qualifications needed to access the next level of education. Time spent in an adolescent mental health unit, a diagnosis of bipolar and the influence of these two amazing teachers laid the foundations of her desire to work with young people.

After starting a family and having a son, Andrew, and a daughter, Holly, she became the youngest foster carer in Leicestershire at just 24 and fostered 50 children over an 18-year period. Alongside this, Alison ran the local youth club, childminded, qualified as a teacher and added daughter Georgina into the mix. With a teaching career of 25 years, Alison started a Facebook group for Health & Social Care teachers during the first Covid lockdown, when she stopped teaching; the group hit 5,000 members in late 2023. Alison is happiest when supporting others; however, behind this inspirational woman there is a husband, Dave, who is her biggest cheerleader! Blessed with friends to guide her, Alison took a leap of faith on her journey as an author, and this is her first book.

Photo credits

p.1 © zinkevych/stock.adobe.com; Fig. 1.4 © Nadzeya/stock.adobe.com; Fig. 1.7 © Reproduced from: Royal College of Physicians. *National Early Warning Score (NEWS) 2: Standardising the assessment of acute-illness severity in the NHS.* Updated report of a working party. London: RCP, 2017. Fig. 1.9 © LIGHTFIELD STUDIOS/stock.adobe.com; Fig. 1.10 © nata-lunata/Shutterstock; Fig. 1.11 © pang_oasis/Shutterstock; Fig. 1.12 © Sherry Young/stock.adobe.com; Fig. 1.13 © WESTOCK/stock.adobe.com; Fig. 1.14 © Government of South Australia; Fig. 1.16 © Motortion Films/Shutterstock; Fig 1.19 © auremar/stock.adobe.com; p.48 © WavebreakMediaMicro/stock.adobe.com; Fig. 2.1 © Edward G. Malindine/Stringer/Getty Images; Fig. 2.3 © JPC-PROD/Shutterstock; Fig. 2.4 © JYFotoStock/stock.adobe.com; Fig. 2.5 © tungphoto/stock.adobe.com; Fig. 2.8 © Flamingo Images/stock.adobe.com; Fig. 2.10 © nimito/stock.adobe.com; p.81 © zinkevych/stock.adobe.com; Fig. 3.1 © An-Maler/stock.adobe.com; Fig. 3.2 © JYFotoStock/stock.adobe.com; Fig. 3.3 © whilerests/stock.adobe.com; Fig. 3.5 © Brian Jackson/stock.adobe.com; Fig. 3.6 © Supak/stock.adobe.com; Fig. 3.7 © steheap/stock.adobe.com; Fig. 3.8 © thephotoholic/stock.adobe.com; Fig. 3.9 & 3.10 © Reproduced from: Royal College of Physicians. *National Early Warning Score (NEWS) 2: Standardising the assessment of acute-illness severity in the NHS.* Updated report of a working party. London: RCP, 2017; Fig. 3.11 © Proxima Studio/stock.adobe.com; Fig. 3.12 © Siberian Art/stock.adobe.com; p.97 © Bangkok Click studio/stock.adobe.com; Fig. 4.1 © themorningglory/stock.adobe.com; Fig. 4.2 © ALAN EDWARDS/Alamy Stock Photo; Fig. 4.4 © samunela/stock.adobe.com; Fig. 4.5 © s4svisuals/stock.adobe.com; Fig. 4.7 © Mouth Care Matters, Health Education England, 2018; Fig. 4.10 © LIGHTFIELD STUDIOS/stock.adobe.com; Fig. 4.11 © sabelskaya/stock.adobe.com; Fig. 4.12a & 4.12b © Reproduced with kind permission of BAPEN; Fig. 4.14 © inspiring.team/stock.adobe.com; Fig. 4.18 © Sebastian Kaulitzki/stock.adobe.com; Fig. 4.20 © lllonajalll/stock.adobe.com; Fig. 4.21 © John/stock.adobe.com; p.142 © Drazen/stock.adobe.com; Fig. 5.1 © Pepermpron/stock.adobe.com; Fig. 5.2 Crown Copyright/OHID in association with the Welsh government, Food Standards Scotland and the Food Standards Agency in Northern Ireland; Fig. 5.3 © sayukichi/Shutterstock; Fig. 5.4 © Mouth Care Matters, Health Education England, 2019; Fig. 5.5 © Gorodenkoff/Shutterstock; Fig. 5.6 © May Thawtar Aung/Shutterstock; Fig. 5.7 © Mathinee srichomthong/Shutterstock; Fig. 5.9 © DC Studio/stock.adobe.com; p.177 © TY Lim/Shutterstock; Fig. 6.4 *l* © Geoff Oliver / Alamy Stock Photo; *r* © SCIENCE PHOTO LIBRARY; Fig. 6.5 © inspiring.team/stock.adobe.com; Fig. 6.6 *l* © Casa nayafana/Shutterstock; *r* © Arthit Premprayot/Shutterstock; Fig. 6.7 ©rob9000/Shutterstock

Text acknowledgements

pp.182–3 The Braden Scale II © 2021 Health Sense Ai. All rights reserved. All copyrights and trademarks are the property of Health Sense Ai or their respective owners or assigns.

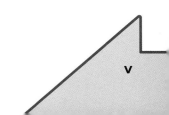

Guide to the book

Content warning

Please be advised that the T Level Technical Qualification in Health (Supporting the Adult Nursing Team Occupational Specialism) does cover topics that some learners may find upsetting. This textbook therefore includes references to domestic abuse, female genital mutilation, self-harm, suicidal feelings and disorders due to mental ill health, within the context of healthcare practice. If you have been affected by any of the topics covered in this book, do reach out to trusted support.

Learning outcomes

Core knowledge outcomes that you must understand and learn. These are presented at the start of every chapter.

Skills outcomes

Core knowledge skills you must understand and practise. These are presented at the start of every chapter.

Key term

Definitions to help you understand important terms.

Reflect

Tasks and questions providing an opportunity to reflect on the knowledge learned.

Test yourself

A knowledge consolidation feature containing short questions and tasks to aid understanding and guide you to think about a topic in detail.

Research

Research-based activities – either stretch and challenge activities, enabling you to go beyond the course, or industry placement-based activities, encouraging you to discover more about your placement.

Practice point

Helpful tips and guidance to help develop professional skills during the industry placement.

Case study

Placing knowledge into a fictionalised, real-life context. Useful to introduce problem solving and dilemmas.

Health and safety

Important points to ensure safety in the workplace.

Assessment practice

Core content containing knowledge-based practice questions at the end of each chapter.

Answers can be found online at: www.hoddereducation.com/answers-and-extras

Healthcare PO1: Assisting with an individual's overall care and needs to ensure comfort and wellbeing

Physical and mental health care is provided by practitioners who are experts in their field. This work is supported by healthcare practitioners who:

▶ meet an individual's needs as identified in a care plan
▶ monitor an individual's signs or symptoms.

The Roper–Logan–Tierney care planning model is one example of a type of nursing model used in healthcare. This model offers an holistic approach that co-ordinates ongoing healthcare intervention and monitors and evaluates the effectiveness of treatment. It ensures that patients receiving healthcare are encouraged to maintain their independence, while having their health needs met.

All nursing tasks must:

▶ meet the rigorous standards of care in the UK
▶ provide a person-centred care package for each patient.

Learning outcomes

The core knowledge outcomes that you must understand and learn:

K1.1 the implications of health and safety regulations, their influence on practice and how they promote person-centred care within the supporting healthcare role

K1.2 the requirements for safeguarding individuals and their wider family/carers and promoting principles to others in practice

K1.3 the requirements for following a duty of care and duty of candour within the scope of the supporting healthcare role

K1.4 required standards, codes of conduct and health and safety including risk assessment relevant to your role in supporting healthcare

K1.5 how to respond to incidents and emergencies relevant to your role in supporting healthcare

K1.6 how to use a range of techniques for infection prevention and control

K1.7 how current best practice and agreed ways of working support healthcare needs

K1.8 how to support individuals' care needs, ensuring privacy and dignity is maintained while recognising the importance of personal health and wellbeing

K1.9 how to interpret individual care plans in order to support a person's health, comfort and wellbeing

K1.10 how to recognise indicators of good physical and mental health

K1.11 the importance of fluids, nutrition and food safety when providing overall care

K1.12 how to recognise the signs and symptoms of a person who is experiencing pain and discomfort and/or whose health and wellbeing is deteriorating

K1.13 how and why to report changes and deterioration when supporting individuals

K1.14 how to safely move and handle people when supporting their care needs using appropriate moving and handling aids

K1.15 the main types of mental ill health and their impact on people's lives

K1.16 how to recognise indicators and limitations in mental capacity and how to respond appropriately in line with local policies and procedures

K1.17 the importance of early diagnosis in relation to cognitive issues

K1.18 the possible signs of mental ill health

K1.19 the possible signs of learning disability

K1.20 factors that may be mistaken for mental ill health

K1.21 how changes in cognition can impact health and wellbeing

K1.22 how to report changes and deterioration in cognition while following appropriate procedures

K1.23 how to support others to report changes and deterioration in cognition

K1.24 how to escalate changes and deterioration in cognition.

Healthcare PO1: Assisting with an individual's overall care and needs to ensure comfort and wellbeing

Skills outcomes

You must understand and practise the following core skills and be able to:

S1.25 safeguard individuals and their wider family/carers if required and promote principles to others in practice

S1.26 implement a duty of care and candour when working with individuals and their families/carers, speaking clearly and confidently using appropriate tone and register that reflects audience and purpose

S1.27 follow all required standards, codes of conduct and health and safety requirements/legislation, including risk assessment, in the healthcare environment

S1.28 maintain a safe and healthy working environment, take appropriate action in response to incidents or emergencies, following local guidelines

S1.29 use a range of techniques for infection prevention and control (for example waste management, spillage, handwashing, use of PPE) and have a thorough understanding of the context of the work

S1.30 provide person-centred care and support to individuals, carers and relevant others

S1.31 provide an effective clinical environment, taking safety into consideration, and promote a good experience for the individual

S1.32 move and handle individuals safely when assisting them with their care needs, using appropriate moving and handling aids

S1.33 assist with individuals' overall comfort and wellbeing

S1.34 recognise issues and deterioration in mental and physical health, report and respond appropriately, supporting others to do so

S1.35 recognise and respond to signs of pain and discomfort in the individual

S1.36 recognise limitations in mental capacity and respond appropriately

S1.37 use appropriate techniques and PPE to ensure effective infection prevention and control in the healthcare environment

S1.38 contribute, record and follow information in care plans

S1.39 promote physical health and mental wellbeing through providing opportunistic advice within scope of role, knowledge and responsibilities.

Working in a person-centred way

Person-centred care is the foundation of good practice. It begins with a positive working partnership between an individual, their informal carers (such as family) and healthcare professionals.

Care needs should be agreed through consultation with all parties and by making decisions that are in the best interest of the person who requires support. Services and professionals should develop a **holistic** care plan that empowers and respects the individual and includes the informal care provided by loved ones.

K1.1 The implications of health and safety regulations, their influence on practice and how they promote person-centred care within the supporting healthcare role

Care planning

The role of the healthcare professional is to contribute to and develop the most suitable care plan to meet the holistic needs of an **individual**.

The **Roper–Logan–Tierney Model** was developed by Nancy Roper, Winifred Logan and Alison Tierney in 1980 and was last edited in 2020. It is most commonly used in nursing and analyses an individual's needs and capabilities in terms of performing everyday tasks. Ideally, these 'activities of daily living' (ADLs) should be carried out independently by the individual or with the least amount of external intervention possible.

The theory is a **biopsychosocial** model and takes into account:

▶ the physical needs of the **patient**, service user, resident or client
▶ the socio-economic and environmental circumstances at their home
▶ the patient's current mental wellbeing.

A patient's capabilities for self-care are measured on a continuum, with 'dependent' and 'independent' at each end of a sliding scale, as shown in Figure 1.1.

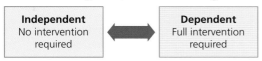

Independent	Dependent
No intervention required	Full intervention required

▲ Figure 1.1 The self-care continuum

The Roper–Logan–Tierney Model lists 12 ADLs, as shown in Figure 1.2.

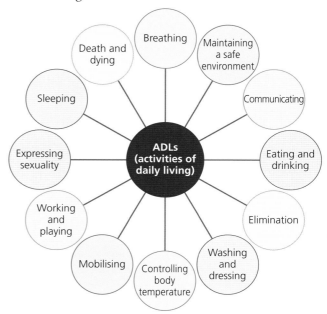

▲ Figure 1.2 The 12 ADLs in the Roper–Logan– Tierney Model

Key terms

Holistic: a way of approaching the delivery of healthcare that considers the whole person, not just the part that requires physical treatment. It also takes into account an individual's intellectual, emotional and social needs.

Individual: a person who may require care, assessment, investigation, support or treatment.

Roper–Logan–Tierney Model: it defines what living means and the daily tasks a person needs to perform. It provides a framework to assess a patient's ability to carry out these tasks independently.

Biopsychosocial: involving the interaction of biological, psychological and social factors.

Patient: a person receiving care, support or treatment.

Care planning assessments analyse an individual's physical impairments and their ability to perform and manage a wide range of ADLs, such as:

▶ getting out of bed
▶ washing themselves
▶ getting dressed
▶ other aspects of life, such as shopping and eating or adequate and appropriate sleep patterns.

Assessments might also be carried out for reasons such as:

▶ to see how medication might reduce a high temperature – a measurement is taken as a baseline assessment, medication is then given, the individual's temperature is monitored and medication is altered until the correct core temperature is reached
▶ to enable a package of interventions and support to be agreed – observation of an individual's ability to carry out ADLs is carried out first.

Care planning should also explore an individual's outlook motivation and **emotional intelligence**, and it should take into account their history and home environment. For example:

▶ Does their **family** provide informal care?
▶ Does the individual have the means to provide essential resources so they can live comfortably?

A person-centred approach seeks to maintain an individual's rights. For this reason, an assessment must include the patient's opinions, wishes and goals, as empowerment is the ultimate objective. A vulnerable individual might reject support and show symptoms of depression, such as self-neglect, disregard for personal hygiene, not eating, and poor physical and mental wellbeing.

Communication

In healthcare, there are frequent verbal, recorded and electronic communications between patients and the various professionals who provide an **integrated service** and work together as a **multidisciplinary team (MDT)**.

The patient has a right to privacy, and their confidentiality must be maintained in line with the Data Protection Act 2018, also referred to as UK GDPR. An individual's emotional security and safety depend on healthcare communications where:

▶ control measures are implemented
▶ information is shared only on a need-to-know basis
▶ records are stored securely.

Failure to comply with legislation covering communications standards in healthcare can have serious implications, from affecting patients' wellbeing to legal action being taken against the **practitioner** or the organisation within which they work. It is good practice to seek guidance when sharing any personal details, even between multidisciplinary professionals; this respects the individual and is in accordance with delivering **person-centred care**.

Duty of care

Healthcare professionals have a duty of care in terms of taking all necessary and appropriate precautions to protect the physical and mental wellbeing of individuals. This is a legal obligation and must be in the best interest of the patient. For example, a check should be in place to monitor a person's capabilities in terms of managing their medication, ensuring they take the right dose at the right time. Once it is clear that this can be carried out independently, this ADL will no longer need supervision or support unless the circumstances change, such as a deterioration in the person's condition.

Key terms

Emotional intelligence: an individual's ability to manage their own emotions and to understand the emotions of the people they come into contact with.

Family: the people identified by an individual as significant and important to them.

Integrated service: various health services collaborating as a multidisciplinary team, enabling them to offer responsive, easily accessible services that meet the population's health needs.

Multidisciplinary team (MDT): a group of professionals from one or more clinical disciplines collaborating to provide the appropriate medical treatment for an individual.

Practitioner: a person appropriately qualified in the practice of an occupation, for example a maternity support worker or a midwife. Practitioners may be registered or unregistered.

Person-centred care: focusing care on the needs, values and preferences of the individual, and ensuring any clinical decisions are guided by these needs, values and preferences.

Risk assessment

Health and safety regulations require a risk assessment to be completed, to evaluate the likelihood of harm when an individual is preparing for or completing a specific task independently. During such assessments, particular attention should be paid to ensuring the safe use of equipment such as mobility aids.

Recorded risk assessments need to be reviewed regularly, as a patient's situation either improves or deteriorates, or if safety concerns have been raised.

Risk assessments must also be carried out for the staff supporting an individual. They must meet the regulations set out in the Management of Health and Safety at Work Regulations 1999. Risk control measures may require that support be given during an activity and will therefore examine the role of the healthcare worker. For example:

▶ coaching a patient in using a bed grab handle
▶ working with a patient with a brain injury who has outbursts of aggression.

In such cases, two members of staff might be required for specific moving and handling tasks, or those with specialist training in therapeutic holding may be required to manage potential aggression and reduce the risk of harm to the practitioners.

The specifics around transporting or escorting patients to appointments, domiciliary (home) welfare visits and the provision of an advocacy service must all be recorded in a risk assessment. Advance care planning looks at preferences and priorities for future care.

Regulatory bodies

In healthcare, there are different levels of regulatory bodies such as:

▶ the Nursing and Midwifery Council (NMC)
▶ the National Health Service (NHS) England
▶ the Care Inspectorate (CI) in Scotland
▶ the Regulation and Quality Improvement Authority (RQIA) in Northern Ireland
▶ the Healthcare Inspectorate Wales (HIW)
▶ the Care Quality Commission (CQC)
▶ the Health and Safety Executive (HSE).

While these bodies have standardised guidelines for healthcare provision, each acts independently to provide care that is safe and of a high quality, always striving to improve these standards. You are probably aware of these organisations and the role they play in overseeing safe, quality practice when delivering person-centred care.

In the UK, healthcare provision is devolved to the four home nations: England, Scotland, Northern Ireland and Wales.

NHS England

In England, the CQC is independent from the government. It regulates and monitors standards in the statutory public and private sectors and provides guidelines. A statutory service is a public service paid for by taxpayers, which is free to use by everyone. Services in the private healthcare sector are paid for by the individual and often offer better facilities with no waiting times. All services, however, are regulated by the CQC in exactly the same way.

The CQC's five standards are:
1 Safe
2 Effective
3 Caring
4 Responsive
5 Well-led.

Services provided by the CQC include care home and hospital inspections. During these:

▶ nursing practices and the delivery of quality clinical skills will be observed
▶ management systems and effectiveness will be checked.

Following an inspection, the CQC will award a grade for each service and publish a report on its findings on its website that can be accessed by the public.

NHS Scotland

There are two separate regulating organisations in Scotland.

The CI regulates individual care services, such as GPs and hospitals. Its work is based on five principles:
1 Dignity and respect
2 Compassion
3 Be included
4 Responsive care and support
5 Wellbeing.

Leadership is regulated by a separate organisation called **Healthcare Improvement**.

As with the CQC in England, all services are inspected. A report will be produced that lists where areas of care are being well provided and also highlights concerns where identified and provides instructions on how to rectify these within a certain timeframe. The purpose is to monitor standards and continuously improve services.

Northern Ireland

In Northern Ireland, the NHS is referred to as **Health and Social Care (HSC)**.

The RQIA inspects and monitors both healthcare and social care provision against four key domains:
- ▶ Safe
- ▶ Effective
- ▶ Compassionate care
- ▶ Leadership.

NHS Wales

The HIW is an independent organisation that regulates healthcare in Wales to ensure that safe, high standards are maintained.

The HIW aims to be a trusted organisation that works to improve healthcare services. Its four stated priorities are to:

1 focus on the quality of healthcare provided to people and communities as they access, use and move between services
2 adapt its approach to ensure it is responsive to emerging risks to patient safety
3 work collaboratively to drive system and service improvement within healthcare
4 support and develop its workforce to enable them, and the organisations they work for, to deliver its priorities.

> ### Research
>
> Choose one of the UK home nations (England, Scotland, Northern Ireland or Wales) to carry out your research.
>
> Your task is to research the principles, standards and focus areas involved in an inspection by a regulatory body. Explore:
> - ▶ what each point means
> - ▶ what influences it has on day-to-day practice
> - ▶ how it promotes person-centred care within the supporting healthcare role.
>
> The websites listed below will help you in your research.
> - ▶ England – Care Quality Commission: **www.cqc.org.uk**
> - ▶ Scotland – Care Inspectorate: **www.careinspectorate.com**
> - ▶ Northern Ireland – Regulation and Quality Improvement Authority: **www.rqia.org.uk**
> - ▶ Wales – Healthcare Inspectorate Wales: **www.hiw.org.uk**

K1.2 The requirements for safeguarding individuals and their wider family/carers and promoting principles to others in practice

Safeguarding legislation

There are seven main pieces of legislation in the UK that aim to prevent harm to adults and maintain their right to live safely and feel secure (see Figure 1.3).

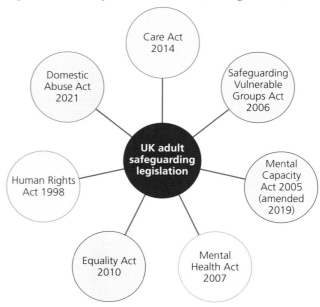

▲ Figure 1.3 The UK's main adult safeguarding legislation

The Care Act 2014

The Care Act aims to safeguard both the **service user** and their care providers.

Part of this legislation – Section 43 – requires every local authority to establish a Safeguarding Adults Board (SAB) for its area. The directive is aimed at all local statutory services responsible for adult provision and the integration of care and support between health and local authorities. It delivers guidance at a strategic level which then filters down to how an individual organisation, such as a stroke unit, implements a safeguarding policy at ground level. For example, having one entrance to a facility that the public can access, which is monitored, and having a clear visitor policy.

> ### Key term
>
> **Service user:** a person receiving or using healthcare services.

Regular reviews are part of the Care Act's safeguarding strategy to monitor working practices. These require all organisations to feed back any issues that are a cause for concern, so that the safeguarding guidance can be continuously improved.

The Care Act includes the six key principles of adult safeguarding (see page 10 for more details).

Safeguarding Vulnerable Groups Act 2006

This legislation prevents people who have a background of criminal behaviour, such as burglary, from working with vulnerable adults. The majority of criminal behaviours may result in a person being considered unsuitable to work with vulnerable adults, and a Disclosure and Barring Service (DBS) check will identify those who should not be in a position of responsibility or have unmonitored access to people who need care.

People working in health and social care roles will frequently work on a one-to-one basis with their service users and be largely unsupervised. With this in mind, pre-employment checks for positions of trust that involve regular and direct contact with vulnerable adults include:

▶ checking references from former employees
▶ shadowing another employee during an induction period.

Once qualified, a nurse, midwife or nursing associate is required to register with their specific regulating body, the Nursing and Midwifery Council (NMC), before being able to work in the UK. Where concerns are raised about a nurse's, midwife's or nursing associate's practice, the NMC will investigate and identify what corrective actions should be taken. In severe cases, this may result in the professional's removal from the register.

Mental Capacity Act 2005 (amended 2019)

This legislation determines whether a person has capacity to make decisions about matters that affect their life and care, accepting that some decisions are unwise. It safeguards and protects the rights of individuals with learning disabilities or degenerative health conditions that affect their cognitive abilities, which may deteriorate over time, helping them make their own decisions and have support that is in their best interest.

There is a complex balance between keeping someone safe, their rights and managing potential risks. For example, a person living with dementia may want

> **Key term**
>
> **Least restrictive:** it refers to practice decisions that support a person's basic rights to freedom, with care actions that interfere with these rights at the lowest level necessary to provide safety.

to shop independently but is at risk of becoming disoriented or confused when out.

▶ In this situation, a decision to support the person must meet physical and emotional safety requirements, with all options analysed.
▶ A mental capacity assessment aims to find the **least restrictive** option to support a person's best interest, allowing them to remain in control of as much as they can.
▶ A balanced approach would see the provision of a care worker to keep the individual company when going to the shops, assisting only when there is a threat of significant harm.

Mental Health Act 2007

The Mental Health Act (MHA) considers all relevant factors in an individual's life:

▶ the impact of mental illnesses
▶ protecting the individual's rights
▶ supporting the implementation of services that best meet their needs
▶ those who care for them
▶ society as a whole.

The MHA ensures that an individual's comfort and wellbeing needs are provided for by presenting clear guidance in relation to professionals, facilities and the extent of services available. For example, an individual can see a psychiatric consultant either as an inpatient or outpatient, and there are community psychiatric nurses often based at GP surgeries who work in the local community. A specialist group of experts form part of mental health crisis teams that are available 24 hours a day, commissioned to monitor people who are on the cusp of requiring urgent care.

Individuals who are experiencing episodes of acute mental ill health are vulnerable and may present a danger to themselves without realising it. This legislation means that the care provided must protect a person who may not realise how vulnerable they are, or who is in denial, or someone who experiences mental ill health but is not aware of this. In most cases, this legislation maintains a person's right to live with a minimally invasive care package and encourages empowerment and security.

The dilemma, however, is that it is also necessary to consider possibilities such as a person who is at risk of suicide, the risk of harm to others or risks to public safety. Should such individuals be kept in a secure hospital facility for treatment, under a court section that goes against the Human Rights Act and the right to freedom?

Equality Act 2010

Originally, there were multiple pieces of legislation in place to protect individuals from discrimination, including the Sex Discrimination Act 1975, the Race Relations Act 1976 and the Disability Discrimination Act 1995. The Equality Act 2010 replaced these Acts, making it a legal responsibility for employers to protect their workforce from discrimination based on nine characteristics. These characteristics are:

▶ age
▶ gender reassignment
▶ being married or in a civil partnership
▶ being pregnant or on maternity leave
▶ disability
▶ race, including colour, nationality, ethnic or national origin
▶ religion or belief
▶ sex
▶ sexual orientation.

Human Rights Act 1998

The Human Rights Act 1998 sets out the fundamental rights and freedoms that everyone in the UK is entitled to. It incorporates the rights set out in the European Convention on Human Rights (ECHR) into domestic British law. Articles that relate to safeguarding in particular are:

▶ Article 2: Right to life
▶ Article 3: Freedom from torture and inhuman or degrading treatment
▶ Article 14: Protection from discrimination in respect of these rights and freedoms.

Domestic Abuse Act 2021

The Domestic Abuse Act supports individuals who are victims of domestic abuse or are survivors of past abuse, including **coercion**. In the case of coercion, although a victim often has a choice, they are under duress and fear the consequences of not complying with demands. The legislation recognises the rights of victims and survivors and the destructive impact of abuse on victims and their families.

NICE publishes guidance on how to recognise and respond to domestic violence and abuse. You can find more information here: **https://www.nice.org.uk/about/nice-communities/social-care/quick-guides/recognising-and-responding-to-domestic-violence-and-abuse**

Domestic abuse can take place between intimate **partners** or between family members.

There are organisations that specialise in providing domestic violence support for women and separately for men. A different skillset may be required, depending on the gender of the person affected by domestic violence (there are more than two genders). Partnership work refers to local solutions carried out between the integrated services and the victim or survivor, who is at the forefront of any decisions made.

When providing person-centred care, a team of professionals will work with a victim to maximise their safety from a basis of empowerment. Accountability refers to contact and communication with a perpetrator that makes it clear that their behaviour has been unacceptable and that they will be held responsible (accountable).

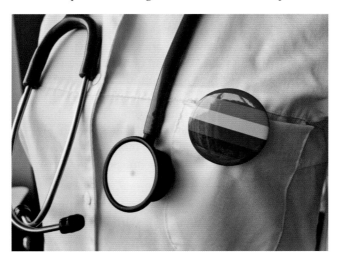

▲ Figure 1.4 Equality is not about treating everyone the same, we are not the same; it is about a provision for all, taking account of people's differences and providing inclusivity

Key terms

Coercion: the practice of persuading someone to do something by using force or threatening them.

Partner: the person considered by an individual to be their life partner.

Research

The Domestic Violence Disclosure Scheme (DVDS) is statutory guidance that enables the police to disclose information where this would protect a member of the public who may be at risk of harm from domestic abuse. It is also known as Clare's Law, after Clare Wood, a woman murdered by an ex-boyfriend who was known to the police as having a history of violence to previous partners.

This means that a member of the public now has the 'right to ask', under a certain set of circumstances (see the DVDS' statutory guidance, section 3), if a person has previously used violence or has a record of abusive offending. A 'right to know' is triggered by the police making a proactive decision to disclose information to protect a potential victim or victims.

► How do these police procedures relate to Article 8 of the Human Rights Act 1998?
► What are the implications of DVDS? How does it influence practice, and how does this promote person-centred care within the supporting healthcare role?

These websites will be helpful for your research:
► Domestic Violence Disclosure Scheme (DVDS): **https://assets.publishing.service.gov.uk/ government/uploads/system/uploads/ attachment_data/file/1162788/Domestic_ Violence_Disclosure_Scheme.pdf**
► Human Rights Act 1998, Article 8: **www.equalityhumanrights.com/human-rights/ human-rights-act/article-8-respect-your- private-and-family-life**

Local policy and procedure

Any organisation caring for vulnerable adults will have a management system in place to implement and review local policy and procedure, such as making disclosure guidelines an integral part of ongoing training.

Figure 1.5 illustrates the policy creation, implementation and review process.

Legislation and regulations can be amended and policies reviewed in order to remain up to date. The process incorporates complaints or issues that have occurred since the previous review. Policies are often reviewed annually to ensure they continue to be fit for purpose.

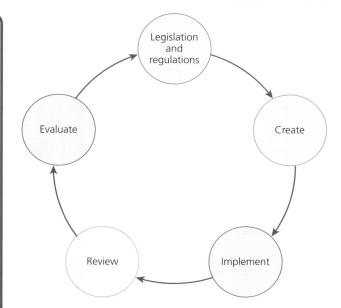

▲ Figure 1.5 The policy creation, implementation and review process

Lines of reporting and raising concerns

Designated Safeguarding Officers (DSOs) are individuals who have undertaken specific training in order to effectively understand the concerns reported and be able to take appropriate action. Usually, concerns that arise with an individual prior to admission, when planning discharge or seeing an outpatient are reported to the local authorities who operate safeguarding teams. It is these teams who then investigate and take action where necessary.

The overseeing DSO will be responsible for investigating when concerns are reported for a patient during their time spent in a healthcare setting. In some cases, concerns are reported to the police, who will also investigate whether any criminal activity may have occurred.

Departmental procedures

Different care services will have particular departmental procedures in place, for example a robust complaints procedure specific to the type of service and service user. A department that specialises in caring for patients who are largely unconscious or have profound or multiple learning disabilities will have a specialist safeguarding policy and procedures for this area of work.

The six principles of adult safeguarding

Enshrined within the Care Act 2014 are six key principles of adult safeguarding (Figure 1.6).

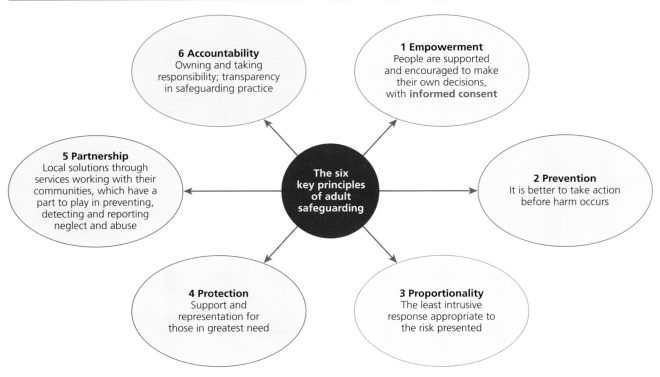

▲ Figure 1.6 The six key principles of adult safeguarding

Test yourself

1 A principle is a foundation of key values. Explain the purpose of the six principles in safeguarding vulnerable adults.

2 Give an example of how a nursing home setting might adhere to each of the 6 principles.

3 Explain how you would train new healthcare professionals to promote the six key principles of safeguarding while they are working with service users and their family and friends.

Key terms

Informed consent: before making a final decision, a person receiving care or treatment has the right to be given all the relevant information about it.

Duty of care: the legal obligation to always act in the best interest of individuals and others to prevent negligence causing harm. It means you should act within your level of competence and not take on anything you do not believe you can safely do.

Duty of candour: the legal obligation to be open and honest with individuals and/or their families about incidents as promptly as possible.

K1.3 The requirements for following a duty of care and duty of candour within the scope of the supporting healthcare role

The similarity between a duty of care and a duty of candour is that they are both legal obligations within any healthcare role.

▶ A **duty of care** refers to your responsibility to act in the best interest of individuals, their health and their welfare when delivering quality care. This includes carrying out only those tasks you are competent to do and not duties outside your job description, training or level of skill.

▶ A **duty of candour** refers to your responsibility to act with integrity and be open and honest with individuals and their families.

When an incident occurs that has the potential to cause harm, or has caused harm, it must be addressed promptly and with transparency to identify what went wrong and the actions that will be taken to resolve it and reduce the likelihood of a repeat. In a situation where wrongdoing has occurred, the person responsible needs to be genuine and convey sincerity, which means you need to understand the difference between expressing regret and apologising:

- Regret is only the expression of sorrow, for example feeling disappointed in oneself.
- Apologising means acknowledging or owning the wrongdoing, so you are taking responsibility alongside an expression of regret.

An apology should never be delivered in such a way that the individual affected by the wrongdoing is expected to offer forgiveness.

The 6Cs

The nursing values known as the **6Cs – care, compassion, competence, communication, courage and commitment** (see Figure 1.7) – were launched in the Compassion in Practice vision and strategy published by NHS England in 2012. They guide practitioners working in the care sector to deliver person-centred care through everyday actions.

These values are at the heart of good practice in nursing, and they are the moral responsibility of individual staff working in a position of responsibility in a care setting, such as a community nurse working with patients in their own homes.

NHS values

NHS England values are principles and strategic values at organisation level that influence facilities, funding and provision of all statutory services.

The National Health Service (NHS) employs more than 1.27 million full-time equivalent staff in England (as of April 2023). Its facilities, provision and staffing must deliver a service that adheres to the six values listed in the left-hand column of Table 1.1. It is the duty of care of the NHS to provide staff with the means and training that will enable them to carry out their duty of care for individuals and to support colleagues.

6Cs - Values essential to compassionate care

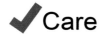 **Care**

Care is our core business and that of our organisations; and the care we deliver helps the individual person and improves the health of the whole community.

Caring defines us and our work. People receiving care expect it to be right for them consistently throughout every stage of their life.

✓ **Compassion**

Compassion is how care is given through relationships based on empathy, respect and dignity.

It can also be described as intelligent kindness and is central to how people perceive their care.

✓ **Competence**

Competence means all those in caring roles must have the ability to understand an individual's health and social needs.

It is also about having the expertise, clinical and technical knowledge to deliver effective care and treatments based on research and evidence.

✓ **Communication**

Communication is central to successful caring relationships and to effective team working. Listening is as important as what we say. It is essential for 'No decision without me'.

Communication is the key to a good workplace with benefits for those in our care and staff alike.

✓ **Courage**

Courage enables us to do the right thing for the people we care for, to speak up when we have concerns.

It means we have the personal strength and vision to innovate and to embrace new ways of working.

✓ **Commitment**

A commitment to our patients and populations is a cornerstone of what we do. We need to build on our commitment to improve the care and experience of our patients.

We need to take action to make this vision and strategy a reality for all and meet the health and social care challenges ahead.

▲ Figure 1.7 The 6Cs: values essential to compassionate care

▼ Table 1.1 NHS values

NHS England	NHS Scotland	NHS Wales	HSC Northern Ireland
The values are: ▶ working together for patients ▶ respect and dignity ▶ commitment to quality of care ▶ compassion ▶ improving lives ▶ everyone counts	There are principles for healthcare patients similar to those applied in England: ▶ a commitment to deliver person-centred care ▶ care and compassion ▶ dignity and respect ▶ openness ▶ honesty and responsibility ▶ quality ▶ teamwork	The core values that underpin the service are: ▶ putting quality and safety above all else ▶ integrating improvement into everyday working ▶ focusing on prevention, health improvement and inequality ▶ working in true partnership with partners ▶ investing in staff	The values jointly represent the principles behind the services that are delivered. The purposes of these are a reflection of the overall culture of its provision, services and professionals: ▶ working together ▶ excellence ▶ openness and honesty ▶ compassion

Table 1.1 shows the values for the NHS and HSC in all four home nations.

Research

Choose one of the UK's home nations to carry out your research.

Your task is to research the NHS values (or Health and Social Care values in Northern Ireland) in detail and produce your own notes. Explore:
▶ what each point means
▶ how it ensures good practice
▶ how these values promote person-centred care within the supporting healthcare role.

Personalisation agenda

The NHS **personalisation agenda** has three broad themes:

1 a person-centred care approach
2 offering greater choice to service users
3 supplying information to service users.

The non-profit organisation Skills for Health was established to identify the skills and competencies required by healthcare workers to enable them to deliver consistent, safe, quality care. This is an ongoing process, with Skills for Health working with regulatory bodies to source feedback on areas to improve in the health sector.

Analysis carried out as part of the personalisation agenda identified skills gaps in:
▶ leadership
▶ advocacy
▶ motivational questioning
▶ ongoing evaluation
▶ commissioning.

Practice points

S1.25 Safeguard individuals and their wider family/carers if required and promote principles to others in practice

A patient has been admitted to a ward following treatment in Accident & Emergency (A&E) for an eye socket fracture (orbital fracture). They are noticeably malnourished, dehydrated and unkempt, and they refused to give any details while they were in A&E.

It is decided that further investigation is required in the shape of a kidney function test, and you have been instructed to take baseline measurements for blood pressure, temperature, oxygen saturates and blood glucose levels.

Demonstrate and explain how you would:
1 monitor signs/symptoms of abuse, record any safeguarding concerns, and escalate if appropriate
2 ensure all the 6Cs of nursing and the eight core values of the Care Certificate are maintained; give examples in context
3 uphold the values of the NHS or the values of the Northern Ireland HSC, and the four overarching principles of the NMC Code of professional standards of practice and behaviour (also known as the NMC Code of Conduct)
4 promote the six principles of adult safeguarding.

It was found that entry-level staff needed to have a broader understanding of what personalisation means, with further training needed in certain aspects of person-centred care. Technical skills gaps that limited existing staff were identified, for example a restricted scope of practice for capable staff who felt they were not challenged at the time or were prevented from moving on to the next stage in their career because the step up to promotion was too big.

Additionally, the area of soft skills required specific training in relation to the communication skills that were needed to demonstrate empathy and convey active listening, and the actions that were needed to demonstrate valuing a person. Developing opportunities for improving soft skills through mandatory and optional further training will increase job satisfaction for employees and raise the standard of care provided.

As a direct result of the 2012 personalisation agenda, NHS England Chief Nursing Officer, Jane Cummings, introduced the 6Cs in December 2017. These play an integral role in ensuring an enhanced patient experience.

Employee appraisals are now more rigorously seen as an important part of a health professional's overall professional development and offer an opportunity to review both current workload and ongoing aspirations for professional growth. Services were also introduced for qualified staff to provide additional support to the workforce, such as independent advocates and access to counselling.

Mental Capacity Act 2005 (amended 2019)

As mentioned earlier (page 7), the **Mental Capacity Act** was implemented in 2005, giving clear guidance on how care for people experiencing mental ill health should be provided. The act was further improved in a **2019 amendment**. A standardised minimum level of care in supporting patients with medical and therapeutic treatments is a multidisciplinary team duty of care. When weaknesses in practice are identified an organisation such as a secure unit has a duty of candour and should seek ways to prevent a recurrence or implement control methods to limit an undesirable impact.

Person-centred care planning

Person-centred care planning means matching the individual who requires healthcare intervention with suitable services and professionals working with them. Every individual with healthcare or wellbeing support needs is entitled to quality care that meets their holistic needs in the most appropriate way, in terms of, for example:
- the location of care provision
- access to care and services
- the convenience of seeing a trained practitioner.

The role of candour in informing practice

If professionals have had to apologise multiple times for similar aspects of care, for example a fall in hospital or the failure to administer a prescribed medication resulting in potential for harm, an investigation is needed. Although certain aspects may be out of the hands of a staff member, the duty of candour has identified issues that need to be addressed.

Whistleblowing

Organisational **whistleblowing** policies are put in place to support the reporting of institutionalised abuse and neglect. It is a legal obligation for every member of staff to report other staff who are neglecting their duty of care, and to take action to safeguard those individuals affected.

One of the most important values in the 6Cs is courage. Senior managers may themselves be involved in a system of abuse and neglect by ignoring malpractice and misconduct. Whistleblowing may not be easy, but whistleblowers are protected and have the right to remain anonymous.

Conflict between rights and responsibility

You will need a similar level of courage to make the right choice when faced with a care dilemma that represents a **conflict between rights and responsibility**. To empower someone but also take away an aspect of choice is not always clear-cut – for example if medication for a mental illness is no longer working and is causing damage to liver function over time, which requires a prescription change, yet the patient has a level of emotional dependency on the drug and their distress is causing an episode of anxiety that is counterproductive to their wellbeing.

> **Reflect**
>
> In a scenario such as the dilemma of a patient who feels an emotional dependency on a medication, and which is a conflict between rights and responsibility, the duty of care is to act in the best interest of the patient.
> - Would the decision involve more than one practitioner and someone acting as an advocate on behalf of the patient?
> - What might be the implications from the patient's perspective?

K1.4 Required standards, codes of conduct and health and safety including risk assessment relevant to your role in supporting healthcare

Care Quality Commission (CQC) 13 fundamental standards of care

The **Care Quality Commission (CQC) 13 fundamental standards of care** state the minimum requirements for an organisation's facilities, leadership, and staff competencies and skills. These standards are all in place to enable the provision of person-centred quality care and to ensure that all services deliver this.

The standards are shown in Figure 1.8.

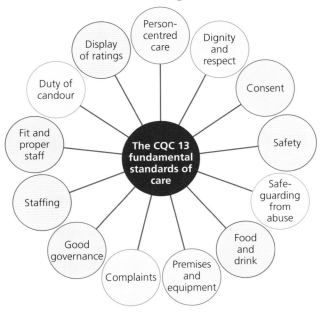

▲ Figure 1.8 The CQC 13 fundamental standards of care

The CQC regulates at an organisational level and inspects every registered healthcare setting in England. As part of its inspections, it undertakes an overview of the service providers, including talking with patients and their families about whether they feel they are receiving a high level of care. Having a formal complaints process that is promoted and that service users are encouraged to use is a helpful tool to find solutions and improvements. Every care setting will have complaints, and when the CQC reviews this area, perfection is not expected; there is a focus on the steps and actions taken to resolve an issue to everyone's satisfaction. The outcome should be recorded to demonstrate the learning that has occurred.

Research

Research any one from: the CQC 13 fundamental standards of care in England, the five principles of the Care Inspectorate in Scotland, the four domains of the Regulation and Quality Improvement Authority in Northern Ireland or the four priorities of the Healthcare Inspectorate Wales. Familiarise yourself with what each standard covers.

The standards and values of NHS England, NHS Scotland, Health and Social Care Trust Northern Ireland and NHS Wales

The standards for these organisations are patient-focused and incorporate the roles of families, carers and frontline staff in delivering care. Patients are encouraged to share their experiences and opinions in the care they receive; this is an important element in feeling valued and listened to. Furthermore, they must be involved in all decisions made about their care, as responsive care considers both physical and emotional wellbeing.

To maintain the standards, staff will hold qualifications and acquire competencies to carry out their duty of care effectively, considering how they would want to be treated if the roles were reversed.

Private healthcare standards

Although non-statutory organisations, such as Bupa, and independent private hospitals are not part of the NHS, in England they must implement the same CQC standards as registrants; however, their services were not given a rating until April 2019. Specifically adapted documentation was published called 'A fresh start for the regulation of independent healthcare', to aid the application of the standards in non-statutory provision.

Occupational standards

The Nursing and Midwifery Council (NMC) has expected standards for the workforce of all of its registrants and **revalidation** is compulsory. National Occupational Standards (NOS) were first approved in 2001 but have evolved over time. Skills for

Key term

Revalidation: a process which all nurses and midwives in the UK must complete to check their competence and maintain their registration with the NMC.

Health is an advocate of and has been influential in setting these standards. NOS describe the knowledge and skills required to undertake particular tasks and set a competency excellence level that directly impacts the scope of practice.

The clarity in the standards leads to the introduction and overhauling of qualifications and training developed by Skills for Health. Entry level and progression is guided by the NOS, which are recommended good practice but are not compulsory.

Organisational codes of conduct

In order to follow the CQC's standards of care, organisations, such as hospitals in England, develop and implement **codes of conduct** through their policies and procedures. This ensures that all aspects of a hospital are held to consistently high standards. A code of conduct will state the expected standards for all departments and clinics, with additional specific guidelines for different departments, such as oncology or the ear, nose and throat team.

Individual risk assessments for patients

Individual risk assessments are carried out in order to ensure health and safety standards are met for both employees and service users. For instance, a patient may be at risk of a fall and measures identified in a risk assessment to prevent or reduce harm to the patient and their supporting staff. Where a person is identified as being at a high risk of falls, equipment may be used to alert the healthcare team to the fact that the person is standing up and attempting to walk unsupported.

Risk assessments for patients with serious mental health conditions will aim to minimise the possibility of actions that might lead to self-harm or suicide. Such assessments are documented and all staff who are in contact with the patient made aware of the measures in place.

A risk assessment for a patient who has aggressive and violent outbursts will inform the procedures used when staff are in contact with them, which could include avoiding triggers, observing early warning signs and ensuring medication is administered at the correct times.

Personal health and safety responsibilities

All employees and volunteers also have a duty to abide by the health and safety guidelines for their own benefit. They must be aware of their responsibilities

and demonstrate their commitment to maintaining the skills and knowledge to adhere to the guidance and safety mechanisms.

For example, a hospice will have its own code of conduct that staff should comply with, which includes self-care, such as debriefing with a senior member of staff or counsellor at regular intervals. The aim of this is to protect the mental wellbeing of specialist staff as a matter of course, and it is also a service that can be requested at difficult times. In order to preserve appropriate professional boundaries and maintain the standard of care while supporting both patient and family, there is mandatory monitoring of wellbeing. The code of conduct could also include following fire evacuation procedures or filling in an accident at work form.

Volunteers have to take part in mandatory training and benefit from the same level of support in this situation as their paid colleagues.

Code of conduct guidance clearly shows the steps to take to stay in line with protocol when dealing with a potential safeguarding issue or a complaint. Any complaint would then be directed at the organisation rather than the individual.

To be deemed fit to practise, professionals must deliver safe and person-centred care. Otherwise, they might be barred from practice in the future, prevented from working with vulnerable adults and have a permanent note added to their DBS file.

Current health and safety legislation

Legislation is implemented in the workplace by employees following protocol as laid out in the organisation's policies. For example:

▶ A record-keeping policy will ensure that documentation (such as a patient risk assessment) is completed accurately, moving, lifting and handling procedures are carried out correctly, and escalation procedures are clear in an emergency.

▶ A safeguarding policy will deliver all aspects of the laws around safeguarding vulnerable groups. An administration of medicines policy will describe the processes of managing medications, taking into consideration all groups of medication, the required storage and disposal processes and the patient's involvement in taking and storing medications independently. It will also detail the actions to be taken where medications incidents have occurred and the importance of reporting such incidents.

Case study

S1.26 Implement a duty of care and candour when working with individuals and their families/carers, speaking clearly and confidently using appropriate tone and register that reflects audience and purpose
S1.27 Follow all required standards, codes of conduct and health and safety requirements/legislation, including risk assessment, in the healthcare environment

Anne, who is living with dementia, is admitted to a surgical ward after investigations into a bowel obstruction that resulted in surgery. Two days later, the patient is dehydrated, the nursing staff having failed to monitor the fluid intake of a patient who does not recognise thirst. In addition, when a relative visits Anne, they notice she is more disorientated and confused than she had been prior to being admitted, and they share their concern with a nurse. The ward has been particularly busy, and the fluid chart has not been kept up to date as instructed.

There is a duty of care breach in this situation, and there will be a system in place for duty of candour to address this error. Appropriate communications will need to take place between the supervising nurse and Anne's visiting relative.

Demonstrate the following:
1 Clarify and define the duty of care and duty of candour as standards.
2 Show your knowledge of one of the following: the relevant CQC fundamental care standard(s), the relevant principle(s) of the CI, the relevant domain(s) of the RQIA, or the relevant priority/ies of the HIW.
3 Describe a risk assessment specifically for patients living with dementia who do not recognise thirst.
4 Explain how dehydration can make confusion worse.
5 Explain the purpose of a fluid intake chart and the robust monitoring of hydration.
6 Compose an appropriate apology.
7 Describe future steps to prevent a recurrence and note how you would reassure the relative.
8 Record the incident of wrongdoing in case there is a formal complaint and disciplinary measures are needed.

K1.5 How to respond to incidents and emergencies relevant to your role in supporting healthcare

Local guidelines

Local guidelines are specific to a clinical area or location. They provide detailed guidance for a specific purpose, such as:
▶ maximum waiting times between a cancer diagnosis and the start of treatment
▶ for rural areas, providing mobile screening or treatment units like those for breast screening or dialysis at home
▶ a hospital's major incidents protocol – for example Significant Emergency (level 1), Serious Emergency (level 2), Catastrophic Emergency (level 3) – all planned and practised
▶ observations using a NEWS2 early warning signs chart, with swift escalation if a patient deteriorates and becomes critical

▶ the government target for all ambulance trusts, which sets a minimum response time of eight minutes for Category 1 calls.

Who should undertake basic life support?

Anyone in a healthcare role may be faced with a patient who stops breathing or chokes. Having basic life support knowledge means you can respond immediately until supported by more specialist professionals. Everyone can undertake basic life support, but it is important for employees to do so within the organisation's procedures. Without a clear order, mistakes and delays can occur when responding to incidents and emergencies, as different professionals jump in to carry out treatments such as cardiopulmonary resuscitation (CPR).

Figure 1.9 shows a group of trainees practising CPR.

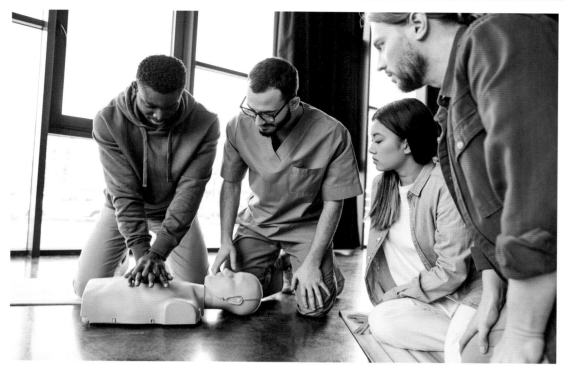

▲ Figure 1.9 A group of trainees practising CPR

Reporting and recording procedures

There will be policies in place with procedures that explain who incidents and emergencies should be reported to. If there is a serious incident, it will need recording with the HSE as part of RIDDOR compliance. These procedures are vital, as misunderstandings between staff can mean a serious concern is not reported to the right person and there is an omission on a patient's records, which could have serious consequences.

Information and data that is recorded before, during and after an emergency or incident can be referred to later if legal action is deemed necessary, and staff with responsibility for receiving reports can be identified and held responsible.

K1.6 How to use a range of techniques for infection prevention and control

Standard infection control precautions (SICPs) are used by all healthcare professionals, in all care settings (for example nursing homes). They are techniques that are used to prevent and control infection, such as a cleaning regime, the restocking and correct usage of personal protective equipment (PPE), and closing a ward if there is an outbreak of diarrhoea and vomiting.

Test yourself

S1.28 Maintain a safe and healthy working environment, take appropriate action in response to incidents or emergencies, following local guidelines

When responding to an incident in the outpatients department, where a patient who is known to have epilepsy falls and has a seizure, explain each action below and give an example of what you would do in these circumstances:

1 Think ahead
2 Stay calm
3 Assess emergency
4 Summon help
5 React within the scope of your role and understand your own limitations
6 Record details if asked
7 Be involved in the debrief and give feedback if required

Key term

Standard infection control precautions (SICPs): basic infection prevention and control measures as part of good practice to reduce the risk of infection transmission.

Maintain good personal hygiene

It is of the utmost importance that you maintain good personal hygiene at work:

▶ Your hair should be clean and tidy – it should be off the collar or tied back.

▶ You should take appropriate care of your nails (see the Hand care section on this page) – and remove nail polish or nail jewellery.

▶ Your uniform should be kept clean and well maintained.

Preventing the transfer or spread of infection can save a life. A patient who is taking immune suppressant medication for an autoimmune condition such as lupus will be particularly vulnerable, as are patients receiving chemotherapy. These individuals expect every measure to be taken to keep them safe from further harm, as part of their care.

▶ Keeping your hair tied up and off the collar reduces the risk of particles of hair falling on to wounds. It also gives a more professional appearance.

▶ Washing your uniform at a temperature of 60°C removes almost all microorganisms.

▶ For patients who are immunocompromised, an otherwise minor infection can cause complications that quickly become life-threatening. If a staff member has even the slightest cold, they should not be in contact with these vulnerable individuals. Infections such as flu and norovirus (a winter vomiting bug) are particularly contagious, and staff should not return to work until their symptoms have cleared. They should also consult their organisation's infection prevention policy.

Handwashing technique

It is very important to keep your hands clean at work (like the surgeon in Figure 1.10). Pathogens can stay on your hands and be transferred to patients easily if the principles of handwashing are not followed.

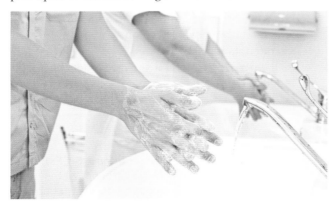

▲ Figure 1.10 A surgeon washing their hands before an operation

> ### Key term
>
> **Gram-negative bacteria (GNB):** bacteria such as E. coli. that are highly resistant to antibiotics and therefore represent one of the world's most significant public health challenges.

The following professional handwashing techniques involve specific steps to maximise infection prevention for all healthcare professionals:

▶ the Ayliffe technique, promoted by the National Institute for Health and Care Excellence (NICE)

▶ the World Health Organization (WHO) 5 moments technique

▶ the WHO/NHS 12-step technique.

The different techniques and their steps are described in Table 1.2.

Remember that no handwashing technique will guarantee the complete removal of a serious multidrug-resistant infection, for instance **gram-negative bacteria (GNB)** such as E. coli. However, while soaps and handwashing may not kill such pathogens, they will reduce the total microbial load, reducing transfer risk.

> ### Research
>
> The most effective way to reduce the spread of E. coli is by proper handwashing. Visit this website and investigate the 12-step technique promoted by the UK Health Security Agency (UKHSA): www.england.nhs.uk/wp-content/uploads/2022/09/nipc-manual-appendix-1-handwashing.pdf

Hand care

A minimum standard of **hand care** aims to focus on places where infections might not be removed by handwashing and eliminate this possibility.

▶ Your **nails** must be kept short and clean, and you must not use nail polish, nail products or artificial nails.

▶ After you have washed them, your hands should be **dried** with disposable paper towels, and you must make no contact with a towel dispenser or with a bin when disposing of them.

▶ If you have any **cuts** they must be covered and sealed with a waterproof dressing.

▼ Table 1.2 Handwashing techniques

Ayliffe technique	WHO 5 Moments for Hand Hygiene	WHO/NHS 12 steps in 60 seconds
▶ Palm-to-palm friction ▶ Palm to palm, fingers interlaced ▶ Back of fingers to opposing palms with fingers interlocked ▶ Rotational rubbing of right thumb clasped in left palm, and vice versa ▶ Rotational rubbing backwards and forwards with clasped fingers of right hand in left palm, and vice versa	▶ Moment 1: before touching a patient ▶ Moment 2: before a procedure ▶ Moment 3: after a procedure or body fluid exposure risk ▶ Moment 4: after touching a patient ▶ Moment 5: after touching a patient's surroundings	1 Wet hands with water 2 Apply enough soap to cover all hand surfaces 3 Rub hands palm to palm 4 Right palm over left **dorsum** with interlaced fingers, and vice versa 5 Palm to palm with fingers interlaced 6 Backs of fingers to opposing palms with fingers interlocked 7 Rotational rubbing of left thumb clasped in right palm, and vice versa 8 Rotational rubbing backwards and forwards with clasped fingers of right hand in left palm, and vice versa 9 Rinse hands with water 10 Dry thoroughly with a single-use towel 11 Use towel to turn off tap 12 Your hands are now safe to use

Personal protective equipment (PPE)

Following meticulous hygiene measures to prevent the spread of infection, the correct application of personal protective equipment (PPE) is then the next step required to continue to prevent cross-contamination from bacteria, viruses and fungi (Figure 1.11).

PPE includes:

- ▶ gloves
- ▶ disposable plastic apron
- ▶ full-body gown
- ▶ goggles/masks
- ▶ headwear
- ▶ footwear.

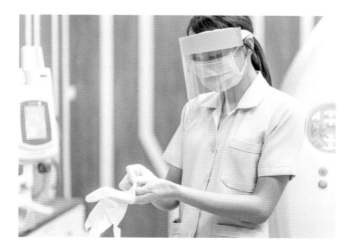

▲ Figure 1.11 The correct type and use of PPE is vital to the prevention of cross-contamination

PPE is classified at four levels, A–D, which dictate the type of kit that should be worn in certain situations. This will be directly related to the type of contact involved and the environment the healthcare professional is working in. For example, a theatre nurse working in a surgery team dealing with significant open wounds will require more PPE than a nurse completing a general ward drugs round. This is because the confined space of a theatre during an eight-hour procedure impacts on the amount of airborne bacteria and viruses transmitted in small respiratory droplets.

Guidance is published on the correct use of **appropriate PPE** for each individual according to **local policy**, the theatre or ward.

Spillage

Blood and body fluids

Blood and body fluids pose a risk to any healthcare professional who may be caring for an infected patient. Blood infections such as HIV and Hepatitis C can cause serious illness, so spillages should be handled with care using the organisational policy of cleaning spillages.

> **Key term**
>
> **Dorsum:** the back of a structure, in this case the hand.

Examples of when blood and body fluids can be spilled include the following:

▶ A patient with norovirus (a winter vomiting bug) may vomit profusely without warning, contaminating floors and furniture. This vomit then harbours the virus which can easily be transmitted to others.

▶ A patient attending the Accident and Emergency department might attend with a serious laceration to their hand which is bleeding profusely. This blood may drip on the floor of the waiting room and pose a risk to others using the department.

Cleaning any spillage requires the wearing of the appropriate level of PPE and following the steps set out in the decontamination policy of the organisation. As a minimum level, gloves and aprons must be worn.

▶ Drops of spilled blood can be wiped clean with a disposable paper towel and then the area should be disinfected thoroughly.

▶ For larger amounts of fluid, the surrounding area and all of its surfaces should also be thoroughly cleaned for potential splashes and splatters, using a hospital-grade disinfectant.

▶ In some cases, a spillage kit will be required. This contains absorbent disposable material which turns the liquid into a solid, so that it can be cleaned up more easily and disposed of in the correct way. The area can then be disinfected and made safe while the surface dries. If the spillage is in an area where someone may walk, a 'wet floor' sign will need to be set up.

Spillage of chemicals and other liquids

Chemical spills are handled in a similar way to body fluids but in most cases, the use of a protective face mask is required to reduce the risk of inhalation. Due to the nature of chemical spills, the decontamination processes for each chemical must be adhered to in order to reduce the risk of injury.

Waste management

To maintain infection prevention levels, **waste management** measures must be strictly adhered to.

▶ **Infectious/hazardous waste** should be collected in a yellow waste bag and incinerated.

▶ **Chemical waste** refers to waste generated from contact with hazardous chemicals or remaining unused chemicals. For example, cytotoxic medications used in chemotherapy treatments and

items that have been in contact with them, such as intravenous bags, tubing and PPE. Specially designated, clearly labelled containers with purple lids are used to collect cytotoxic waste. Waste can also be disposed of in disposal bags that are yellow with purple stripes.

▶ **Safe needle use** (sharps) and the **disposal of scalpels** and other medical equipment that has the potential to cause a puncture wound are closely monitored in healthcare. Sharps bins are collected and disposed of safely by the local council or a licensed biohazard waste disposal company.

Appropriate cleaning regime

All cleaning regimes will follow the six stages of cleaning:

Stage	Task
1	Pre-clean
2	Main clean
3	Rinse
4	Disinfection
5	Final rinse
6	Drying

Cleaning regimes for local areas will clearly lay out the procedures to be followed, presenting them stage by stage. These regimes will vary depending on the area being cleaned.

In a bedroom in a care home, for example, Stage 1 (Pre-clean) may include the removal of visible contaminants or a chemical spray that starts to work on more stubborn contaminants such as dried faeces. In a hospital theatre being prepared for open-heart surgery, Stage 1 (Pre-clean) would be very different and would include cleaning all surfaces in the theatre beginning with higher level surfaces (for example operating lights).

Different workstations and facilities will have specific cleaning substances and sterilising equipment that need to be used. Clear information given on each of these states the competencies and type/level of staff involved with the various local area cleaning requirements. Staff who are using cleaning fluids must be trained in the safe usage and storage as part of the Control of Substances Hazardous to Health (COSHH) regulations.

Practice points

S1.29 Use a range of techniques for infection prevention and control and have a thorough understanding of the context of the work

A patient in the outpatients clinic becomes unwell during a change of dressing and wound check appointment. They tell their friend who is accompanying them that they feel sick but are too embarrassed to tell the nurse changing the dressings. The patient then vomits on the floor.

Demonstrate and describe the following:
1 Appropriate PPE to wear when changing a dressing, and how you would put this on and safely dispose of it.
2 Effective communication to reassure the patient and alleviate stress levels.
3 Spillage steps to take to clean up the vomit on the floor.

Providing overall care

K1.7 How current best practice and agreed ways of working support healthcare needs

Providing everyday care as a healthcare professional means you will be assisting medical staff with care-related tasks.

You will be trained in the correct and safe methods for each task, and will shadow a competent member of staff until you have the skills – communication and clinical – to provide overall care in a safe, person-centred way.

Simple dressings

When applying a **simple dressing**, such as a sticking plaster or sterile pad, you must follow the **aseptic technique** (Aseptic Non-Touch Technique, ANTT) to protect the patient from harmful pathogens entering their body. Handwashing and correct use of PPE are also part of this infection prevention practice. Selecting

Key term

Aseptic technique: the technique that healthcare professionals use to prevent cross-infection during procedures such as dressing changes, wound management, surgery etc.

the most suitable pre-prepared sterile dressing pack will depend on the size and type of wound, and whether a change of dressing is required or an injury needs to be cleaned prior to dressing.

Catheter and stoma care

Urinary catheters can cause urinary tract infections (UTIs), therefore scrupulous attention to hygiene is essential to reduce the risk of this happening. With stoma care, leakages can happen, which require cleaning, as well as daily stoma site washing. To prevent cross-infection, the healthcare professional must wear the correct PPE and ensure that the correct method is used to clean the insertion site.

Correct care of the equipment used for catheterisation should form part of a regular routine (Figure 1.12).

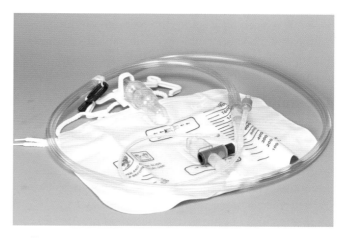

▲ Figure 1.12 Correct catheter care should form part of a regular routine

Personal care and hygiene

Assisting patients with their **personal hygiene** is a core aspect of healthcare. It is essential to maintain patients' privacy and dignity at all times.

Washing and bathing

Washing and bathing offer a good opportunity to perform a full assessment of your patient's skin integrity, which you will learn about in detail in Adult Nursing Performance Outcome 3 (see page 171). It should be done in a dignified way and you should discuss with the patient which aspects of the task they feel they can carry out semi-independently and any preferences they have around such a personal task. Patients who are unable to be moved to a showering facility will require a bed bath. This is washing that takes place in the bed itself, undertaken by two healthcare workers co-operating in the performance of tasks.

Bed baths usually start with the face and neck, then move on to the arms and torso, ensuring the water is changed regularly so that clean water is always used. Legs are washed before toes, and the genitals are washed separately. As soon as an area is dry it should be covered so that the patient does not get cold. Areas that are not being washed need to be kept covered with a dry towel. In order to keep the person at ease, they should be included in all conversations and regularly checked to ensure that they are comfortable and warm. Once the front of the patient's body has been washed, the patient is rolled onto their side so that their back can be washed. Take care not to wet the sheets, which should be changed after the procedure as necessary.

Self-bathing is possible for more able and independent patients. There may be areas that require some assistance, such as washing the hair, but on the whole it will be about acting on the patient's requests for support and referring to any risk assessment documentation for instructions about patient safety.

Dressing

Effective communication is a priority when you are assisting a patient to dress. This particular daily activity can help a person feel empowered and to express themselves. It is good practice to encourage individuals to dress themselves as much as possible. Where this occurs, it is important that they feel supported and not hurried, so it is good practice for you to find other things to do while the person is dressing and being available for them when they need help.

Putting on clothes should be done at the patient's pace; this is especially important if they have joint pain or are recovering from surgery. There are care aids available to help with certain tasks, such as fastening buttons, doing up zips and putting on socks. It may be appropriate for you to offer these and demonstrate their correct use. If putting their arm in a top or cardigan is too painful, you can reassure them that not doing so is acceptable and temporary.

A person must make their own decisions as to what they wish to wear, without being influenced. However, you could offer some information about the weather to assist them in making their choice.

Engaging the patient in conversation that is not related to clothing, as a distraction from dependency, can make dressing a more pleasant experience. Paying a compliment should also have a positive effect. If full

assistance is required this should be delivered in a dignified way, such as first closing the curtains and giving reassurance where applicable.

Toileting

Toileting assistance covers a range of techniques, depending on the patient's mobility and functional control of their bladder and bowels.

Incontinence is the involuntary loss of urine and faeces. The control of these functions requires strength in sphincter muscles which retain and release urine and faeces from the body. The muscles need neurological control to recognise and co-ordinate a voluntary release effectively. There can be a wide range of reasons for incontinence, such as a sudden unexpected urge or stress when exerting. Double incontinence is when an individual is unable to control both their bowel and urinary functions. Depending on the severity of this there is the option of incontinence bags and catheterisation.

A service that addresses an individual's bladder and bowel problems will look at both their physical requirements and the support they need with managing their own toileting. There may be a mobility problem that causes time to be an issue: someone might feel they need to go to the toilet, but the ease with which they can get there means they might not have enough time.

Continence aids must be selected by size and according to purpose; however, you should recognise that a patient might have their own preferences to consider too. There are pads for light urinary incontinence only, for moderate to heavy urine flow, or stretch pants for double incontinence. While faecal incontinence pads are manufactured to contain bowel movements they are not designed to offer a great deal of absorbency. Information is provided with pads and pants to indicate the amount that can be absorbed and required rates of change, as well as measurements and dimensions to ensure that fit is as good and leak-free as possible.

If you are working with an individual who uses continence aids, you will need to maintain a high level of patient personal hygiene for their comfort, to prevent harm to their genitals or skin, and to reduce the risk of urinary tract infections. Being fully prepared with the right PPE and equipment is the first step to changing disposable incontinence absorbent padding.

Patients who are in bed may also be supported to use a commode at the bedside. Bed pans are a least preferred option if someone can be encouraged to get out of bed. This is good psychologically and also from a mobility/ dignity perspective.

Continence care for patients who remain in bed involves the use of bedpans and urine bottles. There is clear guidance on the use of bedpans. This is commonly a two-person healthcare professional task, but sometimes a single healthcare professional may assist a solo nurse with roll movements.

The steps involved on a hospital ward are likely to be as follows:

1 Put on (don) gloves and an apron, and close dignity curtains.
2 Roll the patient, or gently raise their hips, and place a barrier, such as a bed incontinence pad, on top of the bed. Slide the incontinence pad along with a bedpan under the patient's bottom. A bed incontinence pad contains an absorbent layer which draws any spilled urine away from the patient's skin.
3 Position the patient on the bedpan correctly. The deeper portion of the bedpan should be directed towards their toes, and the patient should be centred on the bedpan.
4 Cover the patient with a dignity blanket or bath towel.
5 Raise the head of the bed to a comfortable level for the patient.
6 Leave toilet tissue, dry wipe and wet wipe within reach of the patient.
7 Leave the call light within reach of the patient.
8 If you can safely leave the patient wait nearby, allowing for patient privacy.
9 When the patient signals, return and assist them with hand hygiene care.
10 Gently remove the bedpan using the roll technique and cover the bedpan to avoid contamination of the environment.
11 Assist the patient with **perineal care** where required.
12 Remove the dignity blanket/bath towel and the incontinence bed pad for either disposal or laundry, then help the patient back into a comfortable position.
13 Leave the ward and empty the bedpan, using the ward's bedpan cleaning protocol.
14 Remove (doff) the gloves and apron and dispose of them in the correct receptacle.

A range of equipment is available to assist patients to use the toilet safely.

▶ **Electric hoists** are useful for patients who cannot weight bear, and who are unable to undress or assist in any way. They require sufficient space to manoeuvre safely and are always used by two people for safety.
▶ A **commode** is a chair on wheels with a concealed toilet bowl. It can be moved near a lowered hospital bed or wheelchair, with the brakes applied. An individual can then remove their own clothing and move across to use the toilet with support. It may still be necessary to assist them with low-level perineal care afterwards.
▶ A **mobile toilet frame** can be placed over a toilet, giving additional rails to help patients get on and off independently, with easy access to a call cord in case they have difficulties.

A patient risk assessment must be in place where additional equipment is used so that both the patient and healthcare professional are protected from harm.

Fluids and nutrition

Nutrition and hydration are an essential part of a patient's recovery. In order to maintain and repair body tissue, a diet containing an adequate amount of protein must be consumed. Protein is found in foods such as meat, fish, nuts and pulses. A diet containing sufficient zinc and iron is also important in the healing process.

Zinc is essential for making new skin tissue and to aid wound healing. Iron is responsible for maintaining blood haemoglobin levels, which is essential to healing. Vitamin C assists the absorption of iron from foods. As the body does not store vitamin C, foods containing this nutrient should be consumed daily. Green leafy vegetables and fresh orange juices are a good source of vitamin C. Patients should be encouraged to drink orange juice during a meal and the reason why discussed. Drinking tea while eating is unhelpful, as tea contains tannins, which reduce iron absorption. Patients should be made aware of this.

> **Key term**
>
> **Perineal care:** a cleaning method for genital hygiene to prevent infection; there are different methods for patients of different genders.

In addition to physical difficulties with eating and drinking, certain health conditions, such as dementia, can mean a person lacks the feelings of hunger and thirst. This can be a challenge to patient nutrition in various healthcare settings.

Assisting with fluids and nutrition is a regular support role for the healthcare professional (Figure 1.13) and could include the delivery and recording of fluid and food intake. Food is provided for patients who have filled in a menu choice sheet the day before, and there will be additional meals available for patients who arrive on a ward during the day. Patients who find chewing painful or tiring may prefer softer foods, and patients at risk of choking will sometimes have thickening formula prescribed and added to foods that are too liquid.

Assistive equipment may be used to aid eating and drinking where needed. For example, hot drinks will be served with a lid and, where needed, in a spouted cup with handles. Adapted cutlery with thicker handles that are easier to grip, or with the spoon or fork head turned to reduce the need for a hand/wrist twist can be all the modification that is needed. A plate guard can be added to the outside of a plate to prevent spillage and help with getting food items such as peas onto a spoon.

Suddenly being unable to feed yourself and drink safely is a shock – for example in the case of patients who have had a stroke – and there may initially be a reluctance to engage. Reasons for this could be the extent of the brain injury or the period of time for which these limitations are to be expected. Some patients may prefer a family member to assist, while others prefer a trained healthcare worker independent from any personal ties. The option to protect a patient's clothing using a napkin or serviette will be offered, but spillages on clothing can be laundered.

Talking with the patient is paramount when providing person-centred care, with a particular emphasis on offering choice, privacy, dignity and respect, and recognising people's individuality and desire for independence. Talking while supporting the patient to eat is important – but not to the extent that they are trying to talk to appear polite and eat at the same time. Eating in silence is awkward and there is a fine balance here.

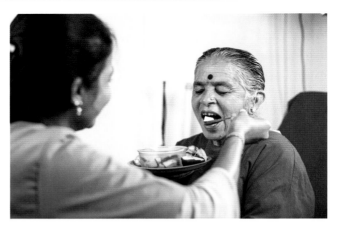

▲ Figure 1.13 Assisting with fluids and nutrition is a regular support role

Reflect

Empowerment when eating means putting the patient in control of what they eat, and when and how they consume their food.

In hospital, *when* patients eat is usually limited to mealtimes.

The choice patients have about *what* to eat is ordinarily limited to what is on the hospital menu. Daily menus will contain four or five choices including options which cater for vegetarians and vegans. There is a separate menu for patients who have allergies. Hospital meals will be carefully created to be nutritious, but patients do not have the extent of choice they would have in their own homes such as having a takeaway or sweets. A patient may wish to ask a relative to bring them alternative foods in but this is discouraged.

How patients eat their food presents a choice too. A patient who wishes, but struggles, to eat independently might progress through a meal very slowly if, for example, they are too weak to chop it small enough to eat. This could mean they take an extended time to eat, and end up eating their food cold. An alternative choice for such a patient could be to ask you to chop the food into smaller pieces and spoon-feed them. This assistance would provide them with warm food more quickly.

▶ What would you like in this scenario if you were the patient – independence or assistance with eating?

▶ Whether a patient eats independently or with assistance, the food will be nutritious and will aid recovery. How could you as a care provider empower a patient in their choices?

Supporting with mobility

When **supporting people with their mobility** you will use specialist equipment set at the right height and which meets their needs in a dignified manner.

- A mobility risk assessment is documentation that is required and can be referred to in order to ensure that the correct level of assistance is provided.
- Movement should be at the pace of the individual. A patient will need time to find their comfortable balance and confidence with any mobility equipment.
- Checking on patients' comfort is good practice in assisting with any mobility tasks, such as asking them if they are ready to be lifted in the hoist. During the early stages of adapting to the mobility changes, effective communication should demonstrate empathy and compassion. Encouragement and reassurance may be all that is needed for some patients; others might need time and patience to adjust, or a conversation that distracts away from what the patient can no longer achieve independently.
- Sitting up in bed takes core muscle usage; it may be an action that can be carried out independently or it might require assistance. Having a firm bedrail to support leverage may assist patients to get in and out of bed independently, or with minimal assistance. For patients who require complete assistance to get in and out of bed, you will need to use a hoist (Figure 1.14) to transfer them from bed to chair, and back again.
- You will assist immobile patients to maintain their personal hygiene through bed baths and bedside washing. As individuals recover, assisting them to sit on a shower chair could support independent washing. Handrails in the shower may be required as a person's health improves; a risk assessment will be carried out to assess the level of risk due to slips and falls, and the necessary support measures will be put in place.
- A patient may have balance issues which mean they require to use a walking frame to stand without support, while others will require assistance to stand, followed by close monitoring. A walking frame is a sturdy piece of mobility equipment on which a patient can lean using both hands, using the frame to bear their weight. Once the patient feels balanced, the frame can be moved a small distance forward by a temporary lift. An occupational therapist is responsible for setting the correct height for the frame and demonstrating its

safe use. They will then check the patient is using it correctly by observation.

- A more suitable mobility aid for some patients is a walking stick. This provides minimal support for balance or can be used to take the pressure off a foot or ankle injury. The height is set and guidance given on safe use. If a patient wishes to have more support than a walking stick but less than a frame, a tetrapod walking stick with four-leg support may be a suitable option. A reasonable amount of arm strength and co-ordination is required for these, so this equipment is not appropriate for all patients.

K1.8 How to support individuals' care needs, ensuring privacy and dignity is maintained while recognising the importance of personal health and wellbeing

Individual care needs

Dignified care means maintaining a patient's privacy while you are carrying out care and treatment tasks and meeting individual care needs, aiming to empower the individual through respectful practice.

Establishing consent

Healthcare consent is when a patient (or their relative with power of attorney) agrees to or gives permission for a medical procedure or clinical task to be carried out. Consent can be given in different forms. Formal written consent will be required for some procedures, such as a surgical procedure. When this is not required, asking for verbal consent before carrying it out or performing any other clinical task shows respect for the patient and gives an opportunity for them to discuss any reservations.

You should not begin any care task without first informing the patient about what the process involves; this applies in particular to personal care tasks. In the majority of cases, you should establish the consent of the patient before performing hypersensitive care duties with compassion. Asking for their consent empowers the patient; asking permission and checking if they are ready to receive any personal hygiene tasks is good practice and shows respect.

- If a patient is unconscious their care plan will highlight the need to address personal hygiene daily and this will be carried out at a time convenient to healthcare professionals, outside visiting times.

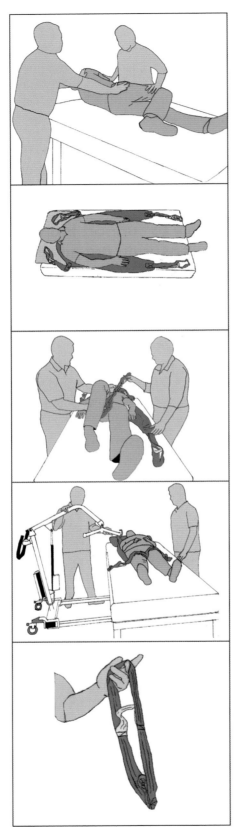

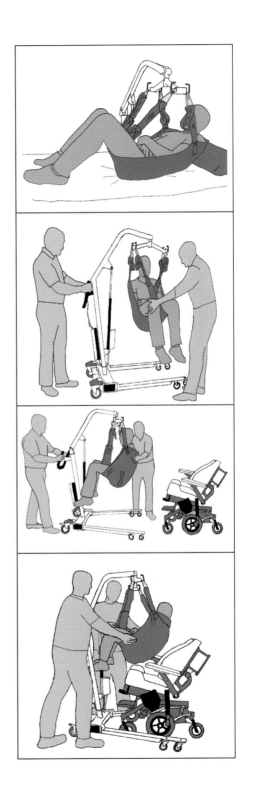

▲ Figure 1.14 Using a hoist safely

▶ In cases where a patient lacks capacity, care is carried out in the person's best interest. For example, for personal hygiene tasks it is expected that health professionals will support this element of care without requiring consent.

▶ Asking a patient about their preference and permission to assist with food at the bedside is appropriate. Assisting with food can mean there are dribbles and potential spillage on a patient's clothing. It may be appropriate to draw the curtains for privacy and to wipe food from around the patient's mouth between mouthfuls to preserve their dignity.

▶ Preparation for a patient before surgery requires a change of clothes into a hospital gown and disposable under garments. Gaining verbal consent prior to assisting with this task and understanding the level of privacy they are happy with is necessary practice.

Respecting cultural differences

Every patient has their own cultural identity. This can be influenced by factors such as ethnicity, geography, education, income, religion, race, sexual orientation, and gender identity or expression. Recognising a patient's uniqueness and individuality encourages them to feel comfortable and able to share what their cultural expectations or needs are.

You need to understand and respect the patient's culture before you carry out any personal hygiene tasks. People from different cultures can have varying opinions on aspects of personal grooming and hygiene, such as the removal of body hair or the frequency of bathing. A conversation should take place with the patient or their relatives regarding their specific cultural needs. Where the patient's usual routine is not in line with the organisation's hygiene and infection prevention policy, you might need to discuss potential risks to the patient's health.

Assisting with personal care and hygiene

Assisting a patient with washing, bathing and toileting, particularly in the case of intimate care tasks like maintaining hygiene in the genital area, calls for a high level of sensitivity and excellent communication skills.

The patient needs to know exactly what is happening and why. Giving an explanation of each step in a procedure and making it clear that they have the right to stop procedures at any point empowers a patient and ensures the experience is as dignified as possible.

If the patient lacks capacity, they may need the support of a relative to reassure them or a Learning Disability Nurse for advice. Any communication barriers need to be identified and overcome. For example, using simplified vocabulary and images can facilitate a patient's understanding and reduce confusion and anxiety.

Assisting with fluids and nutrition

Other healthcare work, such as **assisting with fluids and nutrition**, might include use of a **nasogastric tube** (although this is rarely used in current practice). Nasogastric simply means 'nose to stomach' and the method is used when there is an intestinal obstruction, a problem with swallowing or an issue with premature babies that require a minimally invasive system to monitor their nutrient and fluid intake.

An adult who has had a stroke and is experiencing the symptom of dysphagia (difficulty or discomfort in swallowing), which means they cannot swallow foods without choking, will require tube feeding. This, in combination with other restrictions, can result in an undignified situation. In order to provide empathetic care when assisting with syringe insertion, you must start by closing the dignity curtains surrounding the bed, to protect the patient's dignity, and practise effective communication skills to reduce any negative impact on their emotional wellbeing.

Continual/ongoing care

Ongoing or continual care is often referred to as the care required after the acute phase of the illness has passed. For example, a person who has experienced a stroke will have a person-centred discharge care package. Appointments will be arranged for physiotherapy reviews and speech therapy. The patient's GP will be responsible for close monitoring of blood clotting time, through a blood test called the international normalised ratio (INR), and they will make adjustments to blood thinning medication, commonly warfarin, as ongoing care.

An informal carer, such as a spouse, may not have the capabilities to support their loved one at home. In that case, ongoing care may be in the form of social care in partnership with a District Nurse. Sometimes residential care is the most appropriate choice for safety and ongoing healthcare, even if this is a temporary measure.

Consider communication barriers

Communication barriers can arise in areas such as language, learning and hearing.

▶ Language barriers: a patient who does not speak English, and is not accompanied by a relative who does, will require a translator. A translated leaflet may be all that's needed for you to get consent and explain hospital practices for their care.

▶ Learning barriers: a patient may have difficulty in making themselves understood, for example an individual who has had a stroke or has a physical or learning disability. The use of simplified vocabulary or a picture exchange communication system (PECS) may help you to overcome this barrier.

▶ Hearing barriers: a patient who is deaf could require health professionals to face them when they are talking so that they can lip read. Where possible you should assess the patient's exact communication preferences by consulting them, in order to overcome this barrier. Hearing aids might be required, and you should make sure you speak clearly and do not shout.

▶ The experience of pain, anxiety or distress will alter the ability to communicate, therefore care should be taken to ensure pain is managed well and anxiety alleviated in order to enhance communication.

Communication support for a stroke patient who has aphasia (a complete loss of language) or dysphasia (a partial loss of language) could include written communication or an adult PECS board. This will help overcome problems with making their needs and feelings understood.

The occurrence of a sudden **communication barrier**, or one that is the result of a health condition that is progressive and causing increasing difficulty in conveying messages or asking questions, calls for adaptations and assistive methods that promote dignity in circumstances that are challenging. To overcome such barriers you should, where possible, assess a person's exact preferences for communication by consulting them.

Privacy and dignity

A patient's dignity is the importance and value that they have. Supporting self-respect and self-worth is essential to maintaining a patient's dignity, along with ensuring others treat them with respect. This includes ensuring that they do not feel embarrassed. Treating patients with dignity includes recognising

individuality; what one patient feels comfortable with another person may not. Observing and asking questions to establish the level of comfort conveys compassion, which is important for overall welfare.

An important element of privacy is confidentiality. Privacy is also required for some tasks such as undressing or taking a personal phone call.

Actions that respect a patient's **privacy** and **dignity**, and **reduce anxiety** include:

▶ Closing doors and windows (for example with hospital curtains): closing the door behind a patient who has been escorted for bathing or toileting tasks and being guided by them in terms of the level of assistance they require is good practice which maintains their dignity. Some hospital bays have beds that are visible from a corridor or external window, so actions such as drawing curtains to obscure the view or keep out cooler air may be needed.

▶ Preserving modesty when assisting with bathing (for example a dignity covering): a dignity blanket or towel can be draped over parts of the body that are not being attended to and moved about as a covering that delivers dignified care.

▶ Confidentiality of all information applies to all aspects of care, including hospital notes, patient care records and personal identifiable information such as name, date of birth, address etc. All healthcare workers are bound by a code of confidentiality.

The **age of a patient** may affect their expectations of a healthcare worker's behaviour. You should ask everyone how they like to be addressed, regardless of age.

Test yourself

Explain the methods, actions and communication skills that preserve privacy and dignity when carrying out the following healthcare tasks:

1 simple dressings (such as plasters, sterile pad)
2 urinary catheter care
3 personal care washing
4 personal care dressing
5 personal care bathing
6 personal care toileting
7 removal of soiled bedding and clothing
8 assisting with fluids and nutrition
9 supporting with mobility.

Importance of own personal health and wellbeing

Self-care is important and you will need to manage **your own personal health and wellbeing**. For example, following a twelve-hour shift the regulations generally require that there should be a break of eleven consecutive hours before your next twelve-hour shift. Managing your time well to include adequate sleep between shifts is an important aspect of self-care. When working on a ward you must have a 20-minute break away from your immediate workstation if you are working longer than six hours. Taking the 20 minutes to step away can help with the feeling of burn-out. A senior member of staff will encourage a trainee to engage and share their feelings in a debrief after a particularly traumatic situation involving patient care.

Occupational health

All staff must work within occupational health guidelines. These will include procedures for what to do when something happens at work, such as a needle-stick injury (an accidental stab wound from a used needle). These guidelines will also contain information about mandatory immunisations and how to keep up to date with them.

An organisation's occupational health policy and guidelines will outline the actions that should be taken when a staff member is unwell. Guidelines will outline different actions depending on what the illness is. They will also include who must be contacted in the first instance, how to certificate absence and guidance on when to return to work after an infectious disease.

Mental health

Healthcare professionals should be aware of what mechanisms are in place to support them. Traumatic and upsetting situations can negatively affect mental wellbeing, and time must be built into a professional's daily life to process these events, seek support and attend a professional debriefing where required. It is also important to have a good support network. The NHS has trained Mental Health First Aiders as a point of contact at work.

Practising mindfulness and applying personalised methods to reduce stress levels and achieve a healthy work–life balance promote a healthy mind and lessen the risk factors that contribute to temporary or diagnosed high blood pressure. Mindfulness aims to focus awareness on the present moment. When your mind is overwhelmed, when you are over-thinking, or when stress levels are high, it can be helpful to bring your thoughts to the here-and-now. This can be done, for example, by closing your eyes and listening to your breath as you breathe in and out.

Physical health

Maintenance activities to ensure good physical health, such as getting seven hours' sleep, eating a balanced diet and taking the government-recommended amount of exercise (150 minutes per week), have great importance for overall wellbeing.

If you do not build in time for self-care you are more likely to make mistakes, burn out and become ill, as your immune system is less effective when you are tired or under stress or your diet is poor.

Following extensive research into the impact of stress and tiredness, in 2020 the NHS put together a document called 'Caring for yourself while you care for others: A toolkit for nursing ambassadors to look after their own health.' The document was developed by the health charity C3 Collaborating for Health and brings together advice, links to specific support websites with self-care resources, suggested apps and forums.

The document is well worth reading and includes advice and support in relation to:

▶ physical activity, diet and hydration
▶ mental health, sleep and self-care
▶ supporting nurses and health at work
▶ smoking and alcohol
▶ menstrual health and menopause
▶ caring responsibilities
▶ financial support
▶ bereavement
▶ helping nurses to provide patient care
▶ faith/community groups.

Practice points

S2.12 Support or enable individuals to maintain good personal hygiene

Take part in a bed bath demonstration with a partner or manikin. Narrate the key points as you carry out the task, taking into consideration the importance of communication, privacy and dignity. See also Chapter ANPO2, pages 148–150.

S1.30 Provide person-centred care and support to individuals, carers and relevant others
S1.31 Provide an effective clinical environment, taking into consideration safety, and promote a good experience for the individual
S1.37 Use appropriate techniques and PPE to ensure effective infection prevention and control in the healthcare environment

Madhav is a 40-year-old male who is being treated for bacterial meningitis and has been catheterised due to acute urinary retention. He is conscious but poorly and is showing signs of emotional distress. His wife has questions about his care over the coming weeks. She appears to be in shock. Madhav gives consent for all aspects of his care to be discussed with his wife, to allay her worries and keep her informed. Reassure her by explaining the following:

▶ the organisation's infection prevention procedures (she is aware the cause of the meningitis is bacteria)
▶ how needles are being used in his care (she has read a news report about how a canula was left in a surgical patient in the UK)
▶ how she can visit her husband with their children.

K1.9 How to interpret individual care plans in order to support a person's health, comfort and wellbeing

A care plan will state an individual's preferred care needs. These can be paper documents or electronic systems. Either way, the care recommendations will be recorded in a standardised manner.

Physical needs

The main physical needs are presented in Figure 1.15.

Emotional needs

A care plan does not record how a person feels about necessary assistance – for instance, that they are fiercely independent, have a negative outlook or are having difficulty coming to terms with their diagnosis and not coping with the ADLs necessary to support recovery and maintain independence.

In order to deliver holistic care, those responsible for drawing up a care plan must consider an individual's emotional needs and the effect of the necessary care tasks, which a patient would usually carry out themselves. Reluctance to accept the need for assistance can be addressed in actions and behaviours that improve self-esteem.

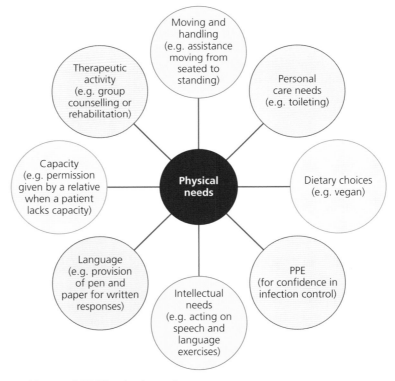

▲ Figure 1.15 Physical needs

Choices

Offering choices wherever possible and giving a person time to choose their preference is empowering. An example of this is consultation about whether they would prefer medication to be administered in liquid or tablet form, and the type of drink they would like to have afterwards.

Independence and dignity

A care plan will state how to maintain independence and dignity in relation to the person's own preference. Healthcare professionals should know to undertake activities in a dignified way, such as closing a curtain before performing a care task. They may need to record in the care plan that the patient prefers to clean her own dentures or deal with her own colostomy bag without anyone else helping.

Social needs

Social needs are very important, particularly in social care. The care plan should record what a person likes to do (such as reading, watching TV, playing music), family members and friends who are likely to visit them and any religious or spiritual activities they like to do.

Supportive relationships

A care plan may note family members who have committed themselves to visiting, but it does not state the frequency of these visits or the emotional connection the patient has with the named people. Some relationships are supportive and others less so, or even damaging. It may not be someone's sincere choice to visit the patient – they may just be doing it out of a sense of duty. There may be protection safeguards in place, so a visit may take place in the communal area rather than the resident's room (in social care, not a hospital). In some cases the visitors may be really important to the patient, but they may also have their own health needs such as dementia or mobility issues.

The time patients and their visitors spend together should encourage the sharing of feelings and provide for the fulfilling of personalised requests, such as bringing in particular sweets or a favourite magazine.

Activity

Physical activity is any movement that raises the heart rate temporarily or strengthens muscles. This can include low-level activities such as chair-based exercises. A patient may benefit from a demonstration or joining in at the start of an exercise task such as arm stretches above the head. Demonstration encourages patients to feel less self-conscious and more motivated. Any exercise releases endorphins (hormones) which can lift a low mood. Making an individual aware of the emotional benefits may encourage participation.

Inactivity does not exercise the heart muscle or the muscles used in gross motor movements. Muscles need to be used in order to maintain their strength and condition, even those of a patient who will not be mobile for several months due to the timescale of their recovery. Without use, joints lose their range of movement and are more likely to be subject to injury, as weakened muscles around the joint are unable to provide the necessary stability when under pressure, such as around the knee when weight is applied by standing.

A physiotherapist will develop an appropriate exercise regime ahead of a patient being capable of mobility, with or without support.

Activity is not restricted to mobility. You will have opportunities to engage patients in social activity during routine clinical tasks. Engaging patients in conversation about themselves or something they are interested in will stimulate their minds.

Engagement

Being part of conversations that take place during a doctor's round, as medical professionals gather around a hospital bed, can lessen anxiety and is a way of acknowledging individuality. The distraction and inclusion will also be beneficial to the patient's mind.

A patient hospitalised with a long-term condition may feel detached and lose connections with life outside the ward. Engaging with the patient by making them aware of a positive news story and encouraging participation in discussions related to this while carrying out care tasks will help support the patient's emotional needs if appropriate.

Cultural and religious needs

Some patients may hold religious beliefs, but even people who are of the same religion may differ – some being more devout than others and interpreting religious texts differently. It is good practice to accommodate and support patients' religious and cultural requirements. For example:
- ▶ A Muslim male who needs to take part in Friday prayers might need to be supported and lowered to a prayer mat, or to have adapted actions enabled that allow some form of participation.
- ▶ Another person of the same religion may accept that this practice will have to be delayed until they have recovered enough to take part without assistance.

Rather than making assumptions, you should consult the patient. This will be empowering, support their emotional wellbeing and comfort them in a situation that can produce insecurities.

> ### Reflect
>
> A 20-year-old biochemistry university student with a supportive friendship group, a boyfriend and a summer placement at a testing laboratory had a stroke. They were home alone and were not discovered for 10 hours. The brain injury is extensive, the right side of the body has partial paralysis, aphasia (reduced ability to understand or produce speech) is present and their vocabulary is limited and basic. For safety they are confined to bed and require formula foods drunk through a straw to address problems with swallowing. Through the use of a communication board they have said they do not want visitors and want to be left to die.
>
> A hospital ward can ensure physical needs are met in a care plan. The patient's expression of feelings conveys almost normal functioning in brain perception and thinking, and a period similar to grief begins.
>
> Naturally occurring opportunities to communicate with this patient come when observation measurements are taken and recorded (for example blood pressure), and during personal care tasks.
>
> ▶ How can compassion be conveyed and sympathy avoided through the use of effective interpersonal skills?
> ▶ What age-appropriate care can be offered in a stroke ward when the other patients are older people?
> ▶ How can care planning include support for intellectual and emotional rehabilitation as well as meeting social needs?

K1.10 How to recognise indicators of good physical and mental health

A patient's physical health deterioration can be monitored from the minute they arrive in a hospital or care home. Mental health concerns may take a little longer to become part of an observed pattern.

Mood

You might notice a subtle change in a patient's **mood** or outlook, such as suddenly becoming disagreeable when they have previously been positive about their treatment and recovery. It's easy to dismiss mood changes and attribute them to an obvious cause without further investigation, but a short conversation with the patient may reveal the root cause, which can then be addressed.

Appetite

Noticeable changes in appetite – such as an individual leaving food untouched or requesting only sweet foods – can be a non-verbal indicator of how they are feeling. Not feeling hungry or thirsty can be a symptom of dementia, so extra attention to this needs to be part of the care plan, to make sure drinks are supplied regularly and the patient is prompted to drink. It is part of good practice when working with a person living with dementia to remind and encourage them to take sips of fluid.

Body language

Body language – for example displaying signs of anxiousness such as fidgeting or lack of eye contact – can reveal whether a person is in pain, anxious or uncomfortable (there is more on this in section K1.12, below). A patient may not want to discuss an aspect of their physical health or may feel that their emotional health is not important enough to share with professionals. You should be alert to such hidden messages as they help to build a picture of an individual, which enables adjustment or additions to a care plan.

Mobility

A patient's motivation to continue physiotherapy exercises designed to improve their mobility can change, suggesting an emotional barrier. In comparison, an obsession with exercise that is impacting someone in a negative way and setting back their recovery is also a mental mindset that is cause for concern.

Normal bodily functions

A patient's bodily functions may deviate from their usual pattern. For instance, withholding of stool or eating less to reduce the amount of faeces that needs to be expelled could be a sign of stress when requiring toileting support, or a way of feeling in control when there is so much that is out of a patient's control. Similarly, refusing to drink can lead to dehydration and increase the risk of urinary tract infections.

Sleep pattern

On average, adults need 7–9 hours of sleep per day. A pattern outside those parameters may be observed and reported. For example, this could be a side effect of a particular medication, which may go unnoticed as the patient does not associate the insomnia with the medication and assumes it's occurring just because they are in hospital and is therefore not worth mentioning.

Personal hygiene

Self-neglect of personal hygiene can potentially be an indicator of low self-esteem, a worsening chronic medical condition or a symptom of depression. Without action, these symptoms could worsen and it will then become more of a challenge to improve them. Observing excessive cleanliness, for example hand washing, could indicate a psychological condition.

K1.11 The importance of fluids, nutrition and food safety when providing overall care

Fluids

Choking occurs when a full or partial blockage to the trachea means that a patient's breathing is impaired or prevented. Fluids are a common cause of choking, as the consistency of the fluid allows liquid to enter the trachea rather than the oesophagus. There are several reasons why an individual might choke when trying to drink fluids:

- ▶ neurodegenerative disease
- ▶ a brain injury caused by an accident or stroke.

Dehydration may complicate a medical problem or slow down recovery, and this can quickly become a serious problem for the patient. An adult is 55–65 per cent water, two-thirds of which is fluids in cells, which means dehydration impacts on all parts of the body and its functions.

A patient who has been experiencing diarrhoea and vomiting prior to being admitted or during hospitalisation may require monitoring of their intake and output of fluids. Dehydration can cause a drop in blood pressure and acute kidney damage, so encouraging the intake of fluids is an important part of managing this condition. Patients who require extensive fluid rehydration or those who are experiencing excessive vomiting and cannot keep down a drink of water may require intravenous fluids and catheterisation, so that fluid balance is closely monitored and kidney function observed. Monitoring **skin turgor** is a simple test for dehydration by pinching a fold of skin on the back of the hand to assess hydration levels. If the skin does not snap back as it should for the patient's age (the older the person, the slower their skin will be to snap back due to natural loss of elasticity) more fluids must be given to prevent damage to the **cytoplasm** level within the cell membrane, a cause of organ failure.

Key terms

Neurodegenerative disease: a group of health conditions where nerve cells do not transmit neural messages as they should and an individual loses normal functioning over time.

Skin turgor: the skin's elasticity and its ability to change shape and return to normal.

Cytoplasm: the material or protoplasm within a living cell.

For some patients, over-hydration is a risk. The kidneys are responsible for water balance as a homeostatic mechanism within the body. A patient with kidney disease may be guided to limit the amount of fluid they consume. Dialysis helps remove excess fluid but will not completely resolve a build-up of fluid retention, usually in the lower legs and hands.

Nutrition

An adequate balance of **nutrition** through a variety of foods supports recovery, such as promoting healing after surgery. Protein, zinc and vitamins – in particular vitamins C and D – help in the healing of bones and skin. If a patient is malnourished it will delay their recovery and compromise their immune system, leading to an intensification of their illness.

A **Malnutrition Screening Tool (MST)** is useful as an initial assessment method. When using one of these you will ask a patient questions about their diet and appetite, and monitor any weight changes. A BMI (body mass index) calculation standardises health risks linked to the amount of body fat a person has, and a care plan will state a person's required nutritional intake in light of this, which may include supplementation to improve their overall health and wellbeing.

Food safety

Food safety is important in order to prevent harm being caused to a patient by consuming food. Harm could include physical contamination, such as a false nail lost in preparation or bacteria or virus being present in the food, which causes food poisoning. Salmonella is a common bacterium which causes food poisoning. It can be found in a variety of foods, including chicken, beef, pork, eggs, fruits, vegetables and even processed foods. Cross-contamination from these raw foods to cooked foods is another way this toxin enters the body.

E. coli is the most serious cause of food poisoning. A 2023 government report stated that there were 6,087 deaths within 30 days of an E. coli infection, indicating a mortality rate of 10.9 deaths per 100,000 population.

Standards of hygiene and cleaning regimes for food workstations must meet **food safety regulations**. Failure to meet the legal standard has the potential to cause a **food poisoning** outbreak, and that is much more dangerous for people who are already vulnerable.

Observing the correct food safety procedures prevents the contamination of foods, which could be responsible for a life-threatening **allergic reaction**. An allergic reaction occurs when a patient's immune system reacts unusually to specific foods. Allergies can be specific, such as sesame seeds, or more general, such as all nuts. The allergic reaction can be mild, such as an individual having itchy skin or hives, or can be acute and rapid, causing anaphylactic shock, which can cause the swelling of the lips and airways and as a result stop breathing.

A food intolerance is not an immune response but can cause an unpleasant reaction to a particular food. Either the food is not digested properly, or it acts as an irritant and causes diarrhoea.

Workstations should have no cross-contamination and should be used, cleaned and monitored in a way that complies with food safety regulations.

As a procedure to avoid cross-contamination, gloves must be removed between touching raw foods (such as meat) and cooked foods. The heat used in cooking food kills food-poisoning bacteria, so uncooked food should not be touched by a glove which could transfer these pathogens to cooked food. Staff will need to remove the gloves correctly and dispose of them safely during cooking and service.

K1.12 How to recognise the signs and symptoms of a person who is experiencing pain and discomfort and/or whose health and wellbeing is deteriorating

Pain is a specific response by the body that indicates there is something wrong. People experience pain in many different ways. Some people have a high threshold for pain in that they can manage their pain well. Others have a low threshold, meaning that they are unable to cope well with pain.

Older people may live with chronic pain and as such do not report additional pain to health professionals

> **Key term**
>
> **Delirium:** a decline in mental state characterised by disorientation, paranoia, hallucinations and agitation.

because they do not see it as being important enough to report.

There are multiple pain assessment tools that can be utilised when monitoring and treating a person's pain. These tools enable the health professional to identify the best approach to pain management – even when the person is unable to articulate the level of pain they are experiencing.

Body language and reactions

A patient's level of consciousness can affect their ability to coherently communicate pain, for instance, a person who is in a state of **delirium** or confusion may not be able to describe the type of pain they are experiencing or locate the origin of that pain. Pain may be the only symptom to indicate a deterioration in a patient's health status, which means monitoring and observing an individual for signs of pain is an important part of your role as a healthcare worker.

▶ People who have injuries that cause paralysis still feel pain. They may not be able to identify where the pain is coming from, but they experience neuropathic pain in varying levels, causing discomfort similar to that experienced by someone with no such paralysis.

▶ An individual with a language barrier could display **body language** that indicates pain, for example **restlessness**, **fidgeting** and **wincing**.

▶ The use of a visual analogue scale (VAS) may be suitable to measure a patient's pain intensity. VAS is a scale from zero to ten which is accompanied by simple outline drawings of a face. Zero is a smiling face and ten shows a face with obvious grimacing and tears. A patient can point to where they think their pain is on the rating scale; this can be repeated to assess any increase or decrease in pain intensity.

Other body language actions, like sharp movements or reactions to touch such as flinching, are easier to spot.

Appearance

Skin colour and appearance alone can signal the possibility of pain. For example, in people with pale skin, vasodilation may cause blood flow to increase at the surface of their skin. The flushed appearance is caused by an increase of adrenergic activity and is usually only temporary. Patients may also present as pale/clammy or nauseous as a result of pain. Such skin colour changes are not so easy to observe in patients who have dark skin, making this type of assessment important so that you do not miss these signs and cues.

Pain assessment tools

Pain is a very personal and individual experience. It is difficult to properly understand what the individual is feeling when they report that they have pain. Pain tools are used for measuring levels of pain when someone is having difficulty expressing what they are feeling. Examples of such tools include:

▶ numeric rating scale (NRS) – the patient rates their pain by a number between 1 and 10
▶ visual analogue scale (VAS) – the patient matches their pain level to colours or smiley/upset faces.

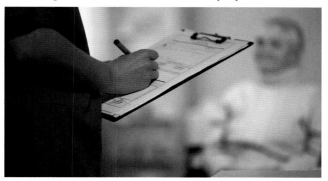

▲ Figure 1.16 Pain assessment plays an important role in treatment decisions

An increasing level of pain is commonly a sign that further assessment is necessary and that treatment needs to be increased or adjusted (Figure 1.16). Monitoring a patient's level of pain over time informs medical practitioners of factors such as how well a medication is working or how inflammation causing pain is reducing over time.

K1.13 How and why to report changes and deterioration when supporting individuals

A nurse is often the first person to notice the changes that suggest a deterioration in health.

How to report

Any changes to a patient's physical health, physiological measurements or appearance while you are carrying out your observations must be reported to a senior colleague and documented in the patients' records. Documentation of physiological and psychological changes are important in that they will

support the health professionals caring for the person to make changes to their treatment on the basis of the changes they are seeing. A report that needs request for immediate action as a result of patient deterioration can be initially verbal but then must be recorded in a timely manner in the medical records of that individual.

Minor changes should be recorded and monitored, so that a picture of the physiological changes is gradually built up. This can then be acted on as directed by the healthcare professional in charge of the person's care.

Why to report

The work pattern changes that take place during a day mean that several healthcare workers will be monitoring the same patient. For this reason, it is important to

Case study

S1.36 Recognise limitations in mental capacity and respond appropriately

Maryam is a 19-year-old patient with Down's syndrome who requires repair surgery for an atrioventricular septal defect (AVSD), which causes blood flow through her heart to not be as it should. This was not picked up when she was a child. Maryam's parents can often recognise changes in her from observing her, and use appropriate communication to clarify points of concern with her, such as the type of chest pain or level of dizziness she is experiencing.

Consent for the operation has been given and you are responsible for Maryam's pre-op care. Working in partnership with her parents will help you gain a more accurate assessment of her current health status to pass on to the team in charge of the patient's care.

You have been tasked with being a point of contact for Maryam and her family, to reduce their anxieties and keep them informed and up to date. Maryam will need adaptations with communication as she lacks capacity and this is a barrier. You have contact details for a trained specialist advocate from the charity organisation Mencap.

Create an information leaflet about AVSD aimed at the parents, and explain it in a role play; the leaflet will act as a stimulus for their questions. Your role is to be factual and offer reassurance about different aspects of the procedure. Reassure the parents that you are listening to them, and that their contributions are valuable. If they have any questions that are beyond your scope of knowledge, you can offer to put these to the specialist medical professional. Leave the leaflet with them so that they can reread it later.

document the care given to the patient and any changes in their health condition. When delivering care it is important to practise continuity of care to accurately highlight patterns, deterioration and improvements. This is a co-ordinated effort by the multidisciplinary team to respond to changes and maintain the most suitable treatment plan to **ensure a patient's care needs are met**.

K1.14 How to safely move and handle people when supporting their care needs using appropriate moving and handling aids

When to move

The Manual Handling Operations Regulations have already formed part of your core learning. There are many different occasions that call for people to be moved safely. For example:

▶ You may need to assist an individual with getting in and out of bed or a wheelchair, after which they may also need assisting to get on the toilet.

▶ A patient who has been sedated or is unconscious will need to be turned at intervals, as decided by the team overseeing the patient's care.

▶ In order to prevent a pressure injury from forming, a patient's position will need to be changed to vary the places where their weight is putting pressure on the surface of their skin and reducing blood flow to the area.

▶ When a patient arrives by ambulance they will need to be moved from the **hydraulic stretchers** to a bed in the Emergency Department.

In the initial phase of care when the patient arrives at hospital, senior members of staff will decide when and how to move them and the staff to be involved, which will often be more than one person. At a later point, a risk assessment will determine the correct method of transfer/movement for each person.

How to move

Risk assessment

The TILE model

Planned or standard patient movement will be preceded by a risk assessment using a model such as the **Task, Individual, Load and Environment (TILE) model**, as shown in Figure 1.17.

Strategies to prevent injury to both staff and patient are examined as part of the risk assessment process,

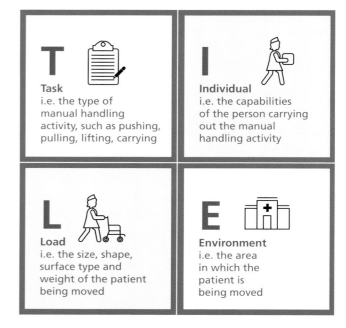

▲ Figure 1.17 The TILE model

starting with any perceived hazards, such as a patient who is confused and may make sudden movements that are unpredictable.

The 5 Manual Handling Principles (5Ps)

Another technique that might be used to guide good practice is the **5 Manual Handling Principles** (5Ps) (see Figure 1.18).

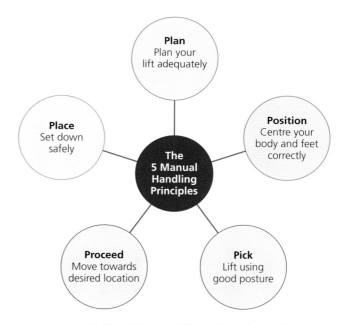

▲ Figure 1.18 The 5 Manual Handling Principles (5Ps)

Key terms

Hydraulic stretchers: stretchers used in medical emergencies that are powered to lift and drop their height, are on wheels for smooth movement, and have side rails and straps to keep a patient safely in position.

5 Manual Handling Principles: the 5Ps guidance on good practice – Plan, Position, Pick, Proceed, Place.

Prepare the environment

The environment where the move is to take place needs to be prepared and you should ensure it is free of trip hazards. Make sure any equipment you will need, such as hoist controls, is to hand and in good working order prior to any use. Thinking about the process before beginning any movement or lifting should help you to assess the risk and remove any hazards before you start.

Encourage active participation

If a patient is able to move themselves safely or has partial movement and can make their way to the side of a mattress, for example, you should encourage them to actively participate and assist with the moving and handling technique you are using. They may wish to put a transfer belt on themselves, position a transfer board and say when they are ready for the move to start, all of which is empowering.

Performing the move

▶ Moving requires a suitable place to grip and you should ensure you **have a firm hold**.

▶ **Keep the weight close to your body, your back straight and your knees bent**.

▶ If a patient does not feel comfortable or is unable to say when the move or lift should start, there

Case study

S1.32 Move and handle individuals safely when assisting them with their care needs, using appropriate moving and handling aids

S1.33 Assist with individuals' overall comfort and wellbeing

S1.34 Recognise issues and deterioration in mental and physical health, report and respond appropriately, supporting others to do so

S1.35 Recognise and respond to signs of pain and discomfort in the individual

You work in a rehabilitation centre and have been supporting two patients, Aamina and Jonathon, for a month. You are to assist in a supporting healthcare role, providing basic physiotherapy and observing/recording signs of pain, discomfort or deterioration. You are to demonstrate your knowledge and skills using a partner, narrating the care you are providing and covering all points in the above four skills criteria.

Some moving and handling tasks will require a second person, so you will need a partner.

It would be an enhanced learning experience if you have your demonstration recorded so you can evaluate your practical demonstration using Gibbs' reflective cycle to identify any areas for improvement.

1   Aamina is a 28-year-old female and is recovering from a car accident. She has no control of her legs due to a spinal injury. Although she has paraplegia she feels pain but cannot identify where it originates.

   ▶ You must assist Aamina to move from her hospital bed to standing for dressing, using a transfer belt then a walking frame for support when putting her trousers on.

   ▶ Once Aamina is dressed you will use a transfer board to assist movement from the bed to a self-propelled wheelchair.

   ▶ Aamina is taking pain medication, but at times when her pain is not managed well additional pain relief is required. You will observe signs of discomfort and report these.

   ▶ The care plan states that progress in social interaction is needed, so you need to encourage contact with society through visitors, the spine injury support group and social media.

2   Jonathon is a 62-year-old male and is recovering from a car accident. He sustained a brain injury and has just arrived at the rehabilitation unit. He is unable to move due to difficulties with co-ordination and balance. While his progress has been positive, there are concerns about small signs of deterioration. Jonathon's wife, Lynda, spends a lot of time at his bedside and must be informed about care tasks and their purpose.

   ▶ You must use a glide sheet to reposition Jonathon for skincare and comfort despite the use of a specialised mattress.

   ▶ You must use a hoist to move Jonathon from bed to manual wheelchair.

   ▶ When his wife is not present you are to support Jonathon at mealtimes, where he needs some assistance.

   ▶ You notice a deterioration in Jonathon's co-ordination meaning he can no longer eat without full assistance. Describe and escalate your concerns appropriately.

must be an **agreed countdown** between all people involved in the move, for example 'move on 3'.

▶ It usually involves at least **two members of staff** to ensure a patient is moved safely.

▶ **Handling aids** and/or **mobility equipment** can be used, depending on the type of movement or lift, for example a transfer belt to support a patient's balance when moving from seated to standing, or a hoist (Figure 1.19).

▶ If you have any concerns about worn or faulty equipment this must be **reported as a maintenance concern** and you should record it.

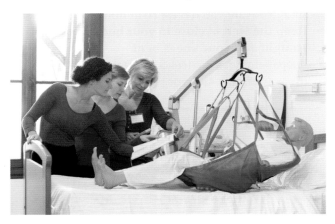

▲ Figure 1.19 Handling aids such as hoists can be used to move and support patients safely

K1.15 The main types of mental ill health and their impact on people's lives

Mental ill health may develop over time or occur suddenly, and to varying degrees of severity. Frequently, people will have a collection of symptoms that do not necessarily neatly fit one diagnosis. For this reason, diagnosis is often 'open', for instance stating that a person has episodes or delusions or is self-harming, rather than specifically labelling the illness.

The main types of mental ill health

There are many different kinds of mental ill health, including:

▶ **mood disorders**, for example depression or bipolar disorder, causing inconsistencies in motivation and self-care during episodes of low mood, or risk-taking behaviours during a bipolar episode, over a period of time

▶ **anxiety disorders**, for example obsessive compulsive disorder (OCD), affecting sleep and functioning, such as being unable to be in close proximity to a doctor without infection prevention measures that are out of proportion

▶ **personality disorders**, for example narcissistic personality disorder, making the patient inconsiderate and unapologetic with other patients

▶ **psychotic disorders**, for example schizophrenia, where a person may be paranoid about being poisoned and will therefore refuse medication and hospital food

▶ **eating disorders**, for example anorexia or bulimia nervosa, leading to secretive behaviour around eating, such as objecting to being observed to ensure food is consumed and not disposed of

▶ **trauma-related disorders**, for example post-traumatic stress (PTS), which has specific triggers that must be identified and strategies implemented to avoid these triggers if possible

▶ **substance abuse disorders** can mean patients' behaviours are unpredictable during withdrawal, and care should be taken that, where possible, re-exposure to the substance is avoided.

The impact of mental ill health

The impact of mental ill health varies from person to person and depends on many factors, such as their support network, whether their employer is understanding and their own willingness to seek help. Each person living with a mental illness will have a collection of symptoms that will vary in their severity – perhaps being continual, occurring in a cycle or in the form of occasional episodes.

Over time some people will find their own managing and coping strategies; others are happy to trial medication and find therapeutic intervention useful. However, there are also people who reject treatment and cannot function properly.

Decision making

The symptoms of mental ill health include making poor choices and a reduced ability to make decisions. For example:

▶ a patient with poor self-worth may refuse to take medication or engage in therapies

▶ during visiting times, an individual could involve a relative in bringing in alcohol or other substances, which must be avoided with the type of medication they have been prescribed

▶ a patient who needs monitoring while medication dosages are being trialled may spontaneously decide to sign a Discharged Against Medical Advice form before discussing potential consequences.

Physical wellbeing

Risk-taking behaviour is any action that has a negative effect on your health, your happiness or other people. This could be direct, such as substance misuse, or indirect, such as being complicit with criminal behaviour of others.

Mental ill health can make a person think only in the short term, for example the next few days and not the longer-term future. The impact of this is not considering the consequences of actions in a few years' time, such as binge drinking and liver damage over time.

Where mental ill health causes self-neglect and self-loathing, destructive behaviours can cause a person to become physically unwell, as they may become malnourished, dehydrated and susceptible to infection.

Emotional and psychological wellbeing

Health psychology is the science of analysing the perspectives that affect people's compliance with treatments, their outlook and whether an individual feels a change in their lifestyle is achievable. Psychological wellbeing can be influenced by mental ill health, but there are other factors that may have an impact too. An individual who is resilient and has self-belief can bring positive actions, compared to an individual with low self-esteem who may be reluctant to believe or comply with advice given about healthy activity.

The **health belief model** states that a person's belief in the personal threat to them from an illness, for example in relation to smoking and cancer, together with their belief in the effectiveness of a recommended health behaviour, for example whether it is worth stopping smoking after 30 years, influences whether they will change their health risk behaviours.

The **theory of planned behaviour** focuses on predicting a person's health compliance intentions, determined by three factors: their attitudes, subjective norms and perceived behavioural control. If a person has family role models who smoke, for instance, this is their norm from which they have developed their attitude. They may believe that change is out of their control, as they know others who have already tried and failed, or they may firmly believe that they need a cigarette and the drive behind this is not a nicotine addiction.

Interactions with others

For a proportion of the people who experience mental ill health, the support they receive brings them closer to family and friends; they feel secure enough to interact with others and sometimes stay in employment, even if it is with reduced hours. A person's engagement with healthcare professionals may be affected by paranoia, lack of confidence or low mood. Certain medications can have side effects that leave a person more easily confused or excessively tired while their body gets used to the drug regimes.

Stigma

Society has reduced the impact of **stigma**, ignorance and judgements experienced by people who are experiencing mental ill health. Low self-esteem may influence a person's compliance with a programme of medication and counselling, as they do not feel worthy or value themselves enough at that time to take preventative measures to support their mental health.

Fear of stigma may influence a person to be reluctant to openly discuss potential symptoms. In addition, certain cultures are not accepting of diagnosed mental illnesses, and people who have pushed themselves to overcome mental barriers to physical activity (such as military veterans) are less likely to seek medical intervention, believing they are weak for not being able to independently change their mindset.

Mental ill health is not always viewed as being as important as physical health, and early signs and symptoms are sometimes ignored until a person requires extensive care or experiences a crisis in their ability to cope with the pressure of mental ill health.

Impact on family and carers

Someone with a mental illness needs to form a support network that gives them an understanding listening ear and opportunities to feel secure during socialising.

The people who form this support network may be friends and family of the patient and they may feel concerned about saying and doing the right thing. That pressure can in turn be felt by the person living with mental ill health, who may already be very likely to feel as if they are dysfunctional and a burden, which can cause strain or deterioration in these relationships.

A patient who does not have friends and family to form a support network, or has become estranged from them, may not have a supportive environment to return to following discharge. For these patients, observing other patients with visitors may contribute to a further deterioration in mental wellbeing.

> ### Key term
>
> **Stigma:** negative perception associated with a particular person or circumstance.

Financial and social impacts

People experiencing mental and physical ill health may find themselves in financial difficulty if they are unable to work. Being able to provide information for the individual around the types of benefits they may be entitled to is an important part of the health professionals' role.

Another symptom of mental ill health may be the development of social phobia or fear of judgement, causing the individual to remove or withdraw themselves from any social contact. Being misunderstood and not having the confidence or words to describe the illness is difficult. The choice is to try to explain their actions or to shy away from the kinds of situation where an individual may be exposed to questions.

K1.16 How to recognise indicators and limitations in mental capacity and how to respond appropriately in line with local policies and procedures

Learning disabilities are usually identified as a child grows, missing developmental milestones, falling behind in terms of interpreting information and behaving in a way that requires adjustments to meet their needs. A deterioration in functioning could be caused by an acquired brain injury or a progressive deterioration due to disease. Some people have fluctuating capacity, which means their decision making can vary and improve during lucid intervals, for example in the case of someone living with dementia.

Examples of loss of capacity may include:
- A person who has severe and unmanaged schizophrenia may make unsuitable or dangerous choices during episodes of delusion or paranoia.
- A brain injury can change an independent adult into one who cannot concentrate, make safe and reasonable decisions or carry out ADL tasks such as managing their finances.
- A patient who experiences symptoms of dementia may lose the power to self-manage at times but have good days (where they need minimal safeguarding support) and bad days (characterised by verbal repetition and increased agitation), meaning their capacity fluctuates.

Mental Capacity Act 2005 (amended 2019)

As we have already seen (page 13), this law protects the rights of people who may find basic information complex and overwhelming, making them vulnerable adults.

Recognising indications and limitations in mental capacity

Indications that a person may lack capacity include:
- **lack of understanding of specific information**, such as the importance of taking medication at a set time, the correct dosage and what the prescription is treating
- **inability to retain information**, for example remembering when to take medication or not forgetting an appointment
- **difficulty in weighing up information** or how to start the process of making a decision, for example whether to have a shower or bath
- **finding it a challenge to communicate a choice**, which takes a level of concentration; thought processing may take longer and feeling there is a pressure to answer might add to a person's stress; someone in this situation may remain quiet or ask the healthcare worker to make the decision for them.

Taking in multiple sensory information can be a challenge, or an impossibility, depending on the level of learning disability: mild, moderate, severe or profound.

Deterioration in someone living with dementia is categorised in stages – early, middle and late – as capacity moves into the lack of capacity phase.

Common symptoms in early-stage dementia include forgetfulness and repeating conversations, difficulty learning new things or following conversations (particularly if it is multi-way communication), poor concentration, limited attention span, or out of character mood swings, including apathy and depression.

Some symptoms in middle-stage dementia can include a further deterioration in thinking and loss of immediate short-term memories; as this progresses, the short-term timeline increases. Patients may no longer manage daily tasks without support and may become unaware of their health condition. Problem-solving steps are sometimes missed, which can cause confusion and distress.

In late-stage dementia there is severe impairment; recognising people, places and objects ceases. Patients lose the ability to speak, to safely eat, to walk and can become doubly incontinent.

How to respond appropriately
Adapt information

You could use simplified language, speak at a slower pace and/or use appropriate prompts to aid an individual's thought processing – for example explaining there is a need for them to take tablets to make them feel better, or giving them the choice to have their medication on a spoon to swallow, prompting them to think about the experience of swallowing or whether they would like a drink with their medication.

The use of images and pictures can be helpful in prompting people to remember information or instigate actions such as eating, drinking, brushing their teeth or using the toilet or shower.

Use of an advocate

Family and formal care providers who know the person best can act as advocates, speaking on behalf of a person who has limited capacity then spending time considering their point of view to ensure they accurately represent their thoughts and opinions, and that these are communicated correctly. An external trained advocate, such as an **Independent Mental Capacity Advocate (IMCA)** or **Independent Mental Health Advocate (IMHA)**, can support a patient where there are complications in family relationships and there is concern that a personal advocate does not have the patient's best interest in mind when care decisions are made.

IMCA is part of the safeguarding process for people who may not be able to keep themselves safe when decision making. In England, IMCAs are appointed by a local authority; in Wales they are appointed by a local Health Board for anyone over 16 who lacks capacity. These advocates are independent and impartially support the person, to ensure their rights are maintained and voice is heard.

An IMHA can support an individual in a range of ways and is an entitlement under the Mental Health Act. They can simply listen to a person's views and concerns; sharing emotions often has a positive effect. Decisions need to be made by a person who is mentally unwell and appropriate support must be offered.

An advocate's role can be to support an individual to explore what options they have and make them aware of rights. This could include providing information which is understandable to help the patient to make informed decisions. They may support a patient to contact relevant people such as estranged family and accompany a person to a care plan meeting or appointments. In some cases, an advocate will speak on behalf of a person, giving their opinion and sharing their wishes and needs when they feel unable to themselves.

Adapt communication

Communication with the individual will need to be adapted. For example, you should start by using the

> ### Key term
>
> ***Asperger's syndrome:*** a developmental disorder that is a form of autism spectrum disorder. Symptoms include difficulties in socialising, misunderstanding sarcasm and social cues, and having behaviours and thinking patterns that can be rigid and repetitive.

name of the person who has **Asperger's syndrome**, to capture their attention and be clear as to who is in the conversation. Respond appropriately at a level that aids understanding, using simplified vocabulary, visual aids or gestures.

K1.17 The importance of early diagnosis in relation to cognitive issues

Identifying signs and symptoms early on will mean an early diagnosis. A gradual decline in mental capacity may start with memory lapses or delusions. Examples of this could be forgetting where everyday objects belong such as keys, or putting items of clothing in unusual places such as the fridge. A memory clinic is a centre where issues with memory will be investigated by specialists. A memory clinic has staff who are experts in working with patients where there are concerns about recall. An early referral to a memory clinic may mean early medical intervention to slow down a decline in cognition.

Episodes of acute mental health decline may be associated with infection such as chest or urinary tract infections. These should be reviewed and treated as soon as possible.

▶ **Formulation and/or adaptation of care plans** is required to support a person's changing needs throughout their life stages and phases.

▶ The sooner a cognitive deficit is noticed and assessments carried out to analyse the causes of behaviours, the sooner **appropriate treatments and support** can be provided.

▶ Introducing an advocate at the early stages of a cognitive deterioration will give time for a relationship to develop. The advocate can get to know the person in times of lucidity, be able to speak on their behalf and guide professionals on how best to communicate with the patient. Getting to know the needs, wishes and preferences of a person who lacks capacity takes quality time. Early involvement is preferable, especially for a person who finds social situations threatening.

K1.18 The possible signs of mental ill health

Symptoms of mental ill health may be visible to the observer, such as those shown in Figure 1.20.

In addition to the signs presented in Figure 1.20, **suicidal thoughts** are rarely discussed by the affected individual and can remain hidden for years. By giving someone opportunities to discuss destructive feelings without pressure, and reassuring them that they will not be judged, you may encourage them to share their

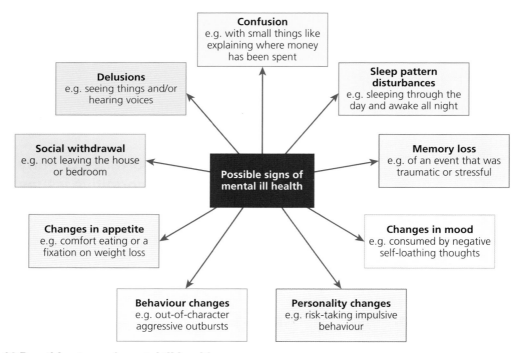

▲ Figure 1.20 Possible signs of mental ill health

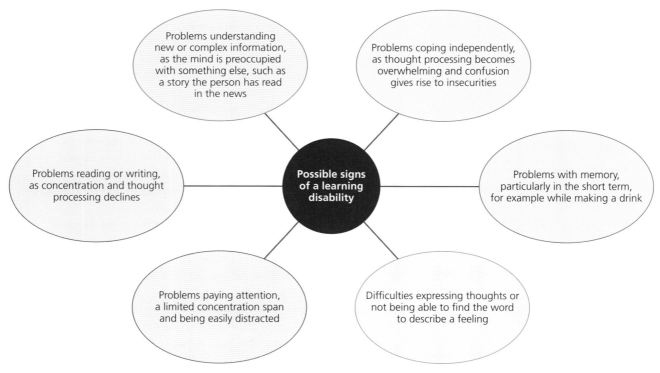

▲ Figure 1.21 Possible signs of a learning disability

feelings. A mental health specialist practitioner, who is independent from an individual's usual social circle, could be the person a patient chooses to tell when they are experiencing suicidal thoughts, or thoughts that relate to them harming themselves in some way.

K1.19 The possible signs of learning disability

Some of the possible signs that a person might have a learning disability are presented in Figure 1.21.

K1.20 Factors that may be mistaken for mental ill health

Marked changes in an individual's usual behaviour, such as distress or anxiety, can be mistaken for symptoms of mental ill health, especially if the person observing them is a family member or friend who is hypervigilant.

External factors

External factors such as diet, exercise and lack of sleep can have an impact on the way an individual feels and behaves. To a greater or lesser extent, these are factors that can be controlled by an individual with support. Other factors, such as the effect of grief or loss, or the use of substances such as alcohol and drugs, can be more difficult to manage.

Lifestyle

The misuse of substances such as alcohol or other drugs is often seen as being symptomatic of the person experiencing mental ill health.

▶ Alcohol and other drugs are often used as a coping strategy and are sometimes described as 'self-medicating'. However, while these substances can enhance a mood, they often contain chemicals that act as depressants; therefore, they can be a contributory factor in the cause of depression in addition, for example, to the damage that excess use of alcohol can cause to the liver.

▶ A recreational stimulant drug is taken by someone who is seeking a high; however, more often than not, this is followed by a natural period of low mood. At some point, there may be a realisation that a substance has become an out-of-control addiction that is damaging to self-image and mood.

▶ Sudden weight loss can cause concern and may be closely linked to the onset of an eating disorder, or it can be a symptom of a physical illness, including overactive thyroid, coeliac disease or cancer.

Life events

An unexpected life event can temporarily give rise to a heightened emotional state. Bereavement, for instance, is a personal journey from loss to the return of normal functioning. Wanting to be alone, a prolonged period of sadness, or appearing unfazed due to denial, could all be viewed as symptoms of depression.

Adaptations from childhood to adulthood

Puberty and the menopause

During puberty, the natural alteration of hormone levels causes physical changes in the reproductive organs. Oestrogen, progesterone and testosterone also lead to changes in mood, as levels of these hormones fluctuate. Although physiological changes during puberty are often similar, they will vary from person to person, and puberty can be a very different experience for two people. For example, a 13-year-old male may experience acne when growing facial hair when another does not. The start of menstruation ranges, on average, between the ages of 10 and 15 years old. For some people in adolescence, hormonal changes are noticeably characterised by outbursts of anger, tears and a distorted perception of a situation.

Individuals experiencing the perimenopause or menopause can have episodes of anxiety in addition to physical effects, such as weight gain due to metabolism changes or loss of libido affecting intimate behaviour. Someone experiencing the menopause may find that they are able to adapt well to changes by, for example, being prepared for short hot flushes. These may occur for roughly four minutes and a person could be prepared by wearing a cardigan which can be removed and put on easily. However, another person's experience of hot flushes may be much more extreme. A hot flush can last for up to an hour and this patient's menopause is more likely to impact on daily life significantly, hindering the ability to work or socialise with confidence.

Sexuality

Sexuality is a personal experience that can be experienced differently from person to person. It is the way people experience and express themselves in a sexual manner. Hormones affect sexual desire, causing an individual's sexuality to become apparent. An individual's sexual desires are not always experienced in the way they expect, which can contribute to a level of confusion and stress over a period of time.

The impact of this can be exhaustion, an increased vulnerability to infections due to a lowered immunity caused by stress and exhaustion, as well as social avoidance.

The healthcare needs of an individual may intersect with their sexuality; for example, a young gay man might need informing of preventative medical treatments to stay healthy while being sexually active. A gay or bisexual woman in a same-sex relationship may feel she wants to think about having a baby in the future and seek information about IVF treatment.

A patient who has been party to bullying or a hate crime may not feel comfortable in sharing their sexuality in a healthcare setting.

Gender identity

During the transformation from child to adult, self-concept develops and an individual's view of gender identity grows, for example affirming gender, changing gender and gender fluidity. This is commonly a time of psychological turbulence and uncertainty, leading to feelings of distress and anxiety in the young person.

In healthcare, it must be acknowledged that the gender of a person cannot be externally read or assumed. Gender identity is what the individual feels, and this may or may not be how they dress, wear their hair, speak or what they call themselves.

As a result of the various ways that society responds to emerging gender realisation, individuals may not feel comfortable expressing their true selves. As such, for reasons including safety, law, comfort and inclusivity, the only way to know the gender of an individual is to ask them.

Low mood and lack of motivation

It is natural for people to experience times of low mood and lack of motivation but these are commonly a temporary state with no root cause or explanation for that mood at that time. Scientists have identified more than 60 different biochemicals that impact on a person's perception and thinking processes.

Delirium and confusion

It is important to identify the cause of delirium rapidly so that treatment can be started, such as fluid replacement or prescribing antibiotics. Getting an early diagnosis for people living with dementia can have a positive impact on their treatment and ongoing quality of life.

The normal ageing process

The human body is made of a complex set of biological systems that age as we get older. This process is a natural part of getting older and, in most cases, there are no visible changes to the way we function as an older adult.

However, when we develop illnesses such as flu or cardiac problems, these will have a bigger impact on an older person, and the symptoms may be more severe as a result of their age and ability to cope physically with their illness.

When we are born, the body consists of more cells than we require, for example we are able to live perfectly well with one kidney or one lung. These are called our 'functional reserves'. As we age, these reserves start to reduce; for example our kidneys stop functioning as well as younger people's kidneys and our lungs become less elastic, meaning we are more prone to getting chest infections. Some of the common changes in older age are changes in sleep patterns and changes in mood.

Changes in sleep patterns

Sleep patterns change as a result of changes in the way we live. Poor sleep quality in older adults can be related to the lifestyle changes that often come with ageing. For example, retirement may lead to a less structured sleep-wake schedule. Other significant life changes, such as loss of independence and social isolation, can increase stress and anxiety, which can also contribute to sleep issues.

Older adults may also experience sleep disturbance during the night as a result of changes to their urinary system, leading to the need to use the toilet more frequently. Certain medication may also impact on the depth and quality of an older persons' sleep patterns.

Changes in mood

Mood changes can be common in older adults, affecting the way they feel, act and think. Although depression is a common problem among older adults, it is not necessarily a normal part of ageing. In fact, studies have shown that most older adults feel more satisfied with their lives, despite having more illnesses or physical problems than younger people. Causes of low mood may include:
▶ medical conditions, such as stroke or dementia
▶ stress, including care-giver stress
▶ chronic pain, a cause of sleep problems.

K1.21 How changes in cognition can impact health and wellbeing

Stress, anxiety and frustration

Although, on the surface, **stress** presents as an emotional state, the associated rise in adrenalin and cortisol speeds up the heart, increases the breathing rate, leads to **insomnia** and, over a prolonged period, lowers the immune system and increases the risk of heart disease.

Anxiety has similar symptoms and may include: a churning feeling in the stomach, palpitations, feeling restless and sweating.

Serious levels of **frustration** can manifest in two ways: either through an outburst of aggression or becoming withdrawn as a coping strategy.

Intellectual wellbeing and social relationships

Factors that impact on the quantity and quality of sleep can cause extreme fatigue, reduce concentration and compromise intellectual wellbeing. Anxiety can make small concerns seem disproportionately large, resulting in a preoccupied mind that is unable to focus on other aspects of life.

Relationships and social wellbeing can be affected. A concerned person who keeps asking someone if they are all right or expects them to explain what is wrong puts pressure on the individual to provide answers that are complex and difficult to explain. The strain on social relationships often leads to avoidance of social situations, which increases concern and leads to further questions.

A supportive network can help with daily tasks, make allowances and reassure their loved one that the impact on cognition can be overcome. Alternatively, feeling isolated, and dealing with confusion and retaining information alone, can increase stress and anxiety, exacerbating the current state and reducing a person's feelings of self-worth.

K1.22 How to report changes and deterioration in cognition while following appropriate procedures

Healthcare professionals need to act promptly if a cognitive change is noticed, following the required procedure (like that shown in Figure 1.22).

K1.23 How to support others to report changes and deterioration in cognition

Working collaboratively with colleagues, family, carers or nominated next of kin

Collaboration between colleagues, family, care givers or a nominated next of kin will help to identify when the individual is experiencing a deterioration in their condition. The observations and opinions of someone who knew the person before they required health intervention can be a useful primary source for reporting any visible and cognitive changes when compared to the patient's usual behaviour pattern. This will help to develop a plan of care to support the individual while they are receiving treatment or support.

Confidentiality and gaining permission and consent to share information must be discussed with a patient to ensure that the regulations of the Data Protection Act 2018 are adhered to. The Act maintains the rights of the patient not to share their personal health details with family, carers or nominated next of kin. Information sharing between colleagues is done so on a need-to-know basis. In cases where only senior staff have the right to information about a patient, there will be a level of electronic security protecting that information so that other staff cannot access it.

Involving informal carers who can act as advocates can be beneficial as a source of feedback, helping

> **Key term**
>
> **Insomnia:** changes in sleep patterns making it difficult to fall asleep, have quality sleep and stay asleep.

| Discuss concerns with an appropriate person as they may already have been reported by others, or the change may be a direct result of a trigger word or situation | → | Record any changes in a care plan, as it could be a possible side effect of a medication that needs to be changed or adjusted | → | Monitor changes, comparing them over a time period, as a pattern may emerge and a trigger point be identified, such as being overtired or hungry, or a particular visitor | → | Inform staff, to alert them during a shift handover that extra vigilance may be required, as well as an increase in interactions as part of an ongoing assessment |

▲ Figure 1.22 Procedure for reporting changes and deterioration in cognition

the smallest signs of deterioration to be picked up. However, not every patient is comfortable with a relative acting as an advocate. This could be because personal information may not always be kept confidential due to the nature of their caring and support role. For example, the patient may wish to receive information about the status of Do Not Attempt Cardiopulmonary Resuscitation (DNACPR) but feel unable to communicate this without causing distress to their informal carer. Support for the patient, including setting out confidentiality boundaries, may be needed to empower a patient in this situation.

Signposting to appropriate specialism

Noticing that an expert assessment is needed can quickly halt a further decline in physical or mental wellbeing, or slow down its effect with appropriate intervention. For example, if a person starts to have an increased level of tremors in their hand movements this could be a sign of interrupted brain functioning, prompting the need for referral for an investigation into a potential neurological disorder.

Delirium may be caused by a temporary bacterial urinary infection. In the community, a GP may prescribe antibiotics for this condition, and the person can then be monitored for a cognitive and physiological improvement.

Providing opportunities to discuss concerns and holding regular multidisciplinary meetings

Regular care plan reviews that involve the presence of or input from medical and therapeutic professionals working in a multidisciplinary team (MDT) provide formal opportunities to discuss concerns on a professional level and involve informal carers where required.

The purpose of the team is to draw together the expertise and experience of specialists in different areas of care. One professional may highlight a concern that the other specialists would not have considered; they may then recommend a new course of treatment. That course of treatment could negatively impact the patient in a way that only a different specialist would be aware of. A discussion of all of a patient's needs and possible avenues of treatment by an MDT allows an appropriate care plan to be formed which enables improved health in all areas for the patient.

The exchange of information at these meetings can be invaluable for patient care, as shared information can flag up the need for more detailed examination by a different medical discipline. What one clinical practitioner views as a decline in functioning another can confirm is an expected change and the start of improvement. For example:

► A patient says their skin graft site is itching. A dermatologist can inform them that cells release a substance that causes inflammation where skin has been removed; this causes itching, which is a sign of healing.

► A mental health professional may conclude that the itching may also be a symptom of a delusional state called parasitophobia, where the patient becomes obsessed with thoughts of insect infestation. This itching is described as 'psychogenic' and can easily be mistaken for a problem with the skin or an allergic reaction.

K1.24 How to escalate changes and deterioration in cognition

Following appropriate procedures

Observation of a person's individual mental state, such as confusion or disorientation, combined with other signs of sepsis, requires the instant involvement of the medical professionals overseeing patient care. In sepsis there is a clear and distinct healthcare pathway to follow regarding deterioration, called the Sepsis Six. There is also a pathway called the National Early Warning Score system that is used to report rapid deterioration (NEWS2).

If a patient's relative reports that they have observed a minor change in thought processing speed, this must be recorded but reporting it to a supervisor is less urgent. Monitoring changes in information retention and processing is important over time but is not an indicator of rapid declining health and the need for critical care interventions.

Recording changes within the care plan

Student nurses will record changes to the care plan from very early on in their training, after the correct education and under supervision. The recording of changes within a care plan will be guided by a supervisor or medical professional.

All changes need to be recorded but will differ on a case-by-case basis. For example, a patient experiencing a symptom of dementia, paranoia and hallucinations may start to refuse to eat their meal. This must be noted and highlighted during a shift changeover or mid-shift huddle as nutrient intake will need to be monitored, especially in the case of patients who have had surgery or require significant wound care. (In all cases, nutritional intake needs monitoring for any patient.)

In this scenario, staff who are working at the time of the next meal round will be aware of the previous refusal and will monitor, and where appropriate encourage, a patient. Alternative food could be offered when there is loss of appetite, and a smaller portion can be less overwhelming, but without reporting a meal refusal the importance of a second missed meal goes undetected.

An underlying cause of meal refusal can be loss of appetite, nausea or the effect of medication.

People living with dementia may simply forget that they need to eat or develop paranoia whereby they believe that food is contaminated or contains poison.

Access to all information regarding changes in physical and emotional wellbeing, and patient understanding, contributes to the most appropriate treatment in a care plan.

Contacting emergency services

There are other emergency services (such as police or fire), and these are equally important within the community. Student nurses are capable of calling ambulance services but will be guided by more senior nurses on duty who will naturally take responsibility for the incident and direct the student.

Case study

S1.38 Contribute, record and follow information in care plans
S1.39 Promote physical health and mental wellbeing through providing opportunistic advice within scope of role, knowledge and responsibilities

Piotr is 72 and has been discharged from medical care following a successful knee operation to correct damage caused by a fall. He has been reluctant to engage with physiotherapy or use a walking frame, as he is a proud man who sees physical impairment as a weakness. Unfortunately, Piotr is unable to leave the hospital since a full assessment into his independence skills has yet to be completed, and he cannot return home without appropriate support and care aids in place. Piotr is upset about the delay in the transfer of care and is moved from the surgical ward to one that specialises in care for older people. He is unable to smoke and drink as he usually does and misses his home life and takeaway food, which he finds frustrating. In addition, his movement is hampered due to being obese.

Demonstrate points from the following skills list using a manikin:
- Document aspects of daily living, for example the urine output or any sleep apnoea concerns.
- Document when moving and handling has taken place, for example using a walking frame to go to the bathroom.
- Document comments from individuals about Piotr's care, for example the fact that he is fixated on going home.

Narrate what you are doing as you go through Piotr's care plan.
- Read the care plan on commencement of duty.
- Implement care as written down in the care plan: daily physiotherapy exercises, independent use of a walking frame when bathing and toileting, independent eating, and self-management of pain relief and high blood pressure medications.
- Discuss with Piotr changes to the care plan to introduce seated exercises to support weight loss strategy, a nutritious diet and calorie intake, cessation of smoking and reduction of alcohol units.

You must encourage social activity and strategies to support Piotr to improve his own physical and mental wellbeing. An opportunistic moment may arise in his care outside a simulation task that enables the delivery of education and advice for improving Piotr's lifestyle choices.

Assessment practice

Your task is to demonstrate the correct procedures involved in delivering a total support care package to meet physical and mental wellbeing needs, maintain standards, health and safety, and report any concerns you may have. You will need a manikin and a partner for moving and handling tasks.

You are to demonstrate your understanding of the Healthcare Performance Outcome 1 knowledge and skills by completing a number of tasks.

During your demonstration you must narrate what you are doing using the correct terminology and explain why you are taking each action.

It would be an enhanced learning experience if you have your demonstration recorded so you can evaluate your practical demonstration using Gibbs' reflective cycle to identify any areas for improvement.

You may refer to notes related to:
▶ the six principles of safeguarding (see page 10)
▶ the 6Cs of nursing (see page 11)
▶ any one from: the CQC 13 fundamental standards of care (see page 14), the five principles of the CI (see page 5), the four domains of the RQIA (see page 6) or the four priorities of the HIW (see page 6)
▶ any one from: the standards and values of NHS England, NHS Scotland, Health and Social Care Trust Northern Ireland or NHS Wales (see page 14).

You are to provide care for an 88-year-old female in a nursing home setting. She has middle-stage dementia, mobility problems due to frailty, cardiovascular disease (CVD), which requires oxygen therapy, and has no family or friends that live close by to visit.

Assist with the following care tasks:
1 Bed bath including oral care
2 Dressing
3 Hoist from bed to chair
4 Feeding and fluids
5 Change of small dressing
6 Observe and report signs of deterioration
7 Introduce a hospital befriending volunteer
8 All communications with the patient must inform in an appropriate manner.

Healthcare PO2: Assisting registered health professionals with clinical or therapeutic tasks and interventions

Working in healthcare requires a co-ordinated team effort, with each professional having a different role and widely ranging responsibilities as experts in their own field. Co-ordinated multidisciplinary teams (MDTs) collaborate to deliver an integrated service, with the person receiving care central to all care activities.

When assisting with tasks relating to patient care, you must work within your scope of practice, level of learning and knowledge.

Like all health practitioners, you will participate in continuing professional development (CPD) to ensure quality safe practice and effective care delivery.

Learning outcomes

The core knowledge outcomes that you must understand and learn:

K2.1 a background and history of the National Health Service (NHS)

K2.2 the scope of your role when assisting registered health professionals

K2.3 clinical tasks, therapeutic tasks and interventions that can be performed

K2.4 the importance of delegation protocols including the Royal College of Nursing (RCN) principles of accountability and delegation

K2.5 the other registered professionals you will work with who can undertake particular clinical and therapeutic tasks

K2.6 your own responsibilities, duties, limitations and scope of practice

K2.7 the importance of the 'Code of Conduct for Healthcare Support Workers and Adult Social Care Workers' in line with local policies and procedures

K2.8 the importance of working in partnership with wider healthcare teams including those in hospital, community care and social care settings

K2.9 the importance of providing relevant information to contribute to clinical handovers between shifts

K2.10 the relevant points of referral for help and advice

K2.11 the importance of gathering individual views and how this influences service provision

K2.12 the ways to identify and escalate opportunities in order to provide a better or more effective service

K2.13 different environments that individuals may be moved to and from

K2.14 the steps taken within discharge procedures

K2.15 how to gather appropriate, relevant and timely evidence to assist in obtaining an individual's history

K2.16 why professional development, personal development plans and using feedback to develop and improve are important.

Skills outcomes

The skills you will need to demonstrate:

S2.17 work with health professionals on clinical and therapeutic tasks and interventions working within scope of role, knowledge and responsibilities

S2.18 gather appropriate, relevant and timely evidence to assist in obtaining an individual's history and review health related data and information

S2.19 handle information in relation to clinical tasks, therapeutic tasks and interventions

S2.20 record, report and store manual and electronic information accurately and legibly in line with local and national policies, keep information confidential, support others to do so and apply these by taking part in audits

S2.21 maintain a record of personal development and training from undertaking CPD

S2.22 use feedback to develop and improve.

The health service and roles and responsibilities when working in health to assist registered professionals

A healthcare professional's role refers to their position within a team and their responsibilities related to the job tasks within their role. For example, a nurse contributes to the planning and provision of care for a patient: their responsibility is to deliver, administer and record a patient's medication, identify, assess and evaluate care delivery, and act as part of the wider multidisciplinary professional team.

A healthcare professional's scope of practice refers to their role and responsibilities according to their level of competence. So, for instance, a trainee nurse will have limitations in their scope of practice compared to qualified registered nurses.

K2.1 A background and history of the National Health Service (NHS)

Background and history

The inspiration, motivation and background behind the UK healthcare service was the population's collective need for a free health service. Before the formation of the NHS, affluent families could afford to pay for medical care but those on a low or no income went without or received charity care. Soldiers returning from the Second World War with all manner of physical and mental illnesses that had developed over time, and who were without family or money, were not always adequately cared for. Voluntary hospitals were established in the eighteenth century but were limited in terms of the services they provided and relied on donations. Rural locations in particular had very few accessible services and professionals, highlighting the divide and inequalities that were present up and down the country.

The history of the NHS begins with its formation on 5 July 1948 by Aneurin Bevan, who was a Welsh Labour Party politician. He vowed to make healthcare accessible to everyone, paid for by taxes, which would be used responsibly.

National Health Service Act 1946

This law was passed in order to improve people's physical and mental health. The legislation was for England and Wales. The other UK nations quickly followed suit, with the National Health Service

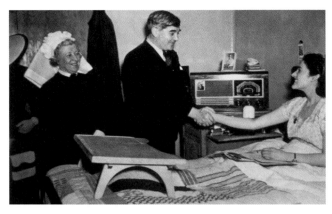

▲ Figure 2.1 Aneurin Bevan, Minister of Health, meeting a patient at Papworth Village Hospital in Cambridgeshire in May 1948; the following July 5th was the first day of the National Health Service

(Scotland) Act 1947 and health services in Northern Ireland created by the Northern Ireland Parliament through the Health Services Act (Northern Ireland) 1948. These original laws have since seen amendments in 1986 and 2006, and were superseded by the Health and Social Care Act 2012 and the Health Care Act 2022.

The legislation evolved to bring together fragmented sections of healthcare and social care to provide continuity in care through organised collaboration. For example, if an older person in residential social care requires medical care as in inpatient and then returns home, integrated services will provide person-centred care using multidisciplinary teams of experts in both fields.

In the late 1990s, healthcare powers were devolved (decentralised and transferred) to the four home nations – England, Scotland, Wales and Northern Ireland – meaning the NHS was no longer one large organisation responsible for the health of the whole of the UK. It split into NHS England, NHS Scotland, NHS Wales and Health and Social Care Northern Ireland. Each home nation has its own regulating organisation to ensure a high standard of care is delivered, monitoring, inspecting and writing reports to which the public has access.

World Health Organization (WHO)

The main purpose of the World Health Organization (WHO), which was established on 7 April 1948, is to promote good health, co-ordinate health affairs for global safety and serve vulnerable people. Its initial priorities were to reduce deaths by malaria,

Key term

Communicable disease: illness spread from one person to another caused by bacteria and viruses.

tuberculosis and other **communicable diseases**, and more recently COVID-19 in 2020.

The WHO funds research into different health concerns across the globe. It gathers statistical data and then researches what can be done to reduce their impact. For example, a study carried out in August 2023 found that 2.2 billion people worldwide have a visual impairment and at least a billion of these cases were preventable. Further research involving 62 countries looked at ways to reduce this debilitating health problem, and a plan was developed with a target date set for 2030.

Source: WHO (2023), 'Blindness and vision impairment', www.who.int/news-room/fact-sheets/detail/blindness-and-visual-impairment

Nursing overseas in developing countries may be something that is of interest to you in the future. There are many ongoing specialist projects that require professional practitioners.

Health and safety

The World Health Organization (WHO) was integral to the global response to the COVID-19 pandemic. The ongoing research it offered to governments and its guidance and advice on the consequences of taking no action informed the decisions made by all countries. As part of the global response to reduce cases of the contagious virus, developing countries were supported financially and supplied with equipment as a co-ordinated effort.

Department of Health

In 1988 the Department of Health and Social Security separated, and the Department of Health was formed. In 2018 the government renamed the department and it became the current Department of Health and Social Care (DHSC).

The governments in the UK's four home nations receive money in the form of taxes paid by the working population. This is then divided up into separate governmental departments that have the responsibility to decide what services are needed and fund facilities run by paid qualified professionals.

Like the WHO, the DHSC funds and supports research into health concerns in the UK population, and politicians are advised by health experts before allocating funding to the most appropriate department for use in health service provision. This is relevant to trainee nurses, as all professionals will be working within recognised frameworks for care, aiming to meet government targets, such as to employ 50,000 more nurses by 2024 (a target set in September 2019).

Despite the different healthcare structures in England, Scotland, Wales and Northern Ireland, there are frameworks, initiatives and research that apply to the whole of the UK, which shape the sector's workforce and vision.

Nursing and Midwifery Council (NMC)

The **Nursing and Midwifery Council (NMC)** was **founded in 2002**, replacing the United Kingdom Central Council for Nursing, Midwifery and Health Visiting (UKCC). This organisation ensures that nurses, nursing associates and the midwifery profession as a whole recognise high standards and practice within the Professional Code of Conduct.

A nurse cannot practise unless they meet the required qualification and training level. The NMC requires all professionals on the NMC register to revalidate every three years. This includes demonstrating that each nurse/nursing associate or midwife has completed the requirements for practice, including undertaking a minimum of 35 hours of continuing professional development (CPD), completing five pieces of reflective documentation, practising over 450 hours and having a professional discussion with another registrant over the preceding three years.

The NMC has a code with clear statements of how a registered nurse/nursing associate or midwife should behave. If a nurse does not meet these standards, they may be referred to the NMC, where an investigation into their practice may occur. Poor clinical practice can lead to a patient or member of the public suffering harm that could have been prevented, and the practitioner could be found guilty of misconduct. The incident, its type and severity will be assessed and appropriate disciplinary measures taken. This is known as a fitness to practise investigation.

Fitness to practise is about keeping patients safe; it is not about punishing nurses. If a nurse makes a one-off mistake it may mean they need retraining, and they will be closely monitored rather than lose their job. A nurse who does not meet the standards, tries to cover up a mistake or does not accept any wrongdoing can be taken off the register, which will mean they then cannot be employed as a nurse. The NMC is the only organisation to place people on the register and also remove them.

National Institute for Health Protection (NIHP)

This organisation was swiftly founded in 2020 as a response to the COVID-19 pandemic outbreak. On 1 October 2021, the NIHP and **Public Health England (PHE)**, which was **founded in 2013**, transferred all health protection functions to the UK Health Security Agency (UKHSA). The UKHSA is responsible for protecting every member of every community from the impact of infectious diseases, chemical, biological, radiological and nuclear incidents, and other health threats. Following research, this organisation attempts to predict various types of health concern, such as trends in children's tooth decay or the rise in obesity rates.

The DHSC funds the UKHSA, which in its role as an executive agency advises the government about future health risks. Public Health Scotland, Public Health Wales (Iechyd Cyhoeddus Cymru) and Northern Ireland's Public Health Agency work closely with the UKHSA to tackle health concerns that cross borders. For instance, in August 2023, a study revealed that one in eight students starting college or university were not vaccinated against four strains of meningococcal bacteria and were therefore vulnerable to meningitis, risking potential long-term disability, serious health complications and the possibility of life-threatening infection. As a result of this, the UKHSA runs a health promotion campaign during college and university freshers' weeks, to educate students and offer the vaccination.

Source: UK Health Security Agency (2023), 'Meningococcal ACWY (MenACWY) vaccine coverage for adolescents in England, academic year 2021 to 2022', www.gov.uk/government/publications/meningococcal-acwy-immunisation-programme-vaccine-coverage-estimates/meningococcal-acwy-menacwy-vaccine-coverage-for-adolescents-in-england-academic-year-2021-to-2022

Health and Care Professions Council (HCPC)

The Health and Care Professions Council (HCPC) was founded in 2003. As a professional regulating organisation that oversees the standards of allied health professionals (AHPs) and **biomedical scientists**, it has a similar role to the NMC.

There are 14 AHP job roles, as shown in Figure 2.2. To practise in the UK, health professionals must register with the HCPC. For the different professional

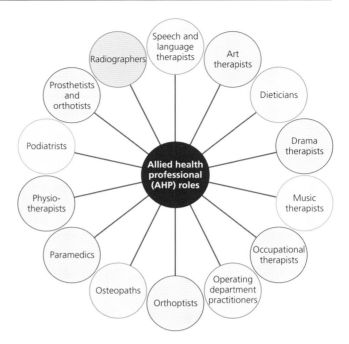

▲ Figure 2.2 The 14 allied health professional roles registered with the HCPC

bodies there is a requirement for CPD and for renewing registration.

NHS structures

Tiered hierarchical structure

In all UK countries the NHS has a tiered hierarchical structure: a leadership-based chain of command that identifies line managers. For example, at the bottom of the NHS pyramid structure, entry-level staff report to supervising staff, and this pattern continues right the way up to the top level: the Chief Executive of the NHS.

Governance describes how an organisation is controlled and managed. It includes a number of aspects including, for example, accountability and leadership. Clinical governance can be defined as a framework through which UK National Health Service (NHS) organisations and their staff are accountable for continuously improving the quality of patient care.

Governance should ensure that healthcare provision meets a quality standard across the UK, addressing health inequalities which statistical data and service user complaints highlight. Where gaps in provision are identified, actions are taken to address these. This includes, for example, the introduction of mandatory training content as part of NMC revalidation.

Governance has a top-down approach. It is everyone's responsibility. It encompasses incidents, complaints, research, audit and education.

Key term

Biomedical scientists: scientists who conduct laboratory testing on fluids and tissue to support diagnosis and treatment of disease.

NHS trusts

In England, the NHS is split into different organisational units, which have specialist functions or serve different geographical areas. In Scotland and Wales these are referred to as Regional Health Boards; in Northern Ireland they are Health and Care Trusts.

Hospital trusts or health boards – sometimes referred to as acute trusts – oversee the running of hospitals in certain areas. For example, Manchester University NHS Foundation Trust is the largest trust in England to date, managing ten hospitals. There are **mental health trusts**, **ambulance service trusts** and **community health trusts** in England, each taking ownership of and managing a specialist provision. The structures differ between the four nations of the UK. They are similar in having a clear structure: who manages and what is managed as a grouping together. Governments change when voting takes place, which means new ideas and initiatives are developed and implemented.

K2.2 The scope of your role when assisting registered health professionals

Scope of your role

Your purpose and function is to assist registered professionals by carrying out activities in a support role with leading qualified staff. The primary qualified staff will have more knowledge, expertise and skills than the entry-level staff who work with them.

An entry-level trainee nurse has a valuable role within the wider team, working within the **scope of their role**; this will include important tasks, such as carrying out observation measurements, supporting patients' personal hygiene and delivering frontline person-centred care. The registered healthcare professional is responsible for ensuring that the tasks delegated are within the education, training and competence of any staff assisting them.

Working to a trained level and being competent to carry out a task

You will need to assist within the limits of your knowledge and particular skill set. As a trainee

> **Key term**
>
> **Scope of role:** range of activities, duties or responsibilities that an employee is reasonably expected to carry out or fulfil within the remit of their job or position.

healthcare worker, you should work within your scope of practice and be accountable for your own actions; this means that you accept, own and take responsibility for your actions, and may need to explain to others why you have taken them.

When working with a registered professional, identify your position when you introduce yourself, as this establishes the competence status to which you are qualified to carry out tasks. A trainee has the responsibility to inform a colleague if they have been instructed to carry out an activity that is not in their scope of practice.

Entry-level trainees will have a portfolio of tasks that they need to observe, will be given an opportunity to participate in and then practise until they are confident about doing them. The process of completing skills competency is continuous, as is the reflective practice for each one. Discussing with a mentor your need for further observations and supportive intervention, or any concerns you might have, is an ongoing aspect of your role. As a trainee healthcare worker, you are responsible for your own learning.

Safeguarding

Safeguarding is within the scope of practice for anyone working in healthcare. For example, a trainee nurse knows to report concerns to a senior member of staff if abuse is suspected and needs investigating. Safeguarding is a legal duty of care and a part of mandatory training.

The value of **courage** in the 6Cs of nursing will be needed when a miscommunication happens in an emergency scenario.

Informing a senior member of staff that you cannot act on their instructions can feel uncomfortable when a colleague requires immediate assistance. However, attempting tasks out of your scope of practice can put a patient at risk and yourself, as a trainee healthcare worker, in a disciplinary situation. For example, dressing a large infected pressure injury that needs to first be checked by qualified staff, who will instruct as to the most suitable wound dressing.

In the above scenario, the relevant statement of the NMC Code is '13 Recognise and work within the limits of your competence', more specifically '13.4 Take account of your own personal safety as well as the safety of people in your care'; this is a safeguarding duty of care. This is likely to be a rare occasion and a dilemma, but being aware of the scope of your practice safeguards patients during an emergency where rapid action is needed to preserve life.

Another example might be where regulations state it is necessary to undertake a two-person moving and handling technique, such as moving a patient from a surgical trolley to a bed. This is a move that must not be carried out by one person, as this can harm the patient and cause musculoskeletal damage to self. If an individual staff member chooses to ignore such regulations, they are accountable, and their action represents misconduct and will be a disciplinary matter. Reporting malpractice or the misconduct of others is the responsibility of all healthcare professionals, both in order to prevent harm to vulnerable patients and as part of maintaining emotional wellbeing and physical health.

Frontline workers have more opportunities to interact with patients and be available to listen to their concerns where required. You should report any patient safeguarding concerns to a line manager, however minor you might think they are; a more qualified person will then take responsibility, investigating further and making their own judgements.

In the interests of safeguarding, registered professional delegation means having a person in authority who transfers a specific task to another competent member of staff.

Whistleblowing

Whistleblowing is when someone who works in an organisation witnesses malpractice – for example emotional abuse of patients, or neglect creating a risk of harm – and reports their concern to an external agency. This may be because reporting a concern to management either has been or will be ignored. Whistleblowing can be anonymous – the whistleblower is protected from retribution by law. Disclosures of wrongdoing can be made to the health trust or the CQC, and the whistleblower's entitlement to protection is set out in the Public Interest Disclosure Act 1998.

Organisational abuse (when a group of colleagues neglect or abuse service users they are paid or volunteer to care for) is rare, but it does occur. For example, in 2011, nine support workers and two nurses at Winterbourne View care home admitted to being involved in the neglect and ill-treatment of residents with severe learning disabilities. Six of those involved were given prison sentences. Without nurses Ashleigh Fox and Terry Bryan reporting this appalling behaviour to the CQC (i.e. whistleblowing), it would have continued.

Knowing points of referral

Knowing when to refer a patient to a more senior colleague and working in partnership with a wider team

of professionals brings continuity of care to a patient. As such, it is often the more junior health professional or student to whom information is disclosed. Opportunities to openly talk to a trainee nurse occur naturally while care is being delivered, and in such cases you as a trainee might gain insights that will benefit both the team and the patient. Effective communication skills help draw out particulars such as a detail the patient did not feel was important or they were afraid to share with someone more senior.

Piecing together facts about potential symptoms in isolation builds a clearer picture, which can improve a treatment plan, modifying or adding aspects to better support a patient. This is integral to good practice and better health outcomes as well as the patient experience. Significant disclosures such as abuse or neglect must be escalated to a more senior member of the team to prevent ongoing harm.

Working as part of a team

Healthcare provision involves working in a team with clear leaders and co-ordination to meet the needs of an individual. Within the team there will be a hierarchy of line managers, and each team member needs to know the name of their supervisor and how to report relevant information.

Organisational and local protocols

An organisation such as an NHS trust or privately funded nursing home will have its own policies and local protocols. For example, a complaints procedure or a mentoring scheme might be slightly different in one hospital compared to another. During an induction at the start of your employment, a supervisor will go through the policies and the managers who oversee them. Departments, such as neurology, are run individually, and specialisms diagnose using specific steps unique to the type of patient illness. Joining a team on rotation will form part of your broader learning, enhancing it and enabling you to have a greater understanding of the differences.

You will have the opportunity to read these policies and refer to them when you need to be clear about your required course of action, for example how to raise concerns if you suspect that a patient is experiencing poor care or how to act in the event of a fire within the building you are working.

Taking part in audits

When you are assisting a registered professional, as a trainee you will be tasked with taking part in audits.

These are part of a process to maintain quality care and performance of colleagues. An audit can be:

▶ local – such as a handwashing audit to check professionals are carrying out the correct process of handwashing

▶ national – such as clinic patient waiting times

▶ specific – such as patient safety.

The information may be used as a measurement and relate to a particular organisational or national target.

Audits have an aim and outcomes, and can take the form of a checklist or rating system involving observation, equipment and appointment details. An audit duty for a trainee nurse could involve:

▶ stock-checking PPE or oral care kits

▶ interviewing patients to separate fact from opinion (An example could be a patient making a complaint against a trainee nurse for not dressing a wound quickly enough. The complaint is part of an audit process regarding the time treatment takes in A&E. The fact is that the trainee nurse could not dress the wound as this is not in their scope of practice; they had to wait for a specialist nurse. The patient's opinion was that they should have dressed the wound, rather than wait for the specialist nurse.)

▶ recording data and findings.

K2.3 Clinical tasks, therapeutic tasks and interventions that can be performed

Clinical tasks

Health professionals working in the clinical area will have a wider range of clinical skills and competencies. Clinical skills will enable the clinician to assess, diagnose, treat and monitor the patient. Clinical skills also encompass non-technical abilities such as communication, empathy and professionalism.

It is essential that health professionals only practice within their knowledge and competence to prevent malpractice and harm being done to the patient.

Working in outpatients or with inpatients will involve you in a wide range of clinical tasks within your scope of practice, supporting and monitoring patients.

Taking samples

Collecting samples is a common task that calls for knowledge and skills of infection prevention, such as labelling correctly and following the correct procedures before the samples are taken to a laboratory to be tested by biomedical science professionals.

Samples of bodily fluids are required to confirm a diagnosis, treatment success or to monitor a condition (Table 2.1 lists different types of sample and how they are collected). Test results will be in electronic form and will sometimes need to be transferred to a written care plan accurately. Samples that are naturally eliminated from the body can be collected by patients themselves, if they are capable of doing so; the task is then recording and labelling. The clinical responsibility for patients who are not fit to safely gather uncontaminated samples themselves lies with the healthcare assistant who is managing continence or working closely with the patient.

▼ Table 2.1 Different sample types and how they are collected

Sample type	Sample collection
Finger prick	Using powder-free gloves, massage the patient's palm, alcohol swab their middle finger and press at the base of the first joint, then lance palm side up. Apply pressure to start blood flow, wipe the first drop and dispose of it (it will be contaminated by the alcohol wipe) and hold finger over tube, massaging from first joint to tip, not touching the blood flowing; alternatively dab blood onto a glucometer strip – this is capillary blood testing. Dress fingertip by applying a small plaster.
Genital fluid	Male: a plastic swab is inserted 1 cm into the urethra after the foreskin has been retracted and, if necessary, cleaned. The swab is gently rotated, removed and sealed in a pot. Female: a plastic swab is inserted 2 cm into the vagina, turned once and left for 10 seconds, then removed and sealed in a tube.
Mucus	A plastic swab is inserted in the nose, both nostrils, roughly to the depth of an index finger, and left for 10 seconds. The swab is put in a sterile tube and sealed.
Semen	Collected by masturbation directly into a sterile container, the entire ejaculated sample needs to be collected for accurate analysis in a lab.
Sputum	A lower respiratory or chest phlegm sample, called sputum, is obtained by deep-coughing and is usually white, yellow or green. Coughing loosens a sputum sample, which is often easiest to collect in the morning. The sample is spat into a sterile container. Sleeping or lying down can build up sputum naturally, causing morning coughing.

Sample type	Sample collection
Stool	Faeces is collected after the natural passing of urine, usual when toileting. A sample can then be captured on toilet tissue and a sterile spatula used to collect a sample that is put in a sterile pot and sealed.
Urine	For sampling, urine is required either first-stream or midstream. It is captured in a sterile pot and sealed. Examples of sample timing instructions can be: after fasting, the first urination of the day, or after a particular substance such as glucose is ingested. A minimum of 30 ml is needed.

Pressure area care

Pressure injuries assessment is covered in Adult Nursing Performance Outcome 1 (ANPO1 K1.9) and grading in ANPO3 K3.4–6. Pressure area care covers skin damage prevention, cleaning and treatment.

Pressure injuries are caused by a lack of blood flow to an area that has weight and pressure on it, usually a joint, heel or bottom. The pressure constricts the surface capillaries so that oxygenated blood does not reach the skin or tissue cells and they start to die off.

The Waterlow pressure ulcer risk assessment tool is used to record the examination results and the potential risk of injury developing is then calculated, which you will learn about in ANPO1.

Prevention of pressure injuries involves movement and the relief of pressure, so that oxygen can access the cells when the pressure point is moved to another area (ANPO3 S3.10). Moving and handling techniques are used to reposition the patient every two to four hours if they are unable to move themselves. Patients who do have the capabilities of movement will be asked and reminded to shift their body weight to a different area, such as moving onto their side or sitting up. Moving the hospital bed to a more upright position, or lowering it, can support the repositioning of areas on the lower back and bottom. The role of a trainee nurse will be to monitor skin integrity and work with a colleague to reposition patients, reporting any concerns.

The Braden Scale (see ANPO1 S1.19, and ANPO3 K3.4 and S3.8) analyses factors that can raise the risk of pressure injuries, such as areas of friction, heels or moisture at incontinence sites. The Braden Scale score calculation highlights the need for clinical action, for example changing incontinence pads regularly, changing bed linen or putting powder on heels to reduce

the amount of heat caused by movement friction. The constant monitoring of patients who are most at risk aims to prevent an injury, but even with all the precautionary measures and clinical skills in place to promote blood flow, these are not guaranteed to be successful.

Public Health England describes a pressure injury as localised damage to the skin and/or underlying tissues as a result of pressure. Pressure injuries are graded according to their severity:

Stage 1: non-blanchable
Stage 2: partial thickness
Stage 3: full thickness skin loss
Stage 4: full thickness tissue loss
Suspected deep tissue injury: hidden under intact skin
Unstageable: undetermined level tissue injury due to slough tissue

Preventing pressure injuries developing or deteriorating is paramount to good patient care. For all stages, specialist pressure mattresses and cushion positioning are used along with a repositioning schedule. Pressure, friction and shear forces should be avoided during repositioning and, depending on the patient's ability to reposition themselves, a schedule of movement may be in a care plan as frequently as every two hours.

Pressure injury stages cannot be reversed, so treatment is a combination of preventing deterioration, infection control and promoting healing. Cleansing the area and wound should use sterile saline, if possible warmed to body temperature. The treatment for different stages detailed in Table 2.2 is guidance only and may not be suitable for every patient situation.

Catheterisation

Catheter passports are currently used in many areas; they are promoted by the NHS, but not all trusts use them. The passport is a document that aims to educate the patient; it is useful to discuss this with the individual who requires a catheter or who is taking on self-care responsibilities.

Inserting a catheter requires additional training, the correct knowledge, the right equipment and the patient's consent.

▶ It is a procedure carried out using the Aseptic Non-Touch Technique (ANTT). The area where the male/female kit is placed, such as a stainless-steel trolley, must be sterile. If you are qualified and it is within your scope of practice, your role would be to insert a catheter tube using a sterile kit.

▶ Catheter bags must be positioned below the bladder, so a patient in bed, for example, will need to have a

▼ Table 2.2 Pressure injury grading and care

	Description	Pressure injury care
Stage 1	Skin in areas where weight-bearing pressure occurs may develop redness when subjected to pressure. A light finger pressure should be applied to see if the skin blanches (goes white) to rule out this redness being a symptom of something else damaging the epidermis. The individual may feel some pain when pressure is applied, and the skin is likely to feel warmer and different to touch from surrounding areas. A pressure injury may be difficult to detect in individuals with darker skin tone; usually its colour may differ from the surrounding area.	The area should be gently washed with soap and pressure avoided by repositioning. The use of equipment, such as a heel pillow and specialist cushioning, to prevent further damage is needed. Transparent hydrocolloid dressing may be appropriate in some cases. Recording treatment in a care plan is required as deterioration could lead to a safeguarding investigation.
Stage 2	Partial thickness loss of dermis is characterised by either an intact shiny blister or a ruptured serum-filled blister surrounded by red-pink wound bed. The blistered area can clearly be seen on darker skin tones.	Saline is used to clean the wound before drying and dressing. Antibacterial creams are used to try to prevent infection, and barrier creams are used to try to stop further deterioration of vulnerable skin.
Stage 3	Full thickness tissue loss occurs and subcutaneous fat may be visible. Slough (a yellow-white liquid) may be present, and the depth of damage can still be seen despite this. There may be some undermining and tunnelling; the depth at this stage varies depending on how much fat is in the adipose tissue over the area under pressure. There is no visible bone and tendons or muscle are not exposed at this point.	The injury will need gentle cleaning and drying, including removing the slough for closer inspection, especially if it appears to have tunnelled. A prescription of antibiotics may be considered and the area sealed with a hydrocolloid dressing. The adhesive of the dressing should not be near any skin affected by the injury. The dressing foam is specialist and absorbs some discharge, with minimal adhesive covering.
Stage 4	Full thickness tissue loss occurs, with exposed bone, tendon or muscle, and a crater-like appearance. Slough or eschar (dead skin tissue) may be present on the deepest part of the wound bed. This stage often includes undermining and tunnelling. Stage 4 injuries can affect a wider area and go into muscle, expose tendons and make osteomyelitis possible.	A gauze dressing may be used as surface dead tissue may come away from the wound when it is removed. Another covering may be applied using a suction device, which creates a vacuum over the wound, speeding up the healing process. Depending on the depth and location minor surgery can be necessary to remove dead tissue, close the wound, or conduct a graft repair using healthy tissue.
Suspected deep tissue injury	Characterised by an area of purple discolouration to intact skin or blood-filled blister, and damage of underlying soft tissue. Deep tissue injury may be difficult to detect in individuals with dark skin tones. The area is painful, firm, spongy, warmer or cooler than adjacent tissue. There may be a thin blister over a dark wound bed or a thin covering of eschar, appearing black or brown in colour with an unpleasant odour.	
Unstageable: full thickness skin or tissue loss	Full thickness tissue loss in which the base of the ulcer is covered by slough which may be different in colour (yellow, tan, grey, green-brown). Until enough slough and/or eschar is removed to expose the base of the wound, the true depth cannot be seen and a stage identified.	

catheter bag hanging stand. Patients who are seated upright will have a bag secured with Velcro to their lower leg to prevent backflow due to gravity.

▶ The tube from bladder to bag must remain straight – kinks and twist will cause a blockage and backflow.

▶ Catheter bags usually have a tap to drain and empty them, assisted by gravity. Measurements of output will need to be recorded.

▶ A larger catheter bag (1 litre) can be used at night and replaced with a day bag (500 ml) in the morning; these need to be emptied when they are two-thirds full.

▶ PPE is worn to clean a catheter area, and a mild soap, sterile or saline solution used to cleanse the genital area where the tube is inserted. If the area is red and looks infected this needs to be reported and recorded.

Venepuncture

Arteries carry oxygenated blood away from the heart. Compared to veins, blood in arteries is at greater pressure since most arteries have thicker walls. Arteries contain sense nerves which mean artery damage is likely to cause pain.

Veins carry deoxygenated blood towards the heart and are easier to locate than arteries as they run superficially.

The pulmonary blood vessels are the exception to this, transporting blood to and from the lungs.

Venepuncture is the process whereby a sample of blood is withdrawn from a vein, usually in the arm. This is an aseptic procedure performed by qualified health professionals usually known as phlebotomists. There are variations when carrying out venepunctures, such as the angle and depth of the needle, the equipment to be used and the method. If they are able, and depending on how good the veins are, the patient can choose which arm is used. Blood samples are captured in tubes and labelled. The tops of blood test tubes are coloured differently depending on what the sample is for (as shown in Figure 2.3). Trainee nurses may be asked to fetch a phlebotomy kit but not to use it themselves.

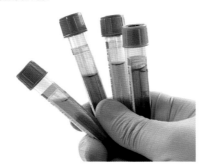

▲ Figure 2.3 A phlebotomy kit for taking blood

Wound care

Wound care varies as recorded in a patient's care plan, for example removing adhesive dressing, assessing wound status, washing or wiping the surrounding area, drying with gauze and using a sterile dressing to cover. If the wound itself requires cleansing, a gentle sweeping motion with a single-use wipe is used, for example, and then the wound is left to dry or gently gauze-dried before redressing. The size, depth and location of the wound, along with infection prevention measures, should all be documented, as they all affect wound care and monitoring assessment.

Urinalysis

This method supports diagnosis and can identify disease or disorder symptoms such as the presence of blood or protein. Urinalysis can be physical, chemical and microscopical. To test urine, a sample of clean or sterile urine is collected and either dipstick-tested immediately or sent for laboratory testing within 24 hours.
- ▶ The clarity of a urine sample must be recorded; urine should be clear and straw-like in colour, not cloudy or visibly pink.

- ▶ A dipstick has a strip with different coloured test areas, and when a substance is detected in the urine these will change colour and can then be compared to a chart.
- ▶ Blood should not be present in urine but can be detected if there is an infection or damage to the bladder or kidneys. Urine can be contaminated by menstrual blood, so it is important to know if this is likely to affect the sample when it is taken.

There are ten chemical patches on a dipstick, which react to different substances in trace amounts. (If necessary, urine can be obtained in a catheter bag for some patients.)

Trace amounts of protein in urine are not usually detected by the strip of chemical patches, so if this appears in large amounts, the test could indicate kidney disease or, in pregnancy, may be a symptom of pre-eclampsia, indicating a potentially serious blood pressure condition.

Glucose should not be present in urine but is a side effect of certain medicines. In cases where no medication is taken it could be a symptom of diabetes.

Ketones are acid chemicals made in the liver when there is insufficient insulin in the blood. They are produced as the body breaks down fat for energy instead of glucose. Ketones are not usually present in urine and may be a symptom of diabetes; a high level can be life-threatening in diabetes as the imbalance in the blood can be toxic.

Electrocardiogram

An electrocardiogram (ECG) records the electrical signal from the contracting of the atria and ventricles by means of a trace (see Figure 2.4).
- ▶ With the patient lying almost flat, ten electrode gel stickers with a foam backing are placed on their ankles and wrists, and in six specific places on their chest.
- ▶ Electrodes are connected to the ECG machine by wires, which pick up the electrical activity and convert it into a trace on the ECG paper; the stickers can be attached with the lead wires already attached.
- ▶ The machine prints out a cardiac trace.

The ECG trace is then analysed, and atria and ventricle contractions measured to detect **arrhythmia**. A patient may be experiencing **angina**, potentially caused by reduced blood flow to the heart muscles.

> ### Key terms
>
> **Arrhythmia:** a problem with the rate or rhythm of the heartbeat.
>
> **Angina:** chest pain caused by reduced blood flow to the heart muscles.

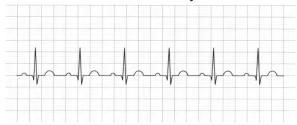

Normal Sinus Rhythm

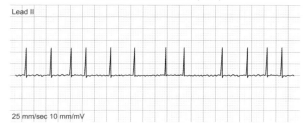

Atrial Fibrillation (AF)

Lead II

25 mm/sec 10 mm/mV

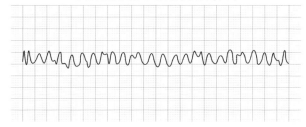

Ventricular Fibrillation (VF)

▲ Figure 2.4 An ECG trace

Taking physiological measurements

A large part of clinical tasks involves taking physiological measurements such as blood pressure, heart rate and temperature. You will learn about initial testing, monitoring, recording and escalating concerns in the next chapter, HCPO3, and have skills assessment while you carry these out using a manikin.

In general, clinical activities are tasks that are documented in a care plan, such as personal care, providing nutrition and hydration, and physiological measurements and monitoring. These tasks are part of assisting the registered nurses and medical professionals who oversee patient care.

Therapeutic tasks
Behavioural therapy

Therapeutic tasks can involve assisting allied health professionals (AHPs), such as art, music or drama therapists and dieticians, with **behavioural therapy** observations. An AHP can specifically request observations of a particular behaviour, or in general, such as regarding a patient's mood stability or motivation. For example:

▶ An adult with a cognitive disability may demonstrate behaviours such as fear or anger, or remain silent, all of which will need to be addressed. As trainee healthcare workers have the most contact with a patient you may be able to spot signs or behaviours that are out of character, which must be reported.

▶ A music therapist may request that signs of stress be monitored and recorded. For example, someone with an addiction may benefit from expressing themselves in lyrics; the AHP will then be able to address concerns with an extra session to support them, to prevent a relapse.

As noted above, because trainee healthcare professionals are in contact with patients more frequently than AHPs, they are likely to have more opportunities to listen to patients and their relatives, and make their own observations. This professional relationship is important, as it often leads to a trusting relationship between the trainee and the patient; it can be less formal than the one they have with your colleagues who carry out assessments in a more formal manner, which means the patient can feel comfortable discussing matters with you. It is important to gain consent to share any information they tell you with a professional if it is deemed necessary.

Physiotherapy

Assisting with physiotherapy tasks is about supporting a patient to recover from a musculoskeletal injury such as a broken hip. Physiotherapists will support the patient to mobilise safely, use their walking frame safely and toilet independently. They will prescribe exercises, checking these are completed correctly.

Occupational therapy

An occupational therapist will make an holistic assessment of the person's living environment for a complete assessment of independence skills, so that the recovering patient can go home with the correct level of support. Mental health occupational therapists assess the stability of a patient, the impact of trauma and coping strategies, while occupational therapists specialising in people with learning disabilities assess a person's independence skills. Whatever the specialist area, detailed and accurate assessments require the support of trainee nurses in their everyday role.

Talking therapies

Talking therapies aim to move a patient forward psychologically into a better place, developing coping strategies and sharing emotional trauma. This is a

> **Key term**
>
> **Talking therapies:** treatments that involve talking to a trained professional, such as a counsellor, about thoughts, feelings and behaviour.

role that also requires assistance, such as educating a patient about what the different therapies are, listening to their questions, worries and doubts, and supporting their understanding of the potential benefits.

Interventions

Interventions are recorded in a care plan and trainee staff have a role to play in supporting documentation. For example, a patient needs to do hand exercises following surgery to repair damage to ligaments, the physiotherapist has recorded the need for these exercises to be completed three times a day, and they will review the patient's progress in one week. However, the patient is not co-operating and believes the injury will sort itself out. It is important to ensure the patient fully understands the need for the exercises, as their hand will have limitations of movement without regular exercise. Providing a prompt, along with encouragement, and the recording of exercise can be the responsibility of trainee staff.

Identifying the need for change

By listening to the patient and encouraging reflection without interference, you might be able to identify the need for a health-related change, such as modifying their diet or handling a suspected toxic relationship. Empathising with a patient who struggles with self-esteem, comfort eating and is obese will mean they feel less judged and more supported in this way. Consequently, this may help with maintaining healthier food choices in the future. An individual in hospital with domestic violence injuries should be treated with compassion; an opportunity may arise to enable the promotion of self-worth and enhance their ability to feel in control without conveying criticism.

Escalation procedure

You will need to recognise when a concern needs to be escalated, and know the procedure to follow. For example, while carrying out physiological clinical tasks a score rating might indicate a deterioration in the patient's condition. This needs reporting immediately to a senior healthcare professional who can take appropriate action.

A trainee healthcare worker may have concerns over potential safeguarding issues. For example, observing grab-mark bruising on the back of a patient's upper arms. This should be reported to a line manager and not investigated by the trainee, who is not a designated safeguarding officer. If a patient disclosed the intent to self-harm, this should be reported to a line manager, even if the patient later retracts their statement. It is important to report this regardless of the patient's change of heart.

Contact emergency services

In an emergency you might need to contact the emergency services such as the crisis team for a patient who talks about taking their own life, or press the call button (Figure 2.5) to raise the alarm and alert senior ward staff to attend immediately for a patient who suddenly deteriorates. Each hospital has its own procedure for this and you should be fully aware of what this is when you start working there.

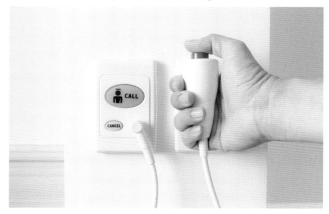

▲ Figure 2.5 The call button can be used to alert senior ward staff if a patient suddenly deteriorates

Changes in care plan

The written and verbal feedback you contribute can help bring about changes to a patient's care plan, meaning that it fits and meets their needs better, and leads to the achievement of better outcomes.

Health promotion

Patients who smoke, drink more than 14 units of alcohol a week or have an unbalanced diet may present an opportunity for **health promotion**. You could provide them with a leaflet or details of volunteer helplines, or have a discussion with them about support groups and share success stories.

Research

The *British Journal of Nursing* article at the following link is directly linked to the teaching of clinical skills in pre-registration nurse education, such as the qualification you are currently studying:
www.britishjournalofnursing.com/content/professional/teaching-clinical-skills-in-pre-registration-nurse-education-value-and-methods

Read the article and consider the following points that arise within it:
▶ Should teaching be shared between one traditional lecturer and one practical educator (teaching current clinical practice) who remains registered?
▶ Why should trainee nursing offer multiple opportunities to practise clinical skills on wards?
▶ What does Miller's pyramid of clinical competency convey?
▶ Why is Peyton's four-step model relevant to knowledge and skills teaching in this T Level Supporting Healthcare OS?

K2.4 The importance of delegation protocols including the Royal College of Nursing (RCN) principles of accountability and delegation

The Royal College of Nursing (RCN) is a professional body and trade union for the nursing profession. A trade union, in simple terms, is a group of professionals that stand together to improve employment conditions; a single employee joins the group, allowing the RCN to represent many people with one voice. Supporting nurses means better patient care, for example in terms of staff–patient ratio and double shift rules, and a role for the NHS Staff Council, which negotiates pay and conditions.

Nurses join the RCN or other unions and pay a monthly fee for access to career advice, counselling and legal support. The RCN provides legal representation in cases of injury, redundancy, dismissals and malpractice investigations. The NMC has fitness to practise misconduct proceedings, and the RCN provides legal representation to the professionals involved. Both organisations have similar principles regarding accountability and delegation, and clear guidelines about what this mean in practice.

Delegation in the best interests of the individual

A supervising manager will instruct staff to complete a particular task, which is called delegation. This must always be in the best interest of the individual receiving care and not performed simply to save time or money. For example, assessing skin integrity is a skill that a registered nurse will be competent to perform but a trainee nurse will not be; delegating this task to a trainee nurse would therefore be unsafe practice for both the patient and the trainee themselves.

Suitable training to perform the intervention

A healthcare support worker must have been suitably trained to perform an intervention For example, they cannot insert a urinary catheter for safe urine collection if they have not completed the relevant training.

At times when the ward is busy, there is the temptation to incorrectly delegate. However, if a trainee does not refuse to complete an activity for which they are not qualified, they are accountable for their own actions. For example:

▶ An individual in the outpatients department is waiting for a change of dressing for their wound. Their blood pressure is taken by a healthcare assistant, but that healthcare assistant does not change the dressing as they are not yet trained in wound care.
▶ The patient is in a hurry, and a qualified member of staff is not available to change their dressing until later. The patient might verbalise their frustrations and put pressure on the trainee to change the dressing.
▶ The trainee must firmly but politely turn down this request, as they will be accountable for any action they take. The whole exchange must be recorded and reported to a supervisor.

Full records of training given/evidence recorded

Whenever learning takes place, it should be recorded and signed off. A full record of training activity, including dates, should be kept as a record of your learning and in order for your seniors to monitor your progress and observe your competencies.

The **National Occupational Standards (NOS)** are approved by the government and involve employers and stakeholders, such as the NHS. The standards are listed in a document that describes the knowledge, skills and understanding that an individual will need to be competent at a job, such as skills for caring. Evidence that your competencies have been assessed should be recorded, and mapped against – and preferably in line with – recognised standards, for example the NOS or the NMC Code.

Guidelines and protocols

An organisation such as a hospital trust will have clear guidelines and protocols in place so that support workers are not required to make stand-alone clinical judgements; training on these procedures is given. Examples of this include an admissions procedure, when a new patient arrives at the ward, or a discharge procedure, when a patient is recovered and considered to be well enough to go home.

The role should be within the job description

During an induction period, the scope of practice should be within the support worker's job description. As the trainee completes each skills competency tasks, following observations and supportive practice, these clinical tasks will increase their scope of practice.

Inform the team that a task has been delegated

Communication must be clear, and the team and any support staff need to be informed that the activity has been delegated. An observer may be required while the delegated task is being completed. The patient will need to be informed and, in some cases, consent should be given for a trainee to be monitored while carrying out a task, such as moving a patient from bed to chair correctly using a hoist or performing a bed bath.

Ensure appropriate supervision for the delegated task

The person who delegates the activity must ensure that an appropriate level of supervision is available and that the support worker has the opportunity for mentorship. The trainee will have a list of competency skills that require development and signing off by a named supervisor. A member of staff who is not part of this process should not delegate a task outside the trainee's level of skills, which they will be aware of. The trainee will have to clarify which stage they are at in their list of skills competency tasks in cases where delegation is not appropriate.

Supervision and feedback levels

The level of supervision and feedback needed depends on the recorded knowledge and competence of the support worker, the needs of the individual, the service setting and the activities assigned. An activity may form part of an assessment or offer an opportunity to practise skills before the formal competency is observed and signed off.

Ongoing development

A healthcare support worker must have ongoing development to make sure their skills competency is maintained. Continual application of knowledge and skills builds confidence and offers opportunities to reflect on progress. This is also essential for safe patient care.

Identify any risks

The clinical task process must be assessed to identify any risks. This will dictate the level of supervision and length of time needed for training.

> ### Test yourself
>
> **S2.17 Work with health professionals on clinical and therapeutic tasks and interventions working within scope of role, knowledge and responsibilities**
>
> You are a trainee nurse on a cardiac ward. You are enjoying this opportunity and considering cardiology nursing as a speciality, so you want to learn and impress your colleagues.
>
> A senior nurse has instructed you to locate an ECG machine, and you are keen and check it has enough paper for a 10-minute examination. The ward is particularly busy and the senior staff member has asked you to apply electrode stickers to the patient and start the device. This is not in your scope of practice.
>
> 1 Which part of the NMC Code of Conduct has not been adhered to by the senior nurse when delegating?
> 2 Which statement in the NMC Code refers to supporting students and colleagues to develop competencies?
> 3 The incident described above had the potential to cause harm. Which statement in the NMC Code refers to acting immediately to put right the situation?

K2.5 The other registered professionals you will work with who can undertake particular clinical and therapeutic tasks

Nurse

Shadowing a registered nurse, and discussing the role's responsibilities and scope of practice, will enable you to observe a wide range of tasks, such as clinical tasks. These include:

▶ **Giving out medication** – for example assisting with handing out patients' prescribed medication as part of a ward medicine round and observing dose and signature requirements.

- **Wound care** – a qualified health professional will be responsible for assessing small wounds or acting on a medical practitioner's instructions to clean and dress a wound. Suitable sterile wound cleaning and wound dressing kits will be used, and as a trainee your role is to locate the correct one and observe its use, and learn how to record the appropriate wound cleaning and care.
- Assisting with **therapeutic activities** such as enabling rehabilitation – for example encouraging, watching and recording the physiotherapy exercises a patient is required to carry out four times a day to restore the range of movement at a joint.

Learning to communicate with an individual effectively before, during and after tasks offers a valuable insight into patient care standards. Working on rotation allows you to experience diverse environments, different types of nursing and specific care tasks to meet a patient's needs, and will be instrumental in helping you to decide on your future specialism.

Doctor

Examining individuals

On average, a GP (general practitioner) spends 55 per cent of their time **examining individuals** in a face-to-face context, while for hospital consultants working in outpatients this figure is lower. Doctors may also assess patients via video-calling and not see them face to face at all.

A doctor may see a patient and request blood tests, which will be carried out during a separate appointment with a phlebotomist. Diagnosis may then be carried out in light of these blood test results and the patient informed by administrative staff. The doctor will electronically inform the designated pharmacy, and the patient can then collect their prescription having had no further contact with the doctor.

Studying a patient's history

The role of the doctor includes **studying a patient's medical history**. Analysing any previous medical contact, treatments and referrals is essential to understanding the current state of the patient's health and wellbeing. An individual may, for instance, have been identified as at high risk of a particular disease, thus indicating a need to observe early warning signs. Electronic records, such as a GP's summary care records, are shared, and information about previous incidences of mental health, allergies and adverse reactions to medications highlighted for immediate attention.

Diagnosing a patient's symptoms

Some illnesses can be **diagnosed** immediately, with clear **symptoms** and straightforward treatment. More complex cases will require referrals to different specialists due to types of symptoms, and co-ordinated collaboration will lead to diagnosis in time. A patient may later mention to you a symptom they had not previously considered important, and your reporting of this information while assisting will provide more precise information to enable an accurate diagnosis – perhaps the final piece of the jigsaw that confirms initial thoughts.

Occupational therapist

- An occupational therapist (OT) is an allied health professional who receives referrals of patients to further **develop a treatment plan** for them, tailored to their needs.
- An OT works with the patient to **arrange support for certain types of activities** so that the desired results are achieved by the patient.
- Time is spent talking with the patient, which is part of a comprehensive assessment to personalise a move forwards, analysing motivation and **agreeing specific goals**.

Physiotherapist

Helping individuals recover

A physiotherapist helps individuals recover from an accident, illness, injury or surgery that impacts on their physical capabilities to live independently. An OT (see above) supports this by working with the same patient to achieve their goal, such as safely making and drinking a hot beverage.

Therapeutic physical exercise sessions

A therapeutic physical exercise session can be supported by a patient's wish to walk unaided and toilet independently. The physiotherapist is knowledgeable about musculoskeletal activities – for example how groups of muscles work together to support joint movement – and will develop an exercise plan to remove joint limitations and improve flexibility and strength.

Using specialist techniques

An example of a specialist technique is electrotherapy, a clinical procedure that directs a small current of electricity from the surface of the skin through to the muscle. Specific damage or pain is addressed by gentle messages to contract the muscle or block normal neural electric signals. In this way the muscle receives better local blood flow and circulation to heal damage, and contraction to help build strength. In cases where pain relief is sought, mild impulses stimulate the body to produce natural pain relievers such as endorphins and to reduce pain signals through sensory neurons to the spine.

Another example is a diagnostic medical sonographer, who carries out ultrasound examinations following a doctor's referral, say to investigate the presence of a cyst or growth, or to see the heart valves in motion. Electronic measurements can be added to a 2D image and recordings seen by a doctor as part of an assessment.

Dietician

Assessing health needs

A referral to a dietician is made where improved health outcomes will be supported by nutrition and hydration or tackling issues with swallowing. This allied health professional assesses an individual's health needs and current diet, discussing their likes and dislikes and cooking skills, and agreeing on a goal they can work towards.

Advising on nutrition issues

These experts in their field can confidently advise individuals on nutrition issues and healthy eating habits. Working in partnership with a patient to plan a gradual change to unhealthy habits, or educating them on the benefits of protein formula smoothies to build weight, are all in the remit of a dietician. A trainee nurse further supports by monitoring a patient's intake and, if appropriate, encouraging them in the change as part of a team effort.

Developing meal plans

When a patient is discharged, a dietician will have developed meal plans, taking barriers and individual preferences into account. At appointments in outpatients or with their GP, a patient's weight is monitored and contact made with the dietician if adjustments or more frequent appointments are needed.

Practice points

S2.17 Work with health professionals on clinical and therapeutic tasks and interventions working within scope of role, knowledge and responsibilities

You will need a manikin for this skills demonstration.

Below are three scenarios relating to different allied health professionals (AHPs) and supporting therapeutic interventions. Your task is to produce a training video for first-year T Level Health students called 'An introduction to clinical and therapeutic tasks and interventions, working with qualified professionals'. Introduce the three tasks below, narrate and demonstrate compassion.

Record your demonstration and evaluate your performance using Gibbs' reflective cycle to identify areas for improvement.

You are a trainee healthcare worker and will support AHPs with therapeutic activities with patients. You will not physically touch the patient; you will encourage and observe, as this is within your scope of practice.

1 A physiotherapist is working with a 60-year-old female with osteoporosis who is ready to use a walking frame. You have been asked to encourage the patient to carry out exercises to increase circulation and build strength and flexibility. Exercises need to be performed ten times at least four times a day. The physiotherapist gives you instructions and guidance regarding the following:
  ▶ ankle exercises, bend up and down briskly
  ▶ buttock exercises, tighten and hold for five seconds
  ▶ thigh exercises, sit up in bed straight-legged, push a knee down into the mattress and tighten thigh muscle, holding for five seconds
  ▶ hip abduction, lying flat, toes upwards and leg sliding outwards then back to the middle.

You are to report to the physiotherapist and orthopaedic doctor, who will record progress.

2 An occupational therapist is working with a patient she wants to toilet independently using a walking frame and a mobile over-toilet frame. The patient can be discharged and return home, as her daughter will move in until she is fully healed.

You have been asked to encourage and observe progress, report to the OT any concerns/progress and record accordingly.

3 A dietician has developed a diet plan that includes foods rich in calcium and vitamin D to help prevent a further deterioration in bone density and aid bone remodelling in a patient's hip. You have been asked to work with the patient to support their understanding of the importance of the diet change and to improve their motivation.

You are to report to the dietician and orthopaedic doctor, giving your opinion on progress.

Health visitor

A health visitor works in the community, often based at a GP surgery. A health visitor is a registered nurse who has spent time working on wards and has had additional specialist training to work in the community and public health nursing. This professional complies with the NMC revalidation process every three years, giving them fitness to practise status. The majority of their workload is working with children aged under five and their parents:

▶ **giving advice to new parents** – working in a clinic at a GP's surgery, a health visitor uses their nursing or midwifery knowledge, for example advising parents how to treat nappy rash or cradle cap

▶ **supporting parents with their children's development needs** – an infant may miss a developmental milestone, for instance speech, and the role of the health visitor is to carry out an initial assessment and refer the child to see a specialist to carry out a more thorough examination

▶ **supporting children with special needs** – parents of children born with a congenital disorder or who have additional physical or cognitive needs can be supported with advice and put in touch with other parents in a similar situation.

Someone who shows symptoms of **postnatal depression** or **postpartum depression** will be referred to adult services for assessment and treatment. A health visitor can also advise and refer a patient for support in other aspects of healthcare such as diet and smoking, and administer vaccinations, for example, as part of their role in public health.

Midwife

Those patients who are pregnant and have an existing health condition will be monitored by an obstetrician, midwives and a specialist. The midwife's role is:

▶ **examining and monitoring pregnant women** – a patient may have had high blood pressure

before pregnancy or take prescribed medication for a mental illness; contact timescales may vary depending on the level of monitoring needed and the additional scans or testing requested

▶ **undertaking antenatal care in hospitals, homes and GP practices** – antenatal (pre-birth) care is generally monitoring the parent and growing baby, abdomen positioning checks, dipstick urine and blood pressure assessments and listening to the baby's heartbeat; any concerns are reported to the patient's obstetrician for more detailed investigation

▶ **carrying out screening tests** – there may be a request for chorionic villus sampling, a procedure where cells are removed from the growing baby's placenta or an amniocentesis fluid sample taken; a maternal-foetal medicine specialist will carry out the sampling, supported by a midwife, using an ultrasound and fine needle.

Assessing care requirements and writing a care plan

Both the midwife team and the specialist consultant will **assess care requirements** and **write a care plan**, including care for the patient's existing health status, such as cardiology monitoring, and supporting the parent-to-be with antenatal care and delivery. Certain complex health conditions will put the patient or developing baby at high risk, for example uncontrolled type 1 diabetes or thyroid disease. Regular outpatient or GP appointments may be necessary to monitor early warning signs and prescribe medication where appropriate.

K2.6 Your own responsibilities, duties, limitations and scope of practice

Responsibilities

In your initial induction period, you will be expected to assess care requirements and contribute to a care plan; this will be observed and feedback given. Once you are fully trained you will be responsible for independently writing detailed and factual notes that contribute to an individual's ongoing care.

Your role is to:
▶ fetch and stock-check sterile kits, such as oral care or items required for a bed bath
▶ prepare the correct equipment, such as locating a clinical observation stand, linen or a suitable sterile catheter kit

> ### Key terms
>
> **Postnatal depression:** a type of depression experienced by parents that impacts on functioning; symptoms are low mood, anxiety and crying, causing concerns for the baby's welfare.
>
> **Postpartum depression:** similar to postnatal depression, but in this case care for the baby is not considered a concern.

▶ practise communication skills by sitting and talking with patients who consent, or reporting a concern to a senior member of staff

▶ observe other professionals' communication skills, such as a registered nurse breaking bad news, if appropriate.

Observations

There are responsibilities and expectations when you are observing a professional perform tasks prior to carrying them out yourself. If you have any questions you should note them down and ask them after the **observation** has finished, and not in front of a patient.

Food and nutrition

An example of a task that could be delegated to you is supporting a patient to eat, ensuring they have access to suitable eating aids such as a spouted cup and being on hand to clear any spillage. A patient may need prompting to hydrate, which can be achieved by you providing them with a drink and sitting with them for company; such observation enhances learning by experience. Food and nutrition are important for healing, which is why working with a patient to achieve a balanced diet is an essential clinical skill to practise.

Following care plans

Your ability to read and comprehend a care plan is knowledge that will be tested by a mentor. Once you have learned this skill, following a care plan will be possible and your confidence in doing so will grow.

Complying with legislation and following codes of practice

During your professional development you will learn to connect procedures for carrying out tasks to the legislation and codes of practice that regulate your work. For example:

▶ NMC Code, statement 3.2, 'recognise and respond compassionately to the needs of those who are in the last few days and hours of life', which you can do by observing a registered professional, who is a specialist in **palliative care** nursing, deliver appropriate care to a terminally ill patient.

> ### Key term
>
> **Palliative care:** care that aims to achieve the best quality of life possible, as actively as possible, until the individual's death from a terminal illness. It is a holistic approach and supports the individual and their family.

▶ NMC Code, statement 8.2, 'maintain effective communication with colleagues' encourages questioning, clarification and seeking reassurance.

▶ NMC Code, statement 11.3, 'confirm that the outcome of any task you have delegated to someone else meets the required standard', means you will participate in a debrief with a supervising registered nurse, and describe the purpose of the actions and necessary skills used and expected in an inspection as part of training.

▶ NMC Code, statement 19.3, 'keep to and promote recommended practice in relation to controlling and preventing infection', refers to making suitable PPE choices, using a sterile small wound kit and educating the patient about the infection precautions required in self-care. This is relevant to the Public Health (Control of Diseases) Act 1984 and Section 2 of the Health and Safety at Work Act 1974.

▶ Health and Social Care Act 2008 Regulations 2014, Regulation 11 protects a patient's right to be given a choice to legally consent to a medical procedure or not; they must be given all the information so the decision is informed.

▶ Contributing to a risk assessment for a patient living with dementia who is volatile and has aggressive outbursts is a legal responsibility to protect employees, under the Health and Safety at Work Act, Section 2. A mental health nurse may be required to wear bite-resistant arm guards to prevent injury, and to work in partnership with two or more staff when carrying out healthcare tasks.

Duties and limitations

Duty of care

You must make sure you are clear about your duty of care, checking to clarify as necessary and being aware of limitations. It is expected that you take time to develop communication skills with patients, reflect on your progress and analyse ways to improve.

Expectations and limitations of your role

Different settings you work in on rotation will have activities that are not appropriate in one location but are in another. Confirming the limitations of your role in a setting such as outpatients or end-of-life care will build your confidence in terms of adhering to your scope of practice.

Safeguarding

Protecting patients from harm is the responsibility of every employee working in the health and social care sectors, and the purpose of clear guidance with regard to scope of practice. Frontline contact, getting to know a patient, gives you a unique opportunity to listen and observe concerning behaviour that may indicate a potential symptom or issue at home. Training in recognising signs of abuse or neglect highlights the importance of reporting a concern. A patient may flinch when you are in close contact, try to hide bruising or dismiss their recent noticeable weight loss, any of which should be brought to the attention of your supervisor and noted.

A safeguarding policy will have procedures that start with informing a supervisor either immediately or in a debriefing, depending on the need for swift action. A patient who may be vulnerable to domestic abuse on discharge or who may have hinted at coercion and retracted a comment can be closely observed at visiting times. Making every effort to provide a supportive environment and convey approachability is everybody's responsibility, as is reporting any suspicions.

Seeking and actioning advice from professionals

Registered nurses and medical professionals are the experts, and you should seek their advice and follow it in your practice.

Scope of practice

There are different aspects to **scope of practice**. You must be:

▶ **trained to carry out the activity** – for example theoretical learning and observing intimate care such as catheter care

▶ **experienced to carry out the activity** – practising intimate care so the competency skills can be signed off and the personal hygiene task can be carried out without being overseen

▶ **permitted to perform the activity** – permission gained from a patient who requires intimate care, with reassuring close monitoring by a supervisor.

Training may be delivered in the form of a set number of observations, which allows experience to be gained before you are signed off to complete a task independently; this is part of good practice.

> **Key term**
>
> **Scope of practice:** sets out the limits of responsibility and ensures individuals do not undertake work outside their level of training or competence.

> **Practice points**
>
> **S2.22 Use feedback to develop and improve**
>
> You have taken part in an observed task where you were asked to support a patient to move from their bed to a walking frame, from the walking frame to lowering onto a toilet frame, toileting and then back to bed. The patient was admitted earlier in the day following a fall and has had two days of diarrhoea and vomiting. They are in pain from musculoskeletal injuries.
>
> You succeed in getting the patient safely to and from the toilet under your supervision; however, you were given five minutes' notice of the task and, under pressure, you omitted handwashing and correct use of PPE. You focused your efforts on assisting with mobility only rather than infection prevention. In addition, you stood in the doorway as the patient used the toilet. Your supervisor feeds back to you that this is an undignified treatment. It has also been noted that you made little effort to inform or reassure the patient using effective communication throughout the task, as you remembered the infection prevention error and this became a distraction.
>
> Your supervisor has asked you to write up your evaluation in your reflective journal, using Gibbs' reflective cycle to take on board their feedback. Include the stages below:
> 1 Description of overall task.
> 2 Feelings: How did you feel before, during and after the task?
> 3 Evaluation: Assess the good and bad aspects of the whole experience. What worked well, and what did not go as well? What were the positive impacts and negative consequences of your actions?
> 4 Analysis: Why did the task go this way? Think about each part, comparing this to how you should have carried out the task professionally, using and demonstrating your knowledge through applied skills in the demonstration.
> 5 Conclusion: What could you have done differently and what did you learn from the experience?
> 6 Action plan: Develop a plan stating what you would do differently when given the same task again.

▼ Table 2.3 Purposes of the CofC

Purpose	Explanation
Clarify the organisation's mission, values and principles	In context, a mission statement is a short explanation of the aim, intention and objectives of the organisation. This serves to inform the general public, employees, service users and stakeholders of the purpose of the facility and provision.
Serve as a reference point	The CofC serves as a reference, helping employees locate relevant documents, services and other resources related to ethics within the organisation. A website will have policies available for public access; Skills for Care has templates and offers guidance to owners and managers of establishments such as hospices.
State expected standards	Individual policies ensure the organisation clearly states the standards workers are expected to meet, supported by training, monitoring and audits. Relevant laws, such as the Care Act 2014 and the Health and Safety at Work Act, are encompassed in the conduct standards requirements, for example the provision of infection prevention PPE, cleaning products, cleaning kit and a COSHH cupboard; the CofC ensures staff practise infection prevention.
Enable role requirements to be checked	An establishment can check its workers fulfil the requirements of their role, behave correctly and take the right course of action in context.
Identify areas for professional development	Competency audits identify areas for continuing professional development (CPD), ensure appropriately qualified staff-to-service user ratios are maintained and prepare managers for a CQC inspection.

K2.7 The importance of the 'Code of Conduct for Healthcare Support Workers and Adult Social Care Workers' in line with local policies and procedures

What is the CofC?

The Code of Conduct (CofC) for Healthcare Support Workers and Adult Social Care Workers sets a standard, a minimum requirement for healthcare support workers, with regard to attitude, behaviours and delivering care with compassion. This CofC is not directly related to a registration like the NMC; it is voluntary and put together by Skills for Care, an organisation funded by the Department of Health and Social Care. An organisation such as a nursing home needs public confidence and to be demonstrating safe, effective, caring and responsive care as laid out by the Care Quality Commission (CQC).

Purpose of the CofC

There are several purposes of the CofC for the organisation, as presented in Table 2.2.

K2.8 The importance of working in partnership with wider healthcare teams including those in hospital, community care and social care settings

Integrated service is a term used to describe the collaboration of health services to deliver a complete package of care. A multidisciplinary team (MDT) brings together professionals who are experts in specific medical fields, such as neurology, with social care professionals, such as social workers in a care home.

▶ In order to collaborate successfully, professionals need a lead practitioner who co-ordinates and oversees care, **utilising leadership and team skills**. Organised teamwork is productive, supports efficient care planning and meets recording requirements. Most partnership and care planning meetings are conducted online instead of face to face due to space constraints, logistics and travel costs. An agenda is circulated before the meeting and each person involved has the option to add any points for discussion at the end of the main agenda. A specialist in one area may wish to bring a point to the attention of others, to contribute to improved MDT planning.

▶ There should be an element of **role modelling** within a department, for example, frontline workers delivering compassionate care with a positive attitude during all aspects of the collaboration with other professionals.

▶ Each professional knows their role and the role of others, which means information can be shared and fed into a single plan using a nursing model of care such as Roper–Logan–Tierney Model's (see page 3) **holistic approach**. The continual review and assessment process will record deteriorations or improvements that impact on a patient's ability to act independently when carrying out ADLs.

▶ The plan will clearly state who is involved, and when and how reviews are conducted, with **effective lines of communication**. There may be parts of the meeting that include information that is on a need-to-know-basis and as such can be conducted in a virtual side room and the content kept from others in the meeting.

▶ A patient who is recovering from a brain and spinal injury will require the collaboration of medical professionals in **supporting efficient care planning and recording**. This ensures all physical and mental health needs are met and the organising of appointments is co-ordinated in such a way that there is the least amount of travel between wards and outpatient clinics. Social care needs will be considered alongside medical needs, which may involve a rehabilitation day care centre, informal carers, support groups and charity-trained advocates. Efficient care planning will have all experts providing person-centred care in a timely, planned manner. Consulting the patient and recording their views alongside all other aspects of professional care will be laid out in a plan accessible to all for reference.

▶ An individual's care plan will need to be clear, involving experts in co-ordinating a care plan that provides **person-centred care**. Care plans are recorded using a standardised template pro forma, making them easily understood across departments, disciplines and workplaces. Trainee healthcare workers will be trained and become familiar with the format by working in partnership themselves.

▶ For trainee entry-level staff, working in partnership provides an understanding of **interagency working** and requires participation from staff who have face-to-face contact with an individual. Observing changes in a patient's behaviour, such as motivation, their engagement in therapeutic intervention and any physical deterioration concerns are examples of responsibilities within a team.

Reflect

S2.19 Handle information in relation to clinical tasks, therapeutic tasks and interventions

Clinical tasks and support with therapeutic interventions are within a registered nurse's scope of practice.

Medical professionals, such as a dermatologist, rheumatologist and psychiatrist, may work together with a patient who presents with red, blistered skin over most of their body. The individual has swollen painful joints, inflammation of the gums, mouth ulcers and says they are tired all the time. When being examined the patient admits to not coping and feeling mentally unsafe. After an investigation, primarily blood tests, the patient is diagnosed with lupus and depression. The rheumatologist and psychiatrist prescribe medication, and a vaccination for shingles and pneumococcal vaccine need to be booked.

A care plan is put together through collaboration, a co-ordinated effort. The information gathered throughout an investigation must be easily available. In this instance, the healthcare worker's effective communication skills lead to the patient opening up, saying they have been made homeless and are in debt. Their lupus symptoms have been severe and they were unable to work. This is then recorded and fed back, so all professionals are aware and social care support is actioned.

The importance of organisational skills when handling information should not be underestimated.

The care plan moving forwards involves therapeutic professionals, a physiotherapist, counsellor and art therapist. A nurse should work with the patient, promoting the work of these professionals, encouraging and motivating. A secondary responsibility is reporting and recording observed behaviours that may or may not be a concern.

Patients with chronic illnesses often have multiple diagnosed conditions and social care problems. In this scenario a care package should involve clinical and therapeutic tasks, working with social care provision, and integrated service person-centred care. The role of the nurse is evident throughout.

1   What are the potential effects of poor communication between professionals and patients?
2   What methods of communication would you recommend: written, electronic or verbal?

K2.9 The importance of providing relevant information to contribute to clinical handovers between shifts

Handover means 'the handover of professional responsibility and accountability for some or all aspects of care for a patient, or group of patients, to another person or professional group, on a temporary or permanent basis' (Bhabra *et al.*, 2007). A shift handover is a specified time that overlaps both shifts, lasting roughly 30–50 minutes, depending on the number of patients, amount and speciality of care and potential demands of the following shift. Continuity of care contributes to a less stressful patient experience.

Source: Bhabra, G., Mackeith, S., Monteiro, P. and Pothier, D.D. (2007), 'An experimental comparison of handover methods', *Annals of the Royal College of Surgeons of England*, 89(3): 298–300.

doi: 10.1308/003588407X168352

Figure 2.6 shows the different elements of an effective handover.

When a patient is moved from the emergency department to a ward, or from one ward to another, there is also a handover procedure. Situation–Background–Assessment–Recommendation (SBAR) is a system used in many hospitals (Figure 2.7). It alerts staff to a need to escalate a clinical problem that requires urgent attention if a patient has suddenly deteriorated towards the end of a shift or while being transported between wards.

During the handover, details might be given about on-call senior staff. A named senior nurse may be overseeing several wards when on shift. Some on-call staff will not be on shift, but their contact details and a time plan of 24-hour availability will be on a rota so that immediate management can be accessed even when they are not physically present at work; for example in an emergency where there is expected to be a large number of casualties (this is known as a major incident).

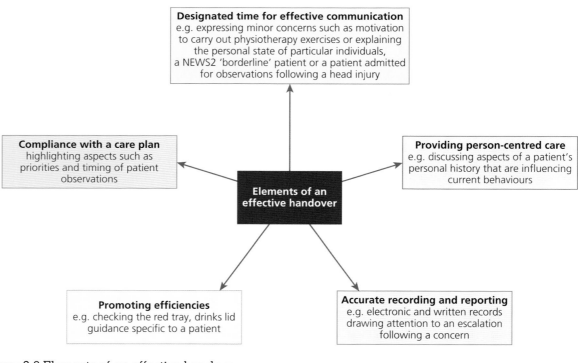

▲ Figure 2.6 Elements of an effective handover

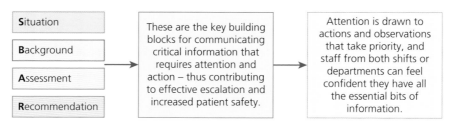

▲ Figure 2.7 SBAR guidance for effective communication during a patient or shift handover

Research

Research the NHS SBAR communication tool:
www.england.nhs.uk/improvement-hub/
wp-content/uploads/sites/44/2017/11/SBAR-
Implementation-and-Training-Guide.pdf

Which of the scenarios below are within the
communication S–B–A–R?

1 'Hello, this is Claudette, from Mahoney Ward.
I'm a registered nurse. We have Mrs Richards in
room 213 and she has suddenly become short
of breath, oxygen sats are now at 89 per cent
with no oxygen, her respiration rate is 23 per
minute, heart rate 112 and her blood pressure is
85/50. She is currently on four litres of oxygen
which increased her oxygen sats to 93 per cent,
breathing rate appears to be increased, she is
confused.'

2 'Would you like me to transfer to ICU? There is
a bed available. Should I increase oxygen to six
litres? Would you like me to contact you again if
she remains like this for more than 10 minutes?'

3 'Mrs Richards was admitted from A&E yesterday
evening at 6 p.m. She has moderate dementia
and had fallen, discovered two hours later
by residential staff who called an ambulance.
A medical realignment was performed in A&E,
there is no skin break and she has a cast on.
Her balance is a concern and she has been
kept in bed with bars up as she is restless.
No relative has visited as yet, due in the
afternoon.'

4 'A dementia risk assessment was carried out on
admissions, Tinetti balance assessment score is
18, BMI is 16, Braden Scale score is 14.'

K2.10 The relevant points of referral for help and advice

Line manager/supervisor

A registered professional may be delegated to observe
a trainee as part of their own training, and to feed back
to the line manager overseeing the progress of both.

Your mentor or supervisor may change due to shifts
and annual leave. A mentoring meeting is held at the
start of any shift and a debriefing at the end. During
your time at work there will be times when clarification
is required, as well as guidance. Being observed is a
matter of course as a trainee. You will be supervised
to start with until you are able to independently
demonstrate your competence.

Designated point of contact

A supervisor or mentor is a designated point of contact
during working hours and often acts as a support
when written assignments are required. They can
offer guidance before the start of assessments and
can signpost further research to support theoretical
knowledge and relevance of applied skills.

Occupational health

If an employment occupational health assessment
is required, it will be carried out by a qualified
occupational health practitioner. (This is not to be
confused with occupational therapy.) The practitioner
will be registered with their regulating body, the
Health and Care Professions Council (HCPC), which
requires revalidation every two years.

The assessment of an employee follows a diagnosis
that needs reasonable adjustments to be made in the
workplace as per the Equality Act 2010. For example,
a trainee with a chronic health condition such as
lupus fatigue will need a risk assessment prior to
employment and any provisions necessary to be made
by the employee, such as a supportive shift pattern that
allows a 'sleep day' and flexibility when the condition
flares up. Lupus can be diagnosed while someone is
working as a healthcare worker, and the employer
or employee can request an occupational health
assessment or referral.

From an employment point of view, the occupational
health professional can advise on adjustments and
discuss what is possible and reasonable. The law
protects an employee from being forced to work as
if they were fully able and supports employers with
appropriate actions.

Regulatory body

A regulatory body such as the NMC or HCPC is able to
give advice and guidance about appropriate education
or training required for a specific role aspiration or
addressing a new challenge. In addition, a regulatory
body can be consulted when there is a concern about
malpractice or misconduct personally/professionally
or with a colleague. It can give clarity and instruction
for a course of action, such as whistleblowing, or
a training course to address a minor incident of
malpractice, for example, how to communicate with
a patient to meet a duty of candour in an incident.

Knowing who to contact before or after an issue arises
is important, and having a meaningful exchange with

the right person will usually resolve any problem or envisaged future difficulty.

K2.11 The importance of gathering individual views and how this influences service provision

In order to benefit from reflective practice and teamwork, professional expert contributions are needed. The voices of service users and stakeholders are usually sought by organisations to improve the service. For example, in England the CQC inspects care homes, hospitals and dentists in order to monitor standards and write reports that can be accessed by the public. It has the authority to set timely targets for improvement and, in worst case scenarios, to shut down an organisation or suspend care. If a service is rated good or outstanding, its next inspection will follow a five-year period; if placed in special measures, improvement targets are set and a reinspection carried out in six months. Similarly, the CI in Scotland writes inspection reports with grades; however, in Northern Ireland, the RQIA has reports without a grading system.

In order for the CQC to make accurate and fair decisions, individuals' views form part of feedback, gathered through interviews, focus groups and surveys. Incidents of formal complaints and how they are handled are reviewed, and even if an outstanding rating is achieved there will be points for improvement. Questionnaires and interviews with managers, employees from different levels and service users are analysed. What is working well and areas of weakness are discussed before a report is written, with the findings based on what has been seen and heard. Constructive feedback is given and follow-up improvements specified, some with an expected timeline for change and outcome target.

Improving practice/identifying good practice

Gathering information identifies good practice that can be shared with other professionals, departments or organisations that need to improve their practice and outcomes (Figure 2.8). For instance:

▶ the booking system used by one consultant is effective in reducing waiting lists, so is shared with another

▶ new technology in one hospital proves to be successful in reducing costs and improving the patient experience; such information is required by managers who control a budget.

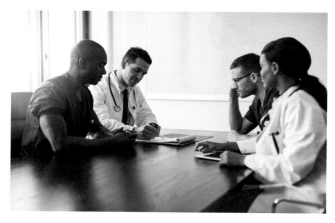

▲ Figure 2.8 Gathering information identifies good practice that can be shared with other professionals

How individuals' views are used to review and adapt services

Feedback from surveying the views of individuals from a range of backgrounds is a practice used to review and adapt services.

Patients and relatives are routinely asked about aspects of their care and their general impressions. Specific questions aim to ascertain a 'patient's eye view' to feed into a service review. Visiting and collaborating professionals may be asked for their contributions as part of the evaluation of current provision and existing staff.

Reviewing a service periodically is standard practice and forms part of an audit process to ensure standards are met in line with a CQC inspection. Sometimes a gap in provision is identified that disadvantages a particular service user group, such as those who live rurally or people from the GRT (Gypsy, Roma, Traveller) community. No service user should be disadvantaged; their rights are protected by the Equality Act and any inequalities in access or provision will need to be addressed.

A service may benefit from being promoted, such as sexual health clinics and others that are not well attended. This will be part of a review to find out if adaptions need to be made or locations changed.

K2.12 The ways to identify and escalate opportunities in order to provide a better or more effective service

Complaints policies and procedures

An organisation will have a **complaints policy and procedures** that are available to the public. A complaint will be received by a senior manager and an investigation carried out. This is explained to the individual who reported the complaint and the outcome shared.

All complaints must be recorded and stages of investigation made clear, along with who is involved and the outcomes, such as a disciplinary action or additional training. A complainant may not feel confident in this system and will then be advised to contact the hospital trust or the CQC, CI or RQIA, for example.

A person who feels aggrieved or mistreated is entitled to complain directly to a regulating body such as the CQC, NMC or Healthwatch. Serious complaints can involve the police and social services if escalation is required, for example serious harm of a patient.

Patient advice services

Support may come from a **patient advice service** such as the Patient Advice and Liaison Service (PALS). Such services offer confidential advice, independent from the NHS, and give information about health-related matters. They can act on behalf of a patient in the role of an advocate, signpost to an expert service such as counselling or provide support with a complaint.

Questionnaires and surveys

Some people prefer to give feedback online; they may have a busy schedule, family commitments or simply prefer technology. Questionnaires and surveys are completed, the information analysed and issues addressed. If a problem is discovered to be occurring repeatedly or information relating to safeguarding identified, an escalation for a formal investigation is an immediate response.

Verbal communication

At outpatient appointments a patient may be asked to give verbal feedback of their opinions on services and their delivery, for example the waiting time and comfort in the waiting room, or whether they felt the appointment was rushed. It may be a relative who responds – as the patient's escort their view is also important. Inpatients will make valid points about care and may have a suggestion as to how one slight change would have made a big difference to them.

This feedback is informal but is often the most honest. Being asked questions means you are on the spot to give an answer, but sharing feelings about a part of the service that has not met a patient's needs is more natural and might be shared more freely. It is good

practice to record verbal feedback, which will then be taken into account when there is a review of a service.

Complaints that require an immediate response can be dealt with swiftly on a ward or department level, but serious grievances will require the involvement of senior staff and the process may take longer. Formal investigations may be required, and feedback from clinicians and healthcare professionals sought, which can take a longer period of time.

Independent regulator

An **independent regulator** is an organisation that is not associated with the service, the professionals or local authorities. It is impartial, avoiding bias and objectively analysing facts, and there are no conflicts of interest. For example, Healthwatch England, established under the Health and Social Care Act 2012, provides guidance to local regional Healthwatch groups. In Scotland the organisation is called Healthcare Improvement Scotland and in Wales the Healthcare Inspectorate Wales; these organisations work in a similar fashion to Healthwatch England.

Healthwatch England feeds back concerns and offers advice to the government's Secretary of State for Health and Social Care, NHS England and local authorities, and must be consulted before the government sets objectives for the NHS. Local Healthwatch groups obtain the views of the public, such as patients and relatives, about their experiences when using services. People are actively encouraged to participate, and the information is written up in a report for Healthwatch England and the relevant regional trust. For example:
▶ The introduction of adolescent wards was a direct response to the public's criticisms of the suitability of hospital treatment for a 17-year-old in a hospital bay with children.
▶ An adolescent on an adult ward is also not appropriate, and anxieties around the two options were fed back to the government and the trust, which funded a ward specifically for the treatment of adolescents.

K2.13 Different environments that individuals may be moved to and from

Transfers within the hospital

Patients can be transferred within the hospital, for example from a surgical ward to a cardiac ward or from

A&E to a ward. Hospital beds can be wheeled along, but a transfer from one bed to another can be suitable if the bed is specialised according to a particular department, for example a patient in a birthing bed in a delivery suite would need to be transferred to a theatre bed if an urgent caesarean procedure was required. Occasionally, if a hospital bed is not available in a specialist ward, the patient will be temporarily admitted onto another ward and transferred as soon as a space becomes available. Ensuring personal possessions, such as a mobile phone, move with the patient is essential and visitors may need to be redirected or informed that their relative has been transferred to a different ward to avoid unnecessary anxiety.

Outpatients can be admitted as inpatients if a consultant feels an immediate response to a condition is needed to prevent deterioration or harm. Outpatients with a planned procedure, such as a small skin graft, will be given an appointment and directed to a day ward, running from 7 a.m. to 3 p.m. On occasion, a patient will require an extended recovery time or a period of close monitoring. In such cases they are moved into a ward as an inpatient. Unexpected admissions in these circumstances can be distressing: a patient is unlikely to have an overnight bag with them or may experience difficulties with car parking arrangements.

Transfers to home

Discharge patients without transport will require a transfer home to be arranged. Bookings like this, for non-emergency transport collection, are funded by the hospital trust. The service is sometimes available through St John Ambulance. NHS Non-Emergency Patient Transport Services (NEPTS) recognises that getting home is more challenging for some people than others and therefore has eligibility criteria. Transport from home to hospital operates with the same criteria, such as older patients who neither drive nor have a relative to supply transport for them, or who have a significant mobility need. Where possible a patient's family can be encouraged to collect them from hospital.

Transfers from secondary to primary care

Discharge arrangements also include transfer care from secondary to local primary care, with appointments with a community nurse to change dressings or a letter to the patient's GP advising of treatment in hospital and medication prescribed for them to take for a period of time at home. Guidance is given to the patient and

symptoms of a deterioration discussed, as well as when to go to A&E or book a same-day appointment with a GP. A consultant can ask the patient's GP to review after eight weeks', monitoring progress or reporting concerns. After a period of time a consultant will sign off a patient who no longer needs the secondary service. If a problem arises after this time, for example a year later, the GP will need to re-refer a patient from primary care services back to secondary.

Transfer between social care settings

A transfer from a social care setting such as a residential care home is a common occurrence. In cases where an ambulance is called for an emergency situation, a care assistant from the care home may escort a patient and stay with them if they are admitted to A&E.

K2.14 The steps taken within discharge procedures

A hospital discharge policy states procedural steps, including administrative responsibilities, reviewing the care in the community package and the transfer from hospital to the patient's usual residence. Effective hospital patient discharge is organised by the staff overseeing a patient's care, handing over to the integrated discharge team when the discharge process is complex.

Section 91 of the Health and Care Act 2022, which was originally enacted as Section 74 of the Care Act 2014, stipulates a duty of care for NHS trusts to involve patients and carers (including young carers) in discharge planning. Discharge to Assess (D2A) was introduced with the aim to free up hospital beds by moving a person who no longer needs an acute bed but still requires care services. Research shows evidence that patients recover faster when they are in an environment of their choice.

Source: The Care Act 2014 Section 74, 'Discharge of hospital patients with care and support' https://www.legislation.gov.uk/ukpga/2022/31/section/91/enacted.

NHS funding supports a person to leave hospital when inpatient care is not necessary. Continued care and assessment will then take place in a different location, which may be a non-acute ward, residential care or community care within a patient's own home. The patient is described as clinically ready, and a multidisciplinary team develops a care package that includes actions to meet health and social care needs. The patient needs to be signed off by each medical professional involved in their care as an inpatient.

Preparation for safe discharge

Prior to this, a senior nurse will have provided the patient and their relative or carer with education and instructions for self-care at home, medication requirements and what appointments to review progress have been made. A leaflet can be given with contact numbers to be used in an emergency or to seek specialist advice, as preparation for safe discharge.

Medication

It is likely that the collection of prescribed medication is required from the hospital pharmacy. Some hospitals have a discharge room or lounge where patients can wait on leaving the ward, and this has the effect of freeing up the bed for a more seriously ill patient. As with all electronic prescriptions there will be some waiting time while a pharmacist receives and **dispenses** medications; however, complex prescriptions, non-standard medication and transport delays can contribute to an extended wait in the discharge lounge which can be frustrating for the patient.

Medication to take out (referred to as TTO medication) will include storage details printed on the box, for example insulin or antibiotic liquids. There may be a need for a **dosette box** with sections to separate days and times with correct dosage.

Equipment

An occupational therapist mobility assessment will indicate what equipment and care aids will need to be in place for a safe return home. A patient may participate in ADL capability assessments while remaining on an acute ward or after transferring to a rehabilitation ward.

Depending on the support out of hospital – informal carers, for instance – equipment for independence will be discussed and trialled for comfort and suitability. Some patients who have a toilet upstairs will need a bed downstairs and therefore access to a commode (stair lifts are not provided by the NHS and must be purchased privately; a person can be eligible for a stair lift grant, but this will not cover all the costs, so support from charities and personal part-payment could be an option). Smaller equipment, such as a shower rail, shower chair and bed grab rails are funded by the NHS. It loans equipment and will expect it to be returned when no longer needed. Each trust or health board runs its own loan scheme, and NHS continuing healthcare eligibility will determine what can be loaned. Integrated care boards (ICBs) assess patients for eligibility to the NHS continuing healthcare service. The British Red Cross also runs a mobility and care aid loan and hire service for people who are not eligible for the NHS scheme, at a small charge. No equipment is given to a patient unless correct and safe usage has been evidenced; mobility and care aids are often accompanied by a leaflet to provide information for the patient and their relative.

Care package

A care package is the result of a multidisciplinary team review that identifies the care needs of the individual. This then translates into funding for the number of care calls that are required per day for the patient and the length of time the care package may be needed.

Effective record-keeping and handover

Three important aspects of effective record-keeping and handover are described in Figure 2.9.

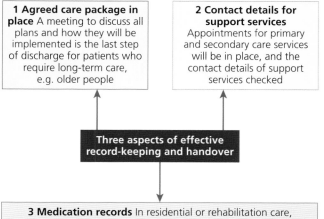

1 Agreed care package in place A meeting to discuss all plans and how they will be implemented is the last step of discharge for patients who require long-term care, e.g. older people

2 Contact details for support services Appointments for primary and secondary care services will be in place, and the contact details of support services checked

Three aspects of effective record-keeping and handover

3 Medication records In residential or rehabilitation care, medication will be stored and dispensed and medication records maintained

▲ Figure 2.9 Three aspects of effective record-keeping and handover

Safe manual handling

A patient who is due for discharge and has mild mobility concerns can be independent with the use of a walking frame and walking sticks. Different walking frames or sticks will be matched to a patient's mobility needs (page 132). For extra stability, a walking stick

(page 132)

Key terms

Dispensing: a process where a qualified pharmacist prepares an order of medication(s) prescribed by a doctor, confirms a patient's details and checks they have understood the instructions.

Dosette box: a tablet organiser with separate compartments for days of the week and time of day, for example morning, lunchtime and evening.

can be a quad walking stick with four feet and height adjusted; these require adequate cleared space since they are wider.

An occupational therapist home visit will risk-assess space requirements and check a patient's understanding of potential hazards. Patients with a moderate mobility issue will be risk-assessed and care plans will include safe manual handling procedure requirements, which could mean a two-person lift to get out of bed, dressing and then being seated. Moving and handling equipment should be in place, for example a transfer belt or mobile hoist – depending on space and need – and the care professional will provide their own PPE at the time of the visit.

Only qualified staff – domiciliary carers within the home or in a residential care home, and healthcare or trainee nursing staff – can move a patient. Provision for this will be in place before a patient is discharged (Figure 2.10).

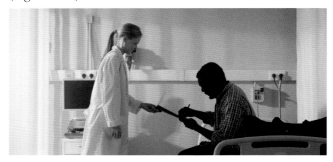

▲ Figure 2.10 Discharging a patient

Preparation for arrival at destination

Carers

Informal carers will be involved in an admission or discharge plan. They are a key person in arrangements such as the collection of prescribed medication from the hospital pharmacy dispenser or in ensuring a patient being admitted is bringing their current medications.

A carer should be informed of factors such as:

▶ any directions the patient needs to follow prior to a hospital follow-up appointment, or further tests that might require the patient to have been Nil by Mouth for a period of time

▶ after discharge, which tablets need to be taken, and any specific requirements such as taking medication with or before food, not eating certain foods with their medication or the times that the medication should be taken

▶ a possible harmful side effect of medication, which needs reporting immediately – the carer will need to be vigilant and observe the patient carefully

▶ dressing regime for any wound/injury aftercare and who is responsible for carrying this out.

Continence aids

Training in the safe use of continence aids such as a commode or incontinence pads (for example the correct size and absorbency) can be a requirement as preparation for a patient's return home. Effective personal hygiene can reduce the risk of infection. The experience and safety of hospital care can make a discharge daunting. Support to adjust to returning home, a direct line and counselling may be offered as part of the discharge package, and recorded in the discharge plan following patient feedback.

Bed availability

The transfer from acute care to specialist rehabilitation can sometimes involve a location far from the patient's home. Lack of bed availability in a specialist unit can cause delays, frustration and anxiety. Preparation for arrival at the destination is helpful for the patient, and informing the relatives of what is needed may mean that specialist equipment such as a hospital bed may be arranged prior to the discharge to make the process safer.

K2.15 How to gather appropriate, relevant and timely evidence to assist in obtaining an individual's history

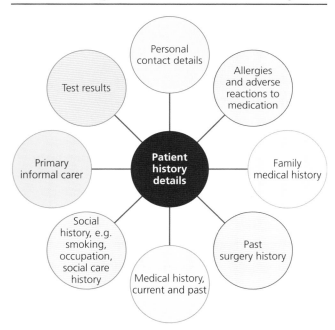

▲ Figure 2.11 Patient history details

At birth a baby is issued with a unique NHS number, which is a method of keeping all patient history

Key term

Guthrie test: a heel-prick capillary test to detect the presence of phenylketonuria markers.

records accessible for that person during their lifetime (the kinds of details that might be included in patient history records are presented in Figure 2.11).

The first entry is often newborn screening results, such as the **Guthrie test**, and childhood vaccination records. In 2005, the government set a target to centralise electronic health records by 2010. The Lorenzo system was part of this national programme and adopted by NHS trusts; however, there were problems that led to mistrust. In light of this, security measures were put in place and the system remains current.

If medical practitioners have access to patient history records, this speeds up accurate diagnosis and treatment. Patient notes are continually being updated, for example recent blood tests and discharge letters. Permission to access records is strictly controlled and a trainee healthcare assistant will not have access. Information governance (IG) has guidelines about how to manage and share information safely and securely. Moving location and changing GP surgery requires the completion of a form, called a family doctor services registration document, with a section where the patient gives permission to trace previous medical records.

Integrated care boards influenced a uniform structure enabling a collaborative system for sharing information between organisations, meeting the regulations of the Data Protection Act 2018. By 2022 patients over the age of 18 had access to all their medical records held electronically, including scanned consultant and written documents. If a person was not born in the UK and is not yet registered – for instance, if they are seeking asylum in the UK – primary care services must still see them.

Qualitative data

Qualitative data includes facts and opinions. Information shared is reliable if it is factual, but patient recollections, professional observations and opinions can be subjective, and therefore less reliable. For example, asking a patient for their views on their quality of life following treatment can be anonymised and the same question asked of others in order to build up a picture. Using a rating system such as 1 for poor and 5 for excellent means data can be compared with ease instead of sifting through patients' written statements, which are harder to analyse.

A person with a positive outlook will give a different account of a side effect to someone who is generally negative and resentful. An opinion may change: an immediate response at the time of a treatment may differ from the recollection a day later when the person is feeling better.

Quantitative data

Patient history includes **quantitative data**, for example on hospital admissions, professional recording of BMI or a medication dosage. This is factual and reliable, as a qualified professional has recorded the details.

For example, a record of a patient's response to medication during an acute illness will indicate the suitability of repeating the same prescription should the illness reoccur. Data related to hospital admissions is used nationally and a financial calculation made for the cost of an overnight stay. This data will be presented in a discussion about the cost of a medication that prevents the need for admission, and the cost of the prescription compared to the cost of an overnight stay.

Sources of information

Reliability may also depend on the source of the information. Past records from qualified professionals should be good, but information might be less accurate from a patient or an advocate.

For example, evidenced-based research findings supported the use of shingles vaccinations for a younger age group: 65 years from September 2023. While people over 70 were deemed vulnerable, further research analysed cases of shingles and their severity in people aged between 65 and 70, resulting in the change of age grouping for this vaccination.

Sources: UK Health Security Agency (2023), 'Shingles immunisation programme: information for healthcare practioners', www.gov.uk/government/publications/shingles-vaccination-guidance-for-healthcare-professionals/shingles-immunisation-programme-information-for-healthcare-practitioners

UK Health Security Agency (2023), 'Introduction of Shingrix® vaccine for the whole programme and expansion of eligible cohorts letter', www.gov.uk/government/publications/shingles-vaccination-programme-changes-from-september-2023-letter/introduction-of-shingrix-vaccine-for-the-whole-programme-and-expansion-of-eligible-cohorts-letter

Patient input sources that are not supported by evidence require careful analysis for their usefulness. For example, a patient who has a learning disability may be asked the date of their last period and be unable to recall this. They may feel pressure to answer and so state, incorrectly, that it was eight days prior to examination. In this case, a decision might be made to carry out a pregnancy test nonetheless, to rule out nausea being morning sickness.

Test yourself

S2.20 Record, report and store manual and electronic information accurately and legibly in line with local and national policies, keep information confidential, support others to do so and apply these by taking part in audits

You are a trainee nurse on a stroke ward, where you are working with the cardiovascular team, speech and language, and physiotherapists. Information needs to be recorded accurately. It must be legible and on the correct forms.

1 What is the role of UK GDPR in storing information?
2 What method is used for safe storage of electronic information?
3 What method is used for safe storage of written information?
4 What method is used to maintain the confidentiality of verbal information?
5 What is sharing on a need-to-know basis?

Case study

S2.18 Gather appropriate, relevant and timely evidence to assist in obtaining an individual's history and review health related data and information

You will need two partners for this demonstration. Your task is to produce a training video with a focus on effective communication.

You are a nurse, asked to gather a patient's history. A doctor is aware of a wrist facture and will require you to provide a logical, coherent written report and a verbal concise summary.

Simulated patient information

Jenny was brought in to A&E by her brother. She has a visible facial cut above her eye and bruising. An X-ray shows a right distal radius fracture. Jenny's brother says she tripped up the kerb and fell, hitting a lamp post.

Jenny:
▶ is flushed and has a temperature, her pulse and breathing rate is fast
▶ has a cough and is wheezy
▶ flinches when her blood pressure is taken, using her left arm
▶ looks nervous and looks at her brother a lot, even when being spoken to
▶ is reluctant to lift up her top – she has a laundry iron shaped second degree burn; it is not covered, and is painful and infected.

Jenny's face shows signs of pain/discomfort.

Her brother answers questions until he is told that Jenny must answer. Jenny does not know her doctor's address; the brother answers for her. Jenny does not own a mobile phone. She is anxious to go home and is dismissive when questioned about the facial bruising, cut and burn.

Jenny says she is 25. She is allergic to penicillin. Jenny has asthma but no Ventolin at home.

When Jenny is taken to an examination room, her brother is asked to remain in the waiting area. Once separated from him, she is able to speak freely: she is able to say her real name is Esme Carter-Large and she is 15 years old. Her 'brother' is her boyfriend. She is in a domestic violence situation.

Clinical tasks and information needed

You must start with an introduction, stating your name and role, and then explain UK GDPR to the patient.

Using dignity curtains, explain privacy. You observe the patient looks nervous. Explain the tests you are going to carry out:
▶ blood pressure 120/70 (left arm)
▶ oxygen saturation 95 per cent

> ▶ temperature 38.5°C
> ▶ breathing rate 24 breaths per minute
> ▶ sounds heard by stethoscope, crackle and wheeze.
>
> You see the burn on the left scapula area.
>
> Get patient history while carrying out physiological measurements; the patient is alert.
>
> The patient's 'brother' answers the majority of your questions; he asks why you need to do so many tests and ask lots of questions.
>
> The patient gets the year of birth wrong – it does not correspond with the age she has given you.
>
> The patient may have a UTI; sample results urine is clear and 7 on the urine colour chart; do not test.
>
> After you have recorded measurements you cannot find any records for the patient on the system and the GP's details given by the 'brother' do not exist.
>
> You do not dress the facial cut.
>
> You put together a report that includes:
> ▶ the medical facts
> ▶ social and safeguarding concerns.
>
> You give your impression of the patient in context, sharing observations.

Personal development

Part of becoming a registered professional is completing training requirements and skills competencies that need signing off by a supervisor. This happens in sequential order and builds up a portfolio that can be regularly reviewed. Reflective practice, assessing current skills and planning next steps is a mandatory part of trainee healthcare work.

K2.16 Why professional development, personal development plans and using feedback to develop and improve are important

Reflective practice using a model, for example Gibbs' reflective cycle or the Atkins and Murphy model, must become a habit; reflection is standard practice in nursing. Self-evaluation starts with analysing why you acted in a certain way, the feelings and thinking behind your action. It also includes a review of what you think you might have done better or will do differently next time.

Discussing a task with a supervisor may be appropriate for feedback; or introspection (self-contemplation) may be more beneficial. The outcome should end at what improvements are needed and how these can be actioned.

Staff appraisal is an opportunity to receive and give feedback, such as in a discussion with a line manager.

Future continuing professional development (CPD) training will support improvements, a move in a different direction or promotion opportunities.

The benefit of working on rotation is that you will be able to get a broader view of different departments, clinics and service user experience.

The NHS encourages progression, such as moving up a pay band. It offers fully funded qualifications, such as for a nurse practitioner to study for a master's degree or advanced nursing practice.

Professional development and using feedback are important as they allow you to assess your skills:
▶ Are they adequate?
▶ Is training and observation needed?
▶ Will practice improve outcomes?

Videoing interactions during clinical practice is a useful way of analysing communication skills, body language and the reaction of the patient, which helps improve self-awareness. Consent must be sought prior to filming patients.

Organisational skills, time management and attention to detail will reduce stress levels at university or college and as a registered professional.
▶ **Assess, identify and develop** personal qualities such as patience, using initiative, confidence and being flexible, which are all suitable characteristic traits for service user care.
▶ **Consider your aims in life** and analyse your progress; this will support your motivation and

self-worth. Setbacks are inevitable and are a good learning opportunity, although at the time they may feel like a failure and your motivation might wane. They provide an opportunity to improve your practice.

▶ **Set goals to realise and maximise your potential:** it is important to set achievable, realistic goals with progress milestones.

▶ **Plan to make relevant, positive and effective choices and decisions for future career development:** reflecting and making a personal development plan will help you to organise your intentions.

▶ **Remain up to date with current practices and national and local protocols:** legislation is amended, as are regulations, and there will be changes to management structures, with evolving technologies impacting on practice, for example a new discharge policy.

The NMC has a student standards framework that applies to all approved educational institutions such as universities. The standards framework for nursing and midwifery education is a document with three sections:

1 Standards framework for nursing and midwifery education
2 Standards for student supervision and assessment
3 Standards for pre- and post-registration programmes, such as for health visitors.

The standards framework helps nursing and midwifery students achieve NMC proficiencies and registration outcomes. All nurses, nursing associates and midwives must practise in line with the requirements of the NMC Code, the professional standards of practice, values and behaviours that registered nurses, midwives and nursing associates are expected to uphold.

Research

S2.21 Maintain a record of personal development and training from undertaking CPD

S2.22 Use feedback to develop and improve

The NMC revalidation requirements include 450 practice hours for nursing, or 900 if revalidating as both a nurse and midwife. In addition, there are 35 hours of continuing professional development (CPD), including 20 hours' participatory learning, for example being observed carrying out a procedure such as wound dressing. The registered nurse needs a minimum of five pieces of practice-related feedback from a work area – this can be a thank you letter from a colleague, a patient or other health professional, an appraisal or a supervisory report. In addition to this, the nurse must have completed five pieces of practice-related reflections, and they must have had a professional discussion recorded with another registered nurse around the reflective pieces.

Recording any learning activity is your responsibility as the trainee healthcare worker. Some tasks may require validation and to be signed off by a supervisor. Figure 2.12 gives an example of a form for recording CPD.

Time/date	Location	Scope of practice	CPD learning or task	Supervisor signed off

▲ Figure 2.12 A sample CPD record form

Click on the following link to explore the NMC information regarding keeping a CPD record, suggested evidence through feedback and standards for registered professionals: **www.nmc.org.uk/revalidation/requirements/cpd**

Your task is to complete four reflective journal activities.

You will have completed two training videos for this chapter's case studies:

1 'An introduction to clinical and therapeutic tasks and interventions, working with qualified professionals' for first-year T Level Health students

2 gathering Jenny's history and collating a logical, coherent verbal report concisely for a doctor.

Now use two different reflection models and identify points to work on as improvements.

1 First, use Gibbs' reflective cycle to review both training videos. Follow these steps:
   ▶ Step 1: Description
   ▶ Step 2: Feelings
   ▶ Step 3: Evaluation
   ▶ Step 4: Conclusions
   ▶ Step 5: Action.

2 Then use the Atkins and Murphy model to review both training videos. Follow these steps:
   ▶ Awareness
   ▶ Describe
   ▶ Analyse
   ▶ Evaluate
   ▶ Identify.

Healthcare PO3: Undertaking a range of physiological measurements

The purpose of observing a patient's welfare and testing their physical wellbeing is to record measurements that can be compared to expected norms. This enables a continual process of monitoring and feedback for medical professionals, which may indicate any early warning signs, for example. During this process, clinical procedure policies must be observed to ensure accurate information that meets infection prevention standards.

Learning outcomes

The core knowledge outcomes that you must understand and learn:

K3.1 the physiological measurements commonly measured by healthcare support workers and the normal range for each measurement in adults

K3.2 why these measurements are taken

K3.3 when these measurements are taken

K3.4 how these measurements are taken

K3.5 how to monitor elimination, nutrition and hydration

K3.6 major factors that influence changes in physiological measurement

K3.7 types of equipment used for measuring physiological states in adults

K3.8 how to check that each piece of equipment is in working order

K3.9 the importance of recording results from physiological measurement tests

K3.10 the purpose of the NEWS 2012 and NEWS2 2017 system

K3.11 how an early warning score is calculated and used

K3.12 reasons for taking and testing venous and capillary blood and other specimens

K3.13 procedures for taking and testing venous and capillary blood and other specimens

K3.14 the policy and current good practices that affect work practice when undertaking physiological measurements

K3.15 why these practices are important.

Skills outcomes

The skills you will need to demonstrate:

S3.16 use physiological measurement equipment correctly

S3.17 record the results of physiological monitoring and measurement using relevant documentation

S3.18 demonstrate the correct process for reporting measurements that fall outside normal levels

S3.19 calculate National Early Warning Scores (NEWS) 2 and escalate findings to a registered health professional where appropriate

S3.20 apply current policy and good practice techniques when undertaking physiological measurement.

Physiological measurements

Physiological measurements give a good indication of a person's health as an initial assessment or as a means of monitoring. Some measurements, such as high body mass index (BMI), can be identified as a risk factor for future health conditions such as diabetes, whereas other measurements can detect an immediate health concern such as high blood sugar levels using a glucometer.

Observation in itself is an opportunity to assess aspects of an individual's health, such as skin colour changes or pupil dilation and reaction, as a measurement. This collection of measurements, once recorded, can build a picture for more senior staff to follow up.

K3.1 The physiological measurements commonly measured by healthcare support workers and the normal range for each measurement in adults

Blood pressure

Blood pressure refers to the force of the blood moving along the arteries. It is measured in millimetres of mercury (mmHg), using a monitor like that shown in Figure 3.1. Systolic is the measurement as the heart beats and is indicated by the number at the top of the fraction, while the bottom number is diastolic, which measures the pressure against the artery walls when the heart is between beats. An adult's healthy normal range for systolic is 90–120 and for diastolic 60–80; however, this is usually lower for a child and higher for an older person due to the differing flexibility and muscle action in their arteries.

Figure 3.2 shows examples of blood pressure readings and the kinds of health problems they might indicate.

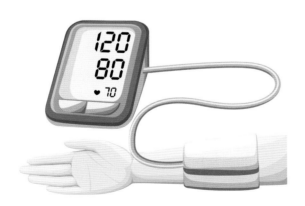

▲ Figure 3.1 A blood pressure monitor in use

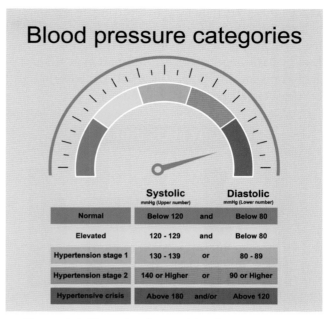

Blood pressure categories

	Systolic mmHg (Upper number)		Diastolic mmHg (Lower number)
Normal	Below 120	and	Below 80
Elevated	120 - 129	and	Below 80
Hypertension stage 1	130 - 139	or	80 - 89
Hypertension stage 2	140 or Higher	or	90 or Higher
Hypertensive crisis	Above 180	and/or	Above 120

▲ Figure 3.2 Chart displaying blood pressure categories

Body temperature

Body temperature is the measurement of how effectively the body can retain or reduce its core temperature. It is measured in degrees Celsius (°C). The adult normal range for body temperature is 36°C to 37.5°C, although this may be a little higher for babies and children.

Respiration rate

A patient's respiration rate is measured by monitoring the number of breaths they take per minute. A normal adult range is between 12 to 20 breaths per minute, but this is notably higher for babies and children.

Heart rate

Heart rate is measured in beats per minute (bpm). A healthy reading for an adult at rest is between 60 and 100 bpm but may be lower for a person who is athletic and physically fit.

Weight and height

BMI is a calculation using weight and height:
- in metric terms, BMI = kg/m², where kg is a person's weight in kilograms and m² is their height in metres
- alternatively, in non-metric format the formula for BMI = weight in pounds divided by a person's height in inches, squared and then multiplied by 703.

These figures are then used to estimate the amount of body fat an individual has, which may indicate the possibility of health complications (Figure 3.3). A healthy BMI range is between 18.5 and 24.9. A figure above or below this range raises the possibility of the presence of a potential health condition.

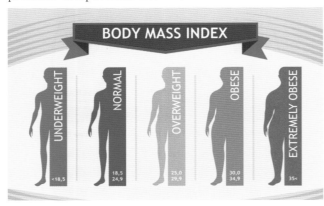

▲ Figure 3.3 Example of a body mass index (BMI) infographic

Urinary output

This is a measurement of the amount of urine a person excretes in one day. It is measured in millilitres (ml) and the healthy adult norm is 800 to 2,000 ml per day. A patient may need closer monitoring for a range of reasons such as chronic or acute kidney disease and, in such cases, urine output would be measured per hour.

Oxygen saturation

This is the level of oxygen in the blood, specifically in the red blood cells. It is referred to as oxyhaemoglobin and is measured as a percentage. Red blood cells contain haemoglobin, which bonds with oxygen, carrying this throughout the body for cellular respiration. A healthy norm is a measurement between 95 and 100 per cent.

Blood sugar levels

This is a measurement that indicates the level of glucose in the blood. It can be taken when fasting and after food has been eaten, due to the **fluctuating readings** in different situations. The results are presented as millimoles per litre (mmol/l), with a healthy level between 4.0 and 7.0. This may differ for people living with diabetes.

Key term

Fluctuating readings: the rise and fall of a numerical amount, such as blood glucose levels.

Research

S3.17 Record the results of physiological monitoring and measurement using relevant documentation

Practitioners refer to a variety of NHS charts to assess risk and record physiological measurements. For example:
- ▶ NEWS2 chart
- ▶ Community Nursing Sepsis Screening and Action Tool
- ▶ 24-hour fluid balance chart, urine output
- ▶ wound assessment document
- ▶ pain score
- ▶ nutritional screening tool, food chart
- ▶ Bristol stool chart
- ▶ BMI
- ▶ peak flow
- ▶ Braden pressure injury risk assessment tool
- ▶ Hospital Rapid Discharge Frailty Assessment Screening Tool document.

Find out what these charts and assessment tool documents are used for and their purpose.

K3.2 Why these measurements are taken

Assessment and information

Physiological measurements form part of an **assessment**, which exists to monitor a specific body function or an overall health status, and will be recorded at the request of a senior healthcare professional. For example, an increase in urine output following an increase of fluid intake indicates an improvement in renal function where a patient has been dehydrated and passing minimal amounts of urine.

These measurements provide **information** on the extent of a disease or disability, which acts as a guide as to what treatment will be most suitable.

Provision and/or response to therapeutic interventions

If a treatment provision and/or response has been administered or trialled, the patient's response must be measured and logged. The data may also be shared to facilitate a multidisciplinary approach and the use of a therapeutic intervention. For example, a consultant may use the data to involve an addiction counsellor, who would also require data on level of liver function deterioration (seriousness) perhaps, say, in the case of a patient with alcoholism. The counsellor represents the therapeutic intervention and an additional element of patient treatment.

> ### Key term
>
> **_Therapeutic intervention:_** a course of action with the intention of managing a patient's physical or mental wellbeing to achieve a positive outcome, with the aim of avoiding the need for further treatment.

Trends and changes in physiology

Continual monitoring, such as hourly testing and observation, can also highlight trends and changes in physiology. For example, pain scale assessment can monitor the effectiveness of pain management medication or form part of an early warning sign assessment where immediate action is required.

Assessments are carried out for different purposes – for example to establish if a patient is well enough and it is safe for them to return home, and what support they would need, such as a frailty assessment (see Figure 3.4). A care plan will include planned timely reviews; however, if there is an unexpected deterioration, a care plan will need to be re-evaluated to ensure it still meets the person's needs.

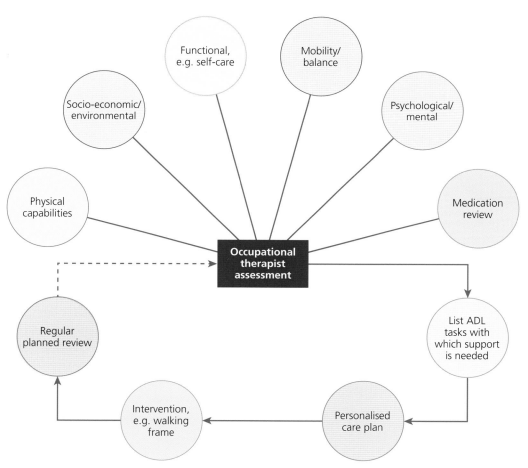

▲ Figure 3.4 Frailty assessment on discharge

K3.3 When these measurements are taken

Measurements must be taken at certain specific times, as shown in Table 3.1.

▼ Table 3.1 When and why measurements are taken

When measurements are taken	Why this is required
Upon arrival to the emergency department or on admission to a ward	Measurements of health form part of a standard assessment when a patient arrives at an emergency department and on admission to a ward, to monitor and look for early warning signs that may mean urgent treatment is needed.
At regular intervals	It may be a requirement to take readings at regular intervals during an individual's stay to observe any deterioration, or an improvement when medication is administered, for example.
Before, during and after a procedure or surgery	A patient may have a planned operation or a need for an emergency procedure or surgery, which requires physiological measurements to be taken before, during and afterwards as standard. Examples include: ▶ checking a haemophiliac's clotting factor levels before any operation ▶ checking a patient's blood pressure.
Back on the ward at certain intervals	Post-surgery, when a patient is back on the ward, monitoring tests may be taken at certain intervals, such as every half hour.
Pre-op clinic	For certain operations and treatments, it may be necessary for an assessment to be carried out days or even weeks in advance of the planned procedure. This allows any actions needed to ensure the person is in a suitable condition for the operation to go ahead, and will be performed in a pre-op clinic.
Post-op monitoring	Examples of post-op monitoring include checking a patient's breathing if they suffer from sleep apnoea (this is when someone's breathing stops temporarily while they are sleeping, possibly due to a high BMI). General anaesthesia can add to risks with apnoea patients and they will need to be monitored closely after operations.

Test yourself

1 A medical professional must check if a medication is negatively affecting a patient's digestive system. What chart would they use?

2 A medical professional will discharge an older patient at the end of the week. What means and assessment forms would they use to inform an occupational health professional of the independent self-care tasks that the patient has completed while they have been an inpatient?

K3.4 How these measurements are taken

A range of small equipment and devices is used to take measurements related to health.

Stethoscope

A stethoscope amplifies sounds, such as the sound of the heart and air intake in different parts of the lungs. If the stethoscope chest piece is in direct contact with the chest wall the sounds of the heart and lungs can be heard. In this way, a leaking heart valve may be detected or an area of the lung that is not receiving any airflow.

Sphygmomanometer

A **sphygmomanometer** is a piece of manual equipment that is used to monitor blood pressure. It consists of an inflatable rubber cuff that is wrapped around the top of the arm and connected to a column of mercury next to a graduated scale. The instrument is pumped by hand to enable the determination of systolic and diastolic blood pressure, by increasing and releasing the pressure in the cuff. It is used in conjunction with a stethoscope to listen to the sound of blood flow while looking at the readings on the manometer (Figure 3.5).

Key terms

Pre-op clinic: an outpatients department that specialises in carrying out tests in advance of a surgical procedure, to measure a person's health and suitability.

Sphygmomanometer: an instrument with a rubber cuff, gauge and inflation bulb, used for measuring blood pressure manually.

It is more common to use a digital blood pressure monitor, which takes a reading automatically. Some people may monitor their own blood pressure at home and are required to inform a health practitioner of their results. There is technology available that permits readings to be sent electronically to a medical practitioner automatically.

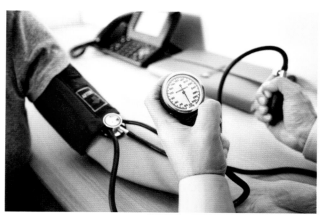

▲ Figure 3.5 Measuring blood pressure using a sphygmomanometer and stethoscope

Thermometer

Thermometers can be electronic and are most commonly inserted into the ear with a disposable probe cover. Such thermometers use **tympanic membrane sensors** and show a reading on a digital display (Figure 3.6).

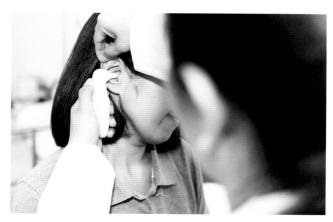

▲ Figure 3.6 Using a tympanic thermometer

Key term

Tympanic membrane sensors: a infrared sensors used to measure body temperature, usually inside the ear.

Pulse oximeter

For oxygen saturation and pulse rate measurement, a pulse oximeter is used (Figure 3.7). It is secured on the fingertip and shines a light through the skin to assess the baseline percentage of oxygen in the blood at any given point.

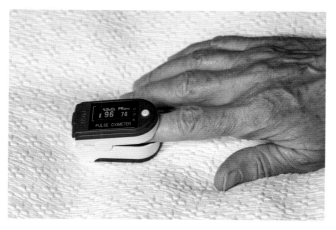

▲ Figure 3.7 Using a pulse oximeter on a finger

Pulse reading

To take a pulse reading manually, a nurse will use a watch with a second hand. They count the number of pulse beats in 10 seconds and then multiply this by six to calculate the pulse rate during a one-minute period.

Blood sugar meter, lancet and test strip

The most common site to test blood glucose levels is the fingertip. A lancet is a short thin needle that is spring-loaded and penetrates the skin, causing blood capillaries at the surface to produce a droplet of blood. This is then touched at the front edge of a testing strip and inserted into the glucometer (blood sugar meter). The level of glucose in the blood droplet will be displayed in seconds. The level is then compared to the range of readings for high, low and a healthy level of blood sugar.

How procedures may need to be adapted for individuals

Depending on the current condition of a patient, there may be a need to adapt the usual ways of taking a recording in order to get the essential measurements. For example, in some cases a pulse oximeter can be used on the ear lobe, such as in the case of serious injury to a person's hands in an industrial accident, or with a person who is confused and keeps removing the oximeter from their finger.

K3.5 How to monitor elimination, nutrition and hydration

Elimination

This refers to body waste measurement and analysis, which require monitoring. This includes the amount of urine excreted, substances detected in the urine, and the colour of urine or bowel motions. The data gathered can be evaluated by using a bowel chart (such as the Bristol stool chart, as mentioned in the Research activity on page 84).

Nutrition

In certain circumstances a food diary may be used to observe nutrient intake, which could also be tested by taking blood samples.

A person may be eating foods that contain a particular nutrient, as evidenced in a food diary, but this is not reflected in a blood test. For example, a patient is eating foods containing calcium, but their blood test shows a measurement below the healthy norm of 8.6 to 10.3 mg/dL. Analysing their food diary highlights a diet lacking in the foods rich in vitamin D required to absorb calcium. Providing information on foods to add to their current diet can inform the patient as to what to eat to improve this situation.

Hydration

Hydration measurement is an important aspect of healthcare. Fluid balance charts are used to record the fluids an individual consumes, for example 20 per cent in foods, an intake in drinks and then the excretion in urine output.

Body measurements

An increase or decrease in BMI forms part of an assessment that focuses on balancing nutritional intake when the patient returns to their home environment and also on nutritional balance for longer-term inpatients.

K3.6 Major factors that influence changes in physiological measurement

There are many factors that will produce changes in physiological measurements, as shown in Table 3.2.

▼ Table 3.2 Factors that influence changes in physiological measurement

Factor	Effect on physiological measurement
Age and weight	An individual's age can influence their measurement readings and this must be given careful consideration. For example, an older person will naturally have higher blood pressure than the expected healthy norms. A person's weight can influence their health. Severe obesity will cause the heart rate to be irregular due to the strain it is under, and an individual who is underweight may have a slower heart rate as their heart muscles have become weaker.
Disease or chronic illness	A chronic illness or disease may cause changing symptoms, which can be detected via monitoring tests. Their severity may require alterations to the treatment plan. For example, genetic inheritance of a condition such as familial hypercholesterolemia (FH) causes high cholesterol levels and the build-up of atherosclerosis in the arteries, increasing blood pressure.
Environment	For example, **hypothermia** and **hyperthermia**, or heat stroke. Outdoor temperatures below freezing point require an individual to dress in clothing that covers their skin and offers warmth. Body movement generates heat; a person who is not suitably clothed and is motionless (for example unconscious) is at risk of hypothermia, indicated by a core temperature below 35°C. In extreme heat, an individual can overheat as the usual homeostasis mechanisms are overwhelmed and their core temperature rises above 38°C. In cases of malnutrition (for example due to neglect or self-neglect), a person who is underweight may have a slow heart rate while seated (bradycardia); however, when they then stand, there may be an abnormally elevated heart rate (tachycardia) compared to the expected norm.
Hydration and nutritional status	Colour and amount of urine indicate hydration levels. Urine colour can be compared to a hydration chart, which gives a good visual representation to aid understanding of a patient's condition. Nutritional status not only looks at the intake of different types of foods but also the body's ability to absorb nutrients in cases where there is a stomach or bowel problem. This requires monitoring at intervals, in case nutritional supplements are needed. For example, during the menopause, the changing levels of hormones impact on enzyme activity and on the body's ability to process vitamin D as it should, causing a deficiency.
Infection	A change in body temperature can be an indication of infection in a patient. An assessment must be made of the baseline data for a patient who has been exposed to extreme cold over a length of time.

Factor	Effect on physiological measurement
Lifestyle	Measurements can change because of lifestyle factors such as the following. ▶ Smoking a cigarette just before a blood pressure reading is taken will cause it to read higher due to nicotine temporarily causing blood vessels to dilate (vasodilation). ▶ Drugs (for example stimulants, or depressants such as caffeine): depending on the amount and the individual, caffeine has an almost immediate effect on blood pressure, causing a high spike; however, this is short term. Cocaine is a stimulant that increases the demand for oxygen, increasing both heart rate and blood pressure while it is in the system. Smoking cannabis also increases the heart rate temporarily but has no significant impact on blood pressure. ▶ Diet: a high-fat diet causes unhealthy cholesterol levels, increased atherosclerosis and elevated blood pressure. ▶ Stress levels (for example due to pressures at work) could cause an increase in heart rate and blood pressure, a psychological stimulus impacting on physiological status.
Medication	▶ Beta blockers act as a block to adrenalin, lowering blood pressure. ▶ Statins slow down the absorption of cholesterol from the diet, so blood vessels are clearer for more efficient blood flow, also lowering blood pressure. ▶ A steroid inhaler opens up airways by reducing inflammation and relaxing constricted airway muscles. This will temporarily improve the oxygen saturation rate. ▶ Paracetamol can reduce a fever by causing interruption in chemical messengers to the part of the brain that controls body temperature.
Mental state	An individual's mental state may cause abnormal blood pressure readings (for example anxiety levels can influence high blood pressure and heart rate readings).

Key terms

Hypothermia: a core body temperature of below 35°C.

Hyperthermia: a core body temperature of above 38°C.

Reflect

White coat syndrome refers to when an individual feels anxious in a medical environment, such as outpatients. Their current mental state can impact on a blood pressure reading. A medical professional may spend more time with the patient in order to allay their worries. However, this may still not be enough to enable a true blood pressure reading to be taken.

Alternatives to offer anxious patients in this kind of scenario include the allocation of a digital blood pressure monitor by their GP for them to take home, with instructions on how to take accurate readings in the morning and evening. This can then be returned to the doctor for analysis. However, one negative that should be considered here is the level of trustworthiness of the patient or their questionable understanding of the requirements, perhaps due to a learning disability or dementia diagnosis.

K3.7 Types of equipment used for measuring physiological states in adults

Various equipment, devices and observations are used to carry out different assessments and general health and wellbeing measurements (see Table 3.3).

▼ Table 3.3 Equipment used for measuring physiological states in adults

Physiological measurement	Equipment
Blood pressure	Sphygmomanometer or digital monitor
Blood sugar levels	Glucometer
Body temperature	Thermometer, ear tympanic or digital
Breathing rate	Observation
Health of respiratory airways	Peak flow device (Figure 3.8)
Monitoring elimination	Observation charts, such as the Bristol stool chart or a fluid output chart
Nutrition and hydration	Observation charts, such as a food diary or a fluid balance chart
Oxygen saturation	Pulse oximeter
Pulse rate	Manual or pulse oximeter
Urinary output	Catheter, measuring jug
Weight/height	Scales, bariatric chair and height stick

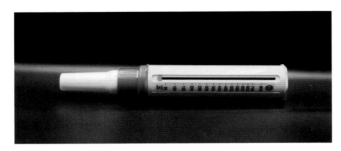

▲ Figure 3.8 A peak flow meter with a disposable mouthpiece

K3.8 How to check that each piece of equipment is in working order

To ensure accurate measurement readings, each device or piece of equipment must be in good working order.

▶ To ensure correct and consistent use, practitioners must follow **manufacturer's instructions**.
▶ Before use, make **visual checks** to look for any signs of wear and tear.
▶ If the equipment appears faulty, then it must be **removed** and **reported** to a line manager. This should be followed by a written report as a record.

Health and safety

Each organisation will have formal documentation for the reporting of wear and tear concerns, and also for when equipment is found to be faulty. There will be procedures in place regarding the immediate cessation (stopping) of use.

K3.9 The importance of recording results from physiological measurement tests

Having accurate, legible recordings of measurement data is vitally important, as it can mean the difference between life and death.

How are results recorded?

▶ At the bedside, readings are mainly recorded manually as a paper-based record. Sometimes these hard-copy records are added to the patient's electronic records for the purpose of ease of access.
▶ Other measurements are always recorded electronically, for example a pre-op assessment.

Why are results recorded?

▶ Physiological measurements recorded at planned intervals will provide evidence to track any changes and deviations from expected patient outcomes.
▶ The record can be easily accessed and is used to inform practitioners who are working as part of a multidisciplinary team (MDT).
▶ They can help build a picture that influences the direction of a treatment plan.

What results are recorded?

The measurement intervals will be decided by a medical practitioner, but they will usually be regular readings.

▶ Close monitoring may require readings be taken every 30 minutes.
▶ A patient in a less serious condition may have health observations taken only every 12 hours.

If a person's results are far from the healthy norms, or if there is an erratic fluctuation in their results, this will determine the regularity of ongoing measurement intervals. Any **deviations from the norm** are flagged up immediately for additional assessment.

Key term

Deviations from the norm: readings that are higher or lower than the healthy norm of the physiological measurement.

K3.10 The purpose of the NEWS 2012 and NEWS2 2017 system

▶ The aim of taking physiological measurements is to determine **how ill an individual is** or how effective the treatment is towards recovery.
▶ Measurements will **inform** the type and speed of treatment or care they receive, or the involvement of a rapid response team, which could be a surgical team who are required to operate on a patient who is actively bleeding.
▶ The recording is added to a **standardised** clinical chart, which is used by both the NHS and private healthcare organisations. Therefore, if a patient is referred to a different practitioner or moves hospitals, for example, all records can be easily analysed in a response to acute illness. This means there are no delays, and a supporting healthcare approach is delivered via a team of specialists and an integrated service.

NEWS key		FULL NAME		
0 1 2 3		DATE OF BIRTH		DATE OF ADMISSION

		DATE										DATE
		TIME										TIME

A+B Respirations Breaths/min

Range	Score		Range
≥25	3		≥25
21–24	2		21–24
18–20			18–20
15–17			15–17
12–14			12–14
9–11	1		9–11
≤8	3		≤8

A+B SpO₂ Scale 1 Oxygen saturation (%)

Range	Score		Range
≥96			≥96
94–95	1		94–95
92–93	2		92–93
≤91	3		≤91

SpO₂ Scale 2† Oxygen saturation (%) — Use Scale 2 if target range is 88–92%, eg in hypercapnic respiratory failure. †ONLY use Scale 2 under the direction of a qualified clinician

Range	Score		Range
≥97 on O₂	3		≥97 on O₂
95–96 on O₂	2		95–96 on O₂
93–94 on O₂	1		93–94 on O₂
≥93 on air			≥93 on air
88–92			88–92
86–87	1		86–87
84–85	2		84–85
≤83%	3		≤83%

Air or oxygen?

	Score		
A=Air			A=Air
O₂ L/min	2		O₂ L/min
Device			Device

C Blood pressure mmHg — Score uses systolic BP only

Range	Score		Range
≥220	3		≥220
201–219			201–219
181–200			181–200
161–180			161–180
141–160			141–160
121–140			121–140
111–120			111–120
101–110	1		101–110
91–100	2		91–100
81–90			81–90
71–80			71–80
61–70	3		61–70
51–60			51–60
≤50			≤50

C Pulse Beats/min

Range	Score		Range
≥131	3		≥131
121–130	2		121–130
111–120			111–120
101–110	1		101–110
91–100			91–100
81–90			81–90
71–80			71–80
61–70			61–70
51–60			51–60
41–50	1		41–50
31–40			31–40
≤30	3		≤30

D Consciousness Score for NEW onset of confusion (no score if chronic)

	Score		
Alert			Alert
Confusion			Confusion
V	3		V
P			P
U			U

E Temperature °C

Range	Score		Range
≥39.1°	2		≥39.1°
38.1–39.0°	1		38.1–39.0°
37.1–38.0°			37.1–38.0°
36.1–37.0°			36.1–37.0°
35.1–36.0°	1		35.1–36.0°
≤35.0°	3		≤35.0°

NEWS TOTAL				TOTAL
Monitoring frequency				Monitoring
Escalation of care Y/N				Escalation
Initials				Initials

Royal College of Physicians

National Early Warning Score 2 (NEWS2) © Royal College of Physicians December 2022

▲ Figure 3.9 NEWS2 2017 observation chart

K3.11 How an early warning score is calculated and used

Physiological parameters

Physiological parameters are measurements that are put together to make an overall assessment of an individual's physical health and wellbeing. A system of scoring six measurements collectively, with zero representing no physiological disturbance and higher scores reflecting greater distance from healthy norms, instantly highlights any immediate action that may be needed.

The six measurements are:
1 respiration rate per minute
2 oxygen saturation, SpO_2: scale 1 (%) and scale 2 on air or oxygen (%)
3 blood pressure systolic, mmHg
4 pulse rate, bpm
5 level of consciousness or new confusion (alert to CVPU: new confusion, voice, pain, unresponsive)
6 temperature, °C.

For example, without oxygen therapy a patient with below 70 per cent oxygen saturation may die. If you are using a NEWS 2012 chart with a patient who is receiving oxygen, in order to maintain a reading of above 95 per cent it will be necessary to add an extra 2 points to the total. The updated NEWS2 2017 observation chart (Figure 3.9) already has scoring for oxygen saturation rates when an individual is receiving air or oxygen.

Calculating the measurement

Each measurement has a numerical score of between 0 and 3, which is then calculated as part of the overall score. This emphasises the seriousness of higher numbers recorded.

Recording the measurement

The NEWS charts are also colour-coded, which gives a visual representation of the severity of a patient's clinical condition (Figure 3.9). The charts are used as a response to acute illness. A score of 0 has no colour and remains white, 1 is yellow, 2 orange and 3 a darker orange colour (Figure 3.10).

Escalation

A medium score of 5 or more, or if one of the measurements scores a 3, is the trigger for immediate escalation to a senior clinician with critical-care competencies for an urgent review.

Chart 1: The NEWS scoring system

Physiological parameter	Score						
	3	2	1	0	1	2	3
Respiration rate (per minute)	≤8		9–11	12–20		21–24	≥25
SpO₂ Scale 1 (%)	≤91	92–93	94–95	≥96			
SpO₂ Scale 2 (%)	≤83	84–85	86–87	88–92 ≥93 on air	93–94 on oxygen	95–96 on oxygen	≥97 on oxygen
Air or oxygen?		Oxygen		Air			
Systolic blood pressure (mmHg)	≤90	91–100	101–110	111–219			≥220
Pulse (per minute)	≤40		41–50	51–90	91–110	111–130	≥131
Consciousness				Alert			CVPU
Temperature (°C)	≤35.0		35.1–36.0	36.1–38.0	38.1–39.0	≥39.1	

National Early Warning Score (NEWS) 2

© Royal College of Physicians 2017

▲ Figure 3.10 NEWS2 scoring system reference

Practice points

Practice points

S3.17 Record the results of physiological monitoring and measurement using relevant documentation

S3.19 Calculate National Early Warning Scores (NEWS) 2 and escalate findings to a registered health professional where appropriate

Patient A

Refer to the NEWS2 chart. You are a nurse working in a busy Accident & Emergency department and have been asked to carry out an early warning sign assessment.

Patient A presents at A&E feeling dizzy and hot, with a respiration rate of 21 per minute, an oxygen saturation of 94 per cent without air or oxygen, blood pressure systolic of 119 mmHg, temperature of 39°C and a pulse of 100 bpm. They are alert and responsive.

1 Calculate the NEWS2 score.
2 What action should be taken after your calculation in this situation?

Patient B

Refer to the NEWS2 chart. You are working with a team who have received a patient brought into A&E by ambulance following an accident.

Patient B has a respiration rate of 10 per minute, an oxygen saturation of 95 per cent and they have been given oxygen on the way to hospital, which is continuing in A&E. Their systolic blood pressure is 98 mmHg, temperature is 37°C and they have a pulse of 44 bpm. They are confused and sometimes unresponsive when questioned.

1 Calculate the NEWS2 score.
2 What action should be taken after your calculation in this situation?

Case study

S3.17 Record the results of physiological monitoring and measurement using relevant documentation

S3.19 Calculate National Early Warning Scores (NEWS) 2 and escalate findings to a registered health professional where appropriate

A limitation of the NEWS2 scoring is that the systolic measurement does not have a score of 1 or 2, as it starts at 3, with a measurement of extreme hypertension recorded above 220 mmHg only. In addition, you may have already noticed that the diastolic measurement is not included.

Tomas is a patient who has scored 5 on the NEWS2 chart. He has a diastolic dysfunction, which research has shown is significant in precipitating heart failure and predicting a health outcome for the individual. Not recording Tomas's reading means that other health conditions may not be detected early.

In addition, Tomas has been in a serious accident and is haemodynamically unstable. This means that he is in shock. Correct analysis of fluid status is therefore made more difficult without the recording of the diastolic mmHg on the NEWS2 chart. Even small delays in accurately assessing this critically ill patient may have a negative impact on any required treatments used to stabilise their condition and improve outcomes.

Do you think making the lead medical practitioner aware of an abnormal diastolic verbally would assist with an accurate diagnosis?

K3.12 Reasons for taking and testing venous and capillary blood and other specimens

A **blood capillary sample** is a smaller volume suitable for certain measurements that can be detected in a blood spot. They are easier to collect and the sampling can be carried out by the patient themselves at home. One benefit of this is that certain readings can be observed immediately, such as inflammatory markers, full blood count, or calcium and iron levels.

Venous specimens have a greater quantity and are used to detect organ, gland and potential disease markers. This type of sampling requires laboratory analysis, such as blood cultures or coagulation tests.

Sampling – such as that using a glucometer (Figure 3.11) – gives a snapshot of a potential symptom that can be used to aid in diagnosis. Single sampling that detects an abnormal reading could indicate a need for further investigation, another sample or other kind of measurement, bringing symptoms together for analysis.

▶ Samples are taken for a number of reasons, such as **monitoring a new or pre-existing illness** or a **pre-op check**.

▶ Following the arrival of test results, a clinician can determine if there is a need for a **treatment plan review** or **further investigative testing**.

▶ The results of a single test may highlight an anomaly, so further different testing or the repetition of a test may be necessary to **clarify a diagnosis**.

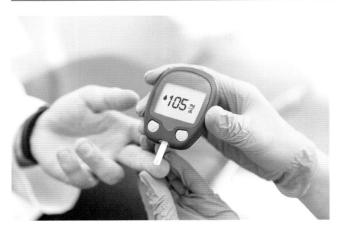

▲ Figure 3.11 A glucometer for measuring glucose levels in blood, used mainly with diabetic patients

K3.13 Procedures for taking and testing venous and capillary blood and other specimens

Venous blood sample

Venipuncture sampling uses different sizes and types of needles, and different angles of insertion. A sample taken from the arm uses tourniquet tightening to temporarily dilate veins so they become more prominent. A needle is used to withdraw blood, the tourniquet is removed and then the needle, while simultaneously using cotton wool or gauze over the injection site to prevent bleeding.

Blood vacutainer sample tubes are colour-coded depending on the testing required, for example purple for a full blood count (FBC).

Capillary blood sample

A **capillary blood sample** takes blood that is closer to an artery, from an arteriole. It is usually a finger prick test such as a blood glucose test.

Other specimens

Other specimens that are gathered for analysis are urine, stool or sputum.
- Some testing can be carried out easily, such as a urine pot dipstick test, whereas other samples will need to be sent to a laboratory for more detailed time-sensitive testing, such as urine culture testing.
- A stool sample is taken using a plastic specimen pot and a specially designed spatula system to collect a small sample that is then sealed automatically. This process can be completed at home with a home test kit and sent to a laboratory in the post, in a specially designed pre-addressed box.

- Sputum (also referred to as phlegm) is a build-up of mucus in the lower lung or lungs and will need to be coughed up, collected and sent for testing as a culture looking at potential bacteria or fungi growth before the most suitable treatment is administered.

Test yourself

1   Give an example of a reason you would complete a capillary blood test.
2   Give an example of a reason you would complete a venous blood test.

Policy and good practice

When carrying out an assessment, good practice such as wearing adequate PPE ensures compliance with infection prevention measures stated in a code of practice under the Health and Social Care Act, which was updated in 2022 following the COVID-19 pandemic.

Disposal of PPE and medical waste will follow an organisational policy that abides by the Environmental Protection Act 1990.

An individual who requires medical care may be vulnerable or lack the capacity to understand decisions made in a care plan. Organisational policies and professional regulations protect everyone's human rights, and there is legislation that dictates safeguarding protocol and aims to prevent discrimination. In a situation where a patient lacks capacity, for example following a brain injury, social care arrangements must be made prior to discharge as part of the duty of care in the Safeguarding Policy. If the patient insists on self-discharging against medical advice, two further policies are relevant. The Equality Policy prevents discrimination on the grounds of disability, in this case a learning disability. A Mental Capacity Act Policy requires an assessment in situations like this and decisions are made in the person's best interest.

K3.14 The policy and current good practices that affect work practice when undertaking physiological measurements

Consent

Informed consent is the term used to describe the patient giving permission for the taking of their physiological measurements. Consent should be obtained before any physical contact is made with the patient. Their decision to give consent must be made voluntarily and free from any pressure or influence. When a patient refuses to give their consent for a procedure, healthcare professionals must give a clear explanation of the importance of the procedure and why it is necessary. A refusal to give consent must be reported to a line manager and recorded. In cases where a patient lacks the capacity to give consent, permission must be given by an approved advocate instead; this could be a member of their family.

Infection control

As with all clinical procedures there is a standard for infection prevention, which includes:

▶ wearing personal protective equipment (PPE)
▶ adhering to standard precautions for hair, nails and handwashing
▶ using approved methods, with sanitised equipment
▶ where appropriate, using disposable equipment such as a thermometer probe cover.

Waste management

Both the PPE and disposable items must follow the organisation's waste management procedures which, in cases of blood tests, will also include sharps (needle) disposal. Follow these guidelines:

▶ Dispose of sharps in a sharps bin.
▶ Put foul linen in a disposable bag.
▶ Dispose of clinical waste in a yellow or black/yellow striped bag.
▶ Dispose of domestic waste in a black bag.

Health and safety

A health and safety policy will cover a range of tasks and situations. Training in the health and safety policy that directly relates to taking observation measurements is mandatory, and you will need to work in line with a risk assessment and standard operating procedure (SOP). The policy will include correct handwashing technique, the use of hand sanitiser between patients, and wearing latex gloves and an apron as well as how they must be donned and doffed.

The policy will also include safe use and disposal of equipment; for example a tympanic thermometer must have a new disposable probe cover, which is disposed of safely after use as part of the standard infection control precautions (SICPs) training.

Data protection

Consent must be given for sharing all personal and identifiable data such as patient details and physiological measurements. These are subject to the Data Protection Act 2018. This ensures patient confidentiality is maintained, and information is stored securely and not open to misuse such as targeted marketing.

A Caldicott guardian is a senior member of staff in the hospital who is responsible for processing health and social care personal data. There are protocols for handling personally identifiable information including, for example, that a patient's relative who does not have their permission to access results from clinical assessments should be prevented from accessing these.

Equality and diversity

If good practice is followed, no individual patient will be disadvantaged compared to another and actions to meet that individual's needs will be taken. For example, a vulnerable adult who may not fully understand what they are giving consent for must be given extra time and support to confirm that they know the extent and purpose of the measurement procedures before any take place.

A relative, medical next of kin, close friend or carer who has the patient's trust can act on their behalf. This is called proxy consent and means that a decision will have been made by the patient to allow their proxy to access their medical records and care plan ahead of treatment. Mental capacity principles must be strictly applied regarding proxy consent, to protect individual's rights.

In some religions it is more appropriate for a patient to be tended to by a professional of the same gender or have a chaperone in place. Leaflets that inform about the different testing a patient may experience can be translated ahead of any procedures. Family members acting as advocates and translators are to be actively encouraged and included to support a patient's understanding and experience.

Human rights

Everyone has rights under the Human Rights Act 1998, and this includes privacy and the right to refuse any observation measurements; this will be incorporated into an organisation's policies.

Safeguarding

Clinical tasks are commonly carried out as one-to-one contact and can involve uncovering skin that is not usually exposed. Rolling up a patient's sleeve to carry out blood pressure measurement could reveal a hidden injury such as a grab bruise, burn or self-harm cuts. Being vigilant and compassionate, especially in the case of a patient who is reluctant to uncover, is important and part of being aware of potential signs of abuse.

Some people may feel comfortable enough to open up and disclose experience of abuse or neglect during the time it takes to carry out observation measurements. If, for instance, you are taking measurements throughout your shifts over the period of a few days, you might be able to build a rapport with the patient. Safeguarding training and protocols act as guidance for the steps you should take in these situations, which must be reported even if the patient asks you to keep the information confidential.

Recording and reporting

All healthcare organisations will have a records management policy that maintains a consistency and standard when recording observation measurements and reporting escalation, for what and to whom.

K3.15 Why these practices are important

Following the relevant policies that apply to the taking of physiological measurements will achieve the results below:

▶ Your good practice will **comply with legislation** (see HCPO1, pages 6–8, for more information on legislation).

▶ Policies and procedures will demonstrate **respect for an individual's right to refuse care**.

▶ Following procedures **reduces the risk of infection** between practitioner and patient, which can lead to cross-contamination to other patients and staff.

▶ It is imperative that the **correct disposal of waste products** follows guidelines (for example disposing of a urine sample container that has been used to gather a urine sample), so there is **compliance with health and safety requirements**.

▶ You will be able to **maintain the patient's confidentiality** on all aspects of their care, including their acceptance or rejection of any healthcare measures. Policies around safeguarding disclosures take a different approach to this – see above.

▶ All organisations will have a records management policy in place and trained staff who fully understand the requirements in the workplace. This establishes a standard for **accurate/correct recording and reporting** procedures, so all practitioners are familiar with these and sources of data are reliable.

Health and safety

Before some physiological measurements are carried out that require patient contact, there are infection prevention mandatory measures that must be observed. It is a statutory requirement to comply with the Personal Protection Equipment Work Regulations 1992 (amended 2022), which include elements such as donning (putting on) and doffing (removing) gloves safely (Figure 3.12).

A records management policy is a document that outlines measures to implement concerning how records are created, written, stored and accessed, as well as when to destroy or archive records.

How to remove glove safely

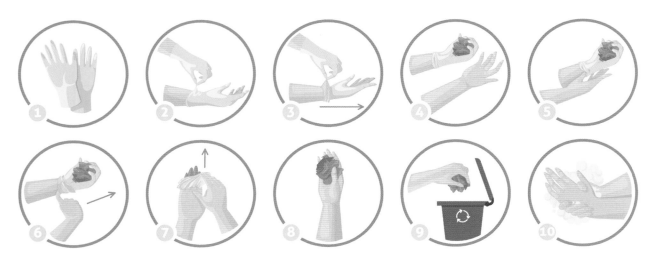

▲ Figure 3.12 An example of operational instructions for safe removal of PPE gloves

Assessment practice

> **S3.16 Use physiological measurement equipment correctly**
>
> **S3.17 Record the results of physiological monitoring and measurement using relevant documentation**
>
> **S3.18 Demonstrate the correct process for reporting measurements that fall outside normal levels**
>
> **S3.19 Calculate National Early Warning Scores (NEWS) 2 and escalate findings to a registered health professional where appropriate**
>
> **S3.20 Apply current policy and good practice techniques when undertaking physiological measurement**

Your task is to demonstrate the correct procedures for the list of physiological measurements below. You must apply all relevant health and safety as good practice. You will need either a partner to take the role of the patient, or a manikin.

During your demonstration, you must narrate what you are doing using the correct terminology and explain why you are taking each action.

As you complete each demonstration, carefully and correctly record all findings gathered from the observation tests on your NEWS2 chart and other relevant charts/forms. Narrate what you would do if early warning scores were over 5.

1 Take the respiration rate using a nurses' watch.
2 Take an oxygen saturation reading.
3 Use both manual cuff and stethoscope and digital sphygmomanometer to take blood pressure readings.
4 Take a pulse rate.
5 Assess the level of consciousness and signs of confusion.
6 Take a temperature reading using a tympanic membrane sensor thermometer.
7 Calculate a BMI and record this.
8 Take a peak flow reading and compare this to norms.
9 Verbally explain how urine output is monitored.
10 Verbally explain your action should any equipment appear worn or faulty.

It would be an enhanced learning experience if you have your demonstration recorded so you can evaluate your practical demonstration using Gibbs' reflective cycle to identify any areas for improvement.

Adult Nursing PO1: Assisting the adult nursing team with clinical skills

To ensure a safe clinical environment for patients and healthcare professionals, there is a foundation of legislation. In addition, there are values and principles as laid down by the NHS regarding the delivery of compassionate person-centred care, expected professional behaviours and an integrated service approach. In order to oversee the standard of care delivery, regulating bodies monitor and advise all registered healthcare services and seek to address shortfalls in care delivery.

Learning outcomes

The core knowledge outcomes that you must understand and learn:

K1.1 the importance of adhering to current legal policy and service frameworks when assisting with delegated clinical skills for adults

K1.2 the relevance of current guidelines, standards, policies and frameworks, set by government, regulatory bodies and delivery partners to ensure core values of care are adhered to when assisting the adult nursing team with clinical skills

K1.3 the range of clinical skills undertaken to promote and support wellbeing in relation to nutrition and hydration in adult nursing

K1.4 the range of clinical skills undertaken to promote and support wellbeing in relation to healthy bowel and bladder function in adult nursing

K1.5 the range of clinical skills undertaken to promote and support wellbeing in relation to mouth care in adult nursing

K1.6 the range of clinical skills undertaken to promote and support wellbeing in relation to mental health in adult nursing

K1.7 the range of clinical skills undertaken to promote and support wellbeing in relation to condition of skin, hair and nails in adult nursing

K1.8 how effective communication skills, including ensuring the most appropriate communication techniques are adopted, support all routine clinical skills when assisting the adult nursing team

K1.9 how the collection of specimens and undertaking individual observations in adult nursing supports a range of risk assessments and clinical assessments undertaken by registered professionals

K1.10 the fundamental principles of moving and handling individuals using evidence-based practice

K1.11 how to safely move and handle individuals using specific moving and handling aids

K1.12 the importance of adhering to agreed ways of working when using appropriate techniques to safely move and handle individuals relevant to their condition

K1.13 when monitoring, recording and supporting the overall care and wellbeing of individuals, the range of equipment and resources used, where to source and how to check them

K1.14 the procedures of how to check emergency equipment

K1.15 the different environments in which clinical skills in adult nursing are undertaken

K1.16 the range of checks to emergency equipment and why these checks are carried out.

Skills outcomes

The skills you will need to demonstrate:

S1.17 adhere to current legal policy and service frameworks when assisting health professionals with clinical skills for adults

S1.18 demonstrate the ability to carry out clinical skills for individuals including clinical assessments and reporting findings

S1.19 support risk assessments for adults and escalate where appropriate

S1.20 demonstrate safe practice when moving and/or positioning the individual for treatment or to complete clinical skills using appropriate moving and handling aids

S1.21 monitor and maintain the environment, equipment and resources when assisting with clinical skills for individuals

S1.22 demonstrate the ability to perform first line calibration on clinical equipment.

Guidelines, policy and service frameworks for adults

In any workplace there is legislation that must be maintained; this comes under the umbrella of the Health and Safety at Work etc. Act 1974. For instance, there are regulations to ensure particular tasks have guidelines that must be adhered to for the safety of staff and anyone who enters the workplace. In healthcare settings there are specific laws and regulations which must be adhered to when working with both adults and children.

The Nursing and Midwifery Council (NMC) is the regulatory body that nurses, nursing associates and midwives need to register with in order to practise. The NMC has a strict code of professional conduct, which provides clear guidance for professional standards of care delivery. There is a wide range of relevant policies, each important for shaping protocols in any clinical setting, such as an infection prevention and control policy. Professional competency frameworks are in place to provide guidance to nursing practice but also reflect the required core competencies of the nursing profession.

K1.1 The importance of adhering to current legal policy and service frameworks when assisting with delegated clinical skills for adults

Compliance is a legal requirement

Compliance refers to the way in which a healthcare setting's policies and procedures ensure adherence to applicable rules and laws. This includes legislation and requirements from the regulatory authorities such as the CQC and NMC. Particular departments have their local specific protocols to ensure compliance; for example, they may have standard infection control precautions (SICPs) training for all staff entering an isolation ward.

A **scope of role** means the range of activities, duties or responsibilities that you as an employee are reasonably expected to carry out or fulfil within the remit of your job or position. A **scope of practice** sets out the limits of an employee's responsibilities, and ensures that they do not undertake work outside their level of training or competence.

▶ Many Band 5 nurses (also referred to as Registered General Nurses) have extensive clinical responsibility, particularly in social care where they

may be in charge of care homes and residents on a daily basis.
▶ A Band 6 nurse is usually in charge of the day-to-day running of wards, or is part of a community nursing team.
▶ The Chief Nurse is usually VSO grade or Band 9 at the least. Matrons and Deputy Associate Chief Nurses and Advanced Paramedic Practitioners are Band 8.
▶ Band 9 can include roles such as directors and chief executives of trusts.

The carrying out and delegation of clinical skills tasks must comply with the law.

Policies in place to protect the individual and healthcare staff

Staffing levels should be at a safe level and staff restricted from working for 11 hours between 12-hour shifts. Employers must comply with the Working Time Regulations 1998, which mean they must not rota staff onto a 13-hour shift, and must provide a 48-hour rest period in a 14-day period of work, which includes overtime shifts.

The NMC Code of Conduct includes statements relating to individuals and healthcare professionals. For example, statement 22.2 states 'keep to our prescribed hours of practice', and 13.4 states 'take account of your own personal safety as well as the safety of people in your care'.

Regulation 13 of the Health and Social Care Act 2008 relates to safeguarding people who use healthcare services when suffering any form of abuse or improper treatment. The Safeguarding Vulnerable Groups Act 2006 requires the implementation of Disclosure and Barring Service (DBS) checks in England and Wales for all new staff and a DBS review for existing staff as part of protecting individuals who are being cared for. The DBS service is the same in Northern Ireland but is called AccessNI. The DBS service is the equivalent of the Protecting Vulnerable Groups (PVG) scheme in Scotland, which is managed by Disclosure Scotland.

Lack of compliance

Nurses who do not comply with legal policies and service frameworks can face consequences, as described in the sub-sections below. For example, statement 20.10 of the NMC Code states 'use all forms of spoken, written and digital communication (including social media and networking sites) responsibly, respecting the right to privacy of others at all times'. There have been a significant number of cases of disciplinary action taken for individuals who have acted inappropriately or not upheld the reputation of the nursing profession.

Source: NMC (2018), 'Read The Code online', www.nmc.org.uk/standards/code/read-the-code-online

Harm to individuals

Guidelines and regulations ensure safe practice. Shortcuts should never be taken, no matter what time pressures there are. For example, moving and handling regulations state that incorrect actions should be avoided. This includes using an under-arm lift, which could cause damage to a patient's shoulder.

Harm can be caused to service users through poor medications practice (most common) and lack of knowledge.

Malpractice investigations

Not adhering to the clear rules in place to ensure physical and emotional safety will give rise to malpractice investigations. These cost time and money, and include the discipline and dismissal of staff. Minor one-off clinical incidents, such as not providing timely pain relief in a treatment plan, are investigated following the duty of candour process, an apology made to the patient, and a review will take place to analyse the likelihood of a repeat incident. If an NMC investigation shows that learning has taken place the employee involved will be considered still fit to practise.

An example of a more serious incident would be a failure to report a disclosure made in conversations while carrying out a clinical task, for example if a nurse taking blood does not report a mother's stated concerns about sexual abuse at the hands of a paternal grandparent which means her daughter, who has learning disabilities, is a vulnerable individual at risk of serious harm. The repercussions of failing to report this disclosure are likely to be that the nurse involved would lose their job and be prevented from being in a job role in care in the future.

In November 2023, The Patient Safety Incident Response Framework (PSIRF) was launched in response to inconsistencies in patient safety responses. This was intended to facilitate learning and improve patient safety. The PSIRF is the NHS's approach to developing and maintaining effective systems and processes for dealing with and learning from patient safety incidents.

Closure of service

A department can be closed for a number of reasons, such as when the regulators find the care to be inadequate. There is a process to go through to give the service time to improve, but if it does not demonstrate improvement in the given time, it can be temporarily or permanently closed.

Departments/units and other services can close as a result of staff shortage, serious environmental concerns and infection prevention processes where an outbreak is active.

Loss of employment

The NMC/DBS/CI can prevent people found guilty of significant misconduct from working with vulnerable service users.

The NMC is the only organisation that can remove someone from the NMC register. The DBS/PVG/AccessNI can put people on a barred list, meaning that they cannot work with adults or children. This can happen for all sorts of reasons.

Prosecution

The NHS or a private healthcare organisation or individual staff can be prosecuted for alleged medical negligence and individual staff prosecuted. From 2020–21, the total cost of compensation claims payment was £2 billion. The Patient Safety Incident Report Framework (PSIRF) aims to make it easier for legal teams to collect data from claims and record any disciplinary action for individuals.

Criminal prosecution may affect the fitness of a nurse to practise. The NMC assesses the seriousness of any incident even if the conduct does not result in a caution or conviction. The NMC aims to uphold the reputation of nursing and take action in cases of neglect, exploitation, assault or direct harm to patients. Prosecutions in a nurse's private life where there is no risk of patient harm may not result in investigation by the NMC but can still be a barrier to new employment.

Research

S1.17 Adhere to current legal policy and service frameworks when assisting health professionals with clinical skills for adults

The NMC Code has four key principles:
1 Prioritise people
2 Practise effectively
3 Preserve safety
4 Promote professionalism and trust.

On its website (nmc.org.uk) it explains how to deliver these. Visit the website and read the statement at the start of each area. Develop a revision resource to reflect this information.

K1.2 The relevance of current guidelines, standards, policies and frameworks, set by government, regulatory bodies and delivery partners to ensure core values of care are adhered to when assisting the adult nursing team with clinical skills

Government, regulatory bodies and delivery partners

Nursing clinical skills are required to meet government, regulatory body and delivery partner standards, policies and frameworks. They aim to uphold a high standard of both physical health and emotional wellbeing, and provide a statutory free service in the National Health Service (NHS).

Most of the patients treated are or have been working and paying National Insurance. In 2022/23, for example, this accounted for 13.25 per cent of their wage. Individuals who are not employed, such as children, older people and those living with significant disabilities, benefit from a free service that enables them to access healthcare.

Private healthcare organisations are subject to the same guidelines. This means a minimum standard of care can be expected by individuals, delivered in suitable facilities staffed by qualified practitioners.

Each of the four countries in the UK has its own healthcare structure. Although these are similar there are distinct differences in terms of regulating bodies, core values and healthcare initiatives, as discussed in HCPO1. In 1990, devolution decentralised government power in the UK, meaning the NHS was no longer one large organisation but was separated into NHS England, NHS Scotland, NHS Wales and Health and Social Care in Northern Ireland.

Department of Health and Social Care (DHSC)

Each of the four nations has its own government ministerial departments:
▶ England and Wales have the Department of Health and Social Care (DHSC), which develops policies for health and adult social care, and oversees the NHS, providing funding from National Insurance taxes for free services.
▶ Scotland has the Scottish Government Health and Social Care Directorates, and the Northern Ireland Assembly has the Department of Health, Social Services and Public Safety, acting in the same role.

Each country then has its own standards and regulating body that monitors and inspects services to ensure a high standard is maintained.

Nursing and Midwifery Council (NMC)

The Nursing and Midwifery Council (NMC) is an independent organisation that regulates standards in the professions of nursing and midwifery. All nurses, nursing associates in England and all midwives must be qualified for registration, with revalidation required every three years.

All registrants adhere to the professional code of conduct: The Code. Where the practice of a nurse, midwife or nursing associate falls below the expected standards:
▶ The NMC may instigate a fitness to practise investigation, and the professional may be required to demonstrate that they have learned from the error or action.
▶ A fitness to practise panel will decide if the professional can continue working, can work with restrictions or should be removed from the register.
▶ The NMC may also suspend a professional during the process of investigation for more serious allegations or where there is a high risk to public safety.

Care Quality Commission (CQC)

In England, the Care Quality Commission (CQC) is independent from the English government and is tasked with regulating and monitoring standards in the statutory and private sectors, and providing guidelines. The CQC's five standards are: Safe, Effective, Caring, Responsive and Well-led. It inspects and grades services according to these standards, writing reports that are accessible to the public.

Healthcare Inspectorate Wales (HIW) monitors NHS services through inspections. It regulates independent healthcare providers using comparable standards to the other regulating bodies, developing policies, organisation guidance and regulations to highlight areas requiring improvement.

Scotland has separate regulating organisations. The Care Inspectorate (CI) regulates 14,000 individual care services in the same manner as the CQC, but leadership is regulated by a separate organisation called Healthcare Improvement.

In Northern Ireland, the Regulation and Quality Improvement Authority (RQIA) regulates services that provide health and social care, according to specific values and strategic goals.

Skills for Care (SfC)

Skills for Care is the strategic workforce development and planning body for adult social care in England. Its role is the effective delegation of healthcare standards, introducing initiatives to support the delivery of social care nursing, and offering guidance on the best practice, tools and resources required to support a high standard of care.

Nurses in social care are experts, with the clinical skills and understanding of patient needs necessary to deliver a high standard of person-centred support. Some examples of social care nurse roles are: learning disability nurse, dementia services, homeless health, and working in partnership with occupational therapy.

Nursing staff working in residential care will be working alongside social care staff who have completed the Care Certificate. The SfC produces workbooks for theoretical and applied competencies that need signing off by a qualified assessor.

Skills for Health (SfH)

Skills for Health is a UK-wide organisation that develops courses to support revalidation and competencies in nursing, providing qualifications to suit all needs and to meet clinical standards in an evolving service. For example, the government acts on research findings that highlight required changes in funding as an initiative is launched to address a need, such as inequality, gender differences in illness among homeless people or the health of patients in a particular city location. Skills for Health develops the additional training necessary to provide the competencies and clinical skills required for such new initiatives, evolving to address this need and ensuring they continue to meet a minimum standard of care. Revalidation requires a minimum of 35 hours of continued professional development and SfH works with the NMC competency requirements.

Guidelines, standards, policies and frameworks

A framework can support a national initiative such as the Public Health Outcome Framework or the 2022 National Framework for NHS Continuing Healthcare and NHS-funded Nursing Care. They incorporate policies to set out clear guidelines in different aspects of healthcare services. Guidelines, standards, policies and frameworks shape the care delivered by nursing, as described in Table 4.1.

▼ Table 4.1 The aims of guidelines, standards, policies and frameworks

Guidelines, standards, policies and frameworks	Purpose	Monitoring of standards	How does it protect people?
Care Act 2014	Safeguards and protects adults from risk of abuse or neglect in social care provision. Care should be personalised, patients offered choices and empowered, working in partnership for their own care.	CQC inspection of care settings has fundamental standards that ensure elements of the Care Act are successfully delivered. Service user complaints are investigated. The regulating body Social Work England monitors individual professional social care workers.	For example, service user care plans are standardised in terms of their content to ensure all aspects of health and social care needs are met, with no omissions. The social worker will be expected to retrain until they are deemed fit to practise or they will be unable to work in social care in the UK.
NHS constitution	The National Health Service Act 2006 and the Equality Act 2010 work to prevent and reduce inequalities in terms of access to healthcare provision. The NHS Constitution protects the rights of patients, the public and healthcare professionals when using NHS facilities. These are set out in constitutional core values and were established in law by Section 1 of the Health Act 2009.	CQC inspection of NHS care settings, such as hospitals. The NMC regulates all nurses, midwives and nursing associates (in England). The General Medical Council (GMC) regulates doctors. The HCPC regulates allied health professionals.	For example, the patient's rights to privacy, confidentiality and to have access to their patient history information. Completion of patient notes must be professional, with no omissions and with provision made for secure storage with password access.

Guidelines, standards, policies and frameworks	Purpose	Monitoring of standards	How does it protect people?
Nursing and Midwifery Council Code and Standards	Maintain a high standard of professional behaviour, which protects the physical and mental wellbeing of patients, nurses and supervisors.	Carries out investigation of reported incidents of malpractice and misconduct. Sanctions range from written disciplinary to striking off the register.	The nurse will be expected to retrain until they are deemed fit to practise or they will be unable to practise as a nurse again in the UK. The number of investigations for the misuse of social media is increasing.
Care Certificate	This is a statutory requirement and a qualification that care workers need to complete within their first 12 weeks of employment. The content ensures all laws and regulations are maintained and a high standard of care is delivered.	The CQC inspects and checks that all staff have completed the Care Certificate. If anyone does not have this evidenced, an inspection report will reflect this and a further 12 weeks allowed for this to be corrected.	To achieve the Care Certificate an element of assessment is carried out, such as observations, a written exam and evidence of theoretical teaching put into practice. Standard 10 relates to safeguarding adults, and care workers will know their responsibilities and role. Standard 14 relates to handling information, and care workers will maintain a service that upholds users' rights to privacy in accordance with the Data Protection Act 2018.
Mental Health Act 2007	This legislation protects the rights of patients who are taken to hospital and kept there for treatment against their wishes. Patients in this position have a right to a second opinion and to challenge the Court Order Sectioning.	The CQC has two roles in regulating the implementation of the Mental Health Act in healthcare work. It monitors all mental health services through care setting inspections and analyses the safe care of patients whose rights are restricted.	For example, the Mental Health Act states that medication can be given without consent when a person is sectioned or under NMC Code, statement 5.2: 'Make sure that people are informed about how and why information is used and shared by those who will be providing care.' This is all part of nursing competencies and clinical skills.

Test yourself

S1.17 Adhere to current legal policy and service frameworks when assisting health professionals with clinical skills for adults

1 The NHS England values have six statements that promote good practice in all statutory healthcare services. List the six statements and give one example of how you would demonstrate each value in a ward situation.

2 The NHS Scotland values have four statements that promote person-centred care. List the four statements and give one example of how you would demonstrate each value in a ward situation.

3 The Health and Social Care Trust (Northern Ireland) has four visions and values. List the four values and give one example of how you would demonstrate each in a ward situation.

4 NHS Wales has five core values in its Values and Standards of Behaviour Framework. List the five statements and give one example of how you would demonstrate each value in a ward situation.

The relevance of guidelines, standards, policies and frameworks when assisting the adult nursing team with clinical skills

The Core Skills Training Framework (CSTF) is a set of standards for statutory and mandatory training for healthcare professionals in the UK. Mandatory CPD includes awareness of the local health and safety policy and awareness of the Control of Substances Hazardous to Health (COSHH) regulations. Without this foundation knowledge, a trainee nurse, for example, could not abide by safety standards set and may cause unintentional harm through ignorance.

▶ This is important learning in your chosen occupational specialism as it ensures a consistent standard of safe and high-quality person-centred care is provided to all individuals. Entry-level trainees must have passed certain assessments in a theoretical setting before being allowed to continue their training in contact with patients. For example, moving and handling certification.

▶ The purpose of this is to **ensure all those providing healthcare**, such as healthcare support workers, physiotherapists and adult nurses, **are trained and competent**. Each organisational policy, for example a hospital's equality, inclusion and diversity policy, will maintain the law, in this case according to the Equality Act. This is also true of NMC Code, statement 1.3, 'avoid making assumptions and recognise diversity and individual choice'. The CQC fundamental standard 'Dignity and Respect' relates to recognising individuality. Abiding by guidelines, standards, policies and frameworks in the workplace means engaging in mandatory training in order to be competent to deliver legal, safe and good practice.

▶ **Failure to follow standards could result in a charge of negligence**, so it is essential that you work within your scope of practice as a trainee or registered nurse and report colleagues who are a concern. Serious misconduct by a nurse will often lead to their being struck off, deregistered and unable to practise again as a nurse in the UK. A guilty verdict in a court case will require the payment of a fine, often a substantial figure, and sometimes even a prison sentence.

Reflect

S1.17 Adhere to current legal policy and service frameworks when assisting health professionals with clinical skills for adults

A trainee nurse must comply with legislation, regulations and policies through good practice. They must work within their scope of role and their scope of practice. Theoretical classroom-based learning is essential, as are activities that give the opportunity to apply this knowledge in day-to-day working.

You have learned about health and safety, safeguarding legislation, the NMC Code and national standards – for example, NHS England standards (see this webpage for further details: www.gov.uk/service-manual/service-standard) – and you are aware of how regulations govern the clinical tasks and standards in nursing.

You have knowledge about professional behaviours, leadership and working as a team to deliver a safe minimum standard of care.

The Occupational Specialism assessments look specifically at this knowledge through your demonstration of these skills and your reflection on how you provided quality care.
▶ What is the significance of practising interpersonal skills for addressing an incident where your duty of candour is needed?
▶ What is the importance of reporting malpractice, misconduct, faulty equipment and facilities that fail to meet internal control safety standards?

Guidelines and policies in relation to performing basic life support (BLS)

There are different **options available for undertaking basic life support (BLS) training**.

Standard 12 of the Care Certificate covers knowledge about administering BLS training. Its guidance follows the DRABCD action plan: Danger, Response, Airways, Breathing, Call 999/Circulation, Defibrillation.

The Resuscitation Council UK has set guidelines for first aiders for different emergency situations:
▶ safe management of an incident, solo or co-ordinating in cases of multiple casualties, calling emergency services
▶ dealing with an unresponsive breathing casualty, including the recovery position

- dealing with an unresponsive non-breathing casualty, steps in cardiopulmonary resuscitation (CPR) and chain of survival
- dealing with a choking casualty, both mild and severe, back slaps and abdominal thrusts
- using an automated external defibrillator (AED) and how to locate the nearest unit.

To find your nearest AED, visit **www.defibfinder.uk**

BLS training is mandatory for registered nurses. The correct **sequence of steps** for adult basic life support is as follows:
1 Safety first
2 Check responsiveness
3 Check and open airway
4 Check breathing
5 Deliver breaths
6 Check circulation
7 Deliver chest compressions.

Additional items are available and may be included, such as a self-inflating bag:
- A bag valve mask (BVM), known as an Ambu bag, or generically as a manual resuscitator or self-inflating bag, is a hand-held device used in hospitals to provide positive pressure ventilation to patients who are not breathing or not breathing adequately.
- The air is forced into the patient in the same way as with BLS, avoiding lip contact for infection prevention.

Practice points

S1.17 Adhere to current legal policy and service frameworks when assisting health professionals with clinical skills for adults

You will need a CPR manikin to use in a CPR demonstration. Your task is to produce a training video where you narrate what you are doing and the purpose of each action.

The Resuscitation Council UK has a sequence of steps that serve as prompts, represented by an acronym for basic life support care. Start your video by explaining these.

It also has a seven-step guide to carrying out CPR. Use the manikin to demonstrate and narrate each step for an audience of Year 11s who are interested in studying T Level Health.

Evaluate your practical demonstration using Gibbs' reflective cycle to identify areas for improvement.

Routine clinical skills most relevant for adults

Clinical skills cover the broad range of competencies required in nursing to build a relationship and carry out tasks that manage, monitor and inform, to ensure the most suitable treatment and care plan meets an individual's holistic needs. These encompass skills that range from gathering a patient's history all the way through to care after death procedures.

Learning through theory and then observation is the beginning of your building such abilities; you will then carry out supervised tasks with guidance, and will eventually be safe to practise without supervision.

K1.3 The range of clinical skills undertaken to promote and support wellbeing in relation to nutrition and hydration in adult nursing

The NMC Code states that 'The fundamentals of care include … making sure that those receiving care have adequate access to nutrition and hydration, and making sure that you provide help to those who are not able to feed themselves or drink fluid unaided.'

Source: NMC (2018), 'Read The Code online', www.nmc.org.uk/standards/code/read-the-code-online

70 per cent of all patients admitted to hospital are malnourished in some way. There is a strong focus on nutrition and hygiene for healing, and in most health and social care organisations, mealtimes are protected.

Nurses and student nurses play an important role in the provision of diet and fluids. They work closely with dietitians to make sure appropriate dietary provisions are made.

Provision of food and drink appropriate to the individual's condition and preferences

The responsibility for nutritional care has not always been clear but its importance is, and **food and drink must be provided** that is **appropriate to the individual's condition and preferences**. Blood tests can detect nutritional deficiencies, and medical investigations into digestive dysfunctions, such as villi biopsies, can highlight problems with absorption.

Patient dietary planning is based on the following key principles:

► adequate
► balanced nutrients
► calorie energy control
► nutrient density
► moderation
► variety.

Dietary needs

Once a nutritional health need is identified, a diet plan will aim to provide for a particular need and in some cases dietary supplements will be prescribed.

The texture of foods needs to be considered for patients who are finding chopping food and/or chewing it a challenge. Foods are identified as 'soft diet' on hospital menus which patients may choose for a number of reasons. This could be:

► a patient with a mouth sore from wearing dentures.
► a patient with difficulty swallowing. The NHS adopted the International Dysphagia Diet Standardised Initiative (IDDSI) in April 2019 for patients with swallowing difficulties. The purpose was to consistently use terminology and definitions to describe texture modified foods and thickened drinks in different healthcare settings. The IDDSI framework consists of a continuum of eight levels (0–7) identified by labels, numbers and colour codes to assist with identifying food consistencies easily. The standardised descriptors ensure consistent production and testing of thickened drinks and texture modified foods for patients. The level of thickening will vary, as identified in a care plan, but trial and monitoring may be needed as abilities can fluctuate depending on factors such as fatigue or stress.
► **bariatric patients** recovering from gastric band surgery will require a liquid diet, and others who are fed via nasogastric tube will have formula feeds at regular intervals.

Hospital food provision can come as a shock for individuals whose usual calorie intake exceeds

> ### Key term
>
> **Bariatric patient:** an individual who has a BMI greater than 30 and is classified as obese.

3,000 calories and, for example, whose usual diet contains a large amount of processed and takeaway foods on a daily basis. On hospital menus, healthy options and high-energy foods are coded to distinguish between them, and patients are educated about meal options that would best serve their needs.

Personal preference is considered, with vegetarian and vegan options provided and a menu that changes daily. A vegetarian meal will not include meat or fish, and a vegan meal will not contain any animal products, including eggs, milk and honey. A patient may need reassurance that a meal meets their dietary requirements, so it is helpful if the person serving the food has knowledge of the main ingredients.

Inpatients place an order for next day, but new arrivals and day patient wards will have a small selection available at mealtimes.

Cultural/religious requirements

The UK National census figures from 2021 indicate 46.2 per cent of the population in England and Wales are Christian; 6.5 per cent identify as Muslim; 1.7 per cent as Hindu; 0.9 per cent as Sikh; 0.5 per cent as Jewish; and 0.5 per cent as Buddhist. The Equality Act 2010 prevents discrimination on the grounds of religion and to some extent cultural beliefs. The National Standards for Healthcare Food and Drink 2022 set standards that NHS services respond to, which ensure dietary needs are met for patients and staff.

The eight standards are:

► Organisations must have a designated board director responsible for food (nutrition and safety) and report on compliance with the Healthcare Food and Drink Standards at board level as a standing agenda item
► Organisations must have a Food and Drink Strategy which considers religions and cultures
► Organisations must ensure that they have access to appropriate catering dietetic advice and support
► Organisations must have a nominated food safety specialist to ensure Food Safety Act 1990 standards are maintained
► Organisations must invest in a high calibre workforce and improved staffing, and they must recognise the complex knowledge and skills required by chefs and food service teams in the provision of safe food and drink services. This knowledge must include the provision that meets religious and cultural needs.

▶ Organisations must be able to demonstrate that they have an established training matrix and a learning and development programme for all staff involved in healthcare food and drink services

▶ Organisations must put steps into place to monitor their food waste, manage any waste produced and take action to reduce the food waste produced in all areas: plate waste, production waste and unserved food

▶ Organisations must have suitable food and drink solutions for all staff over a 24/7 service period.

Respecting cultural food preferences will be in a care plan, but the finer details on specifics can be best obtained through talking with the patient and their relatives. For instance, a patient who is Jewish will require kosher beef, lamb, poultry, and fish served with fins and scales. Kosher food is prepared according to specific rules of the Jewish religion.

Dietary planning

Dietary planning is undertaken in collaboration with individuals, wherever possible, and professional colleagues, beginning with medical requirements. Dietitians are allied health professionals who use scientific information about nutrition and food and apply this into healthcare dietary advice. They communicate guidance in terms that are understood by an individual, delivering impartial advice about nutrition and health. Dietitians advise about food-related problems and treat disease and ill health, such as intolerance, irritable bowel syndrome (IBS) and diabetes. For example:

▶ A patient who has type 1 or 2 diabetes will require meals that are low in carbohydrates as these increase blood glucose levels; patients with a high BMI will need a reduced daily calorie intake.

▶ If a patient has had **colostomy** or **ileostomy** surgery they will have a stoma bag and while they are healing will need a liquid diet and thereafter adjustments for the individual, following trial and error, until the foods the individual needs to omit from their diet are identified.

▶ A texture modified diet is most commonly needed for patients who have experienced a stroke or have a progressive neurological disorder such as Parkinson's disease or motor neurone disease (MND).

▶ Elderly patients and those who are living with middle- or late-stage dementia may need a modified diet if their chewing force has deteriorated or they have swallowing difficulties (dysphagia).

Psychologically, a patient's outlook, motivation and resistance to change will form part of an assessment and a personalised plan to meet their holistic needs.

> ### Key terms
>
> **Colostomy surgery:** an operation to divert the end of the colon through an opening, usually in the mid- to lower abdomen, called a stoma.
>
> **Ileostomy surgery:** an operation to divert the end of the small intestine, the ilium, through an opening in the mid-abdomen.

Setting unrealistic targets for diet change is damaging; talking with the patient about what they believe they can manage has better outcomes. A gastroenterology surgeon who has patients with Crohn's disease, for example, or oncologists treating patients with bowel cancer, will have advice about a suitable diet to sustain recovery.

Appropriate equipment

The prevalence of malnutrition in UK hospitals reported over the last 15 years ranges from 13 to 40 per cent, with many patients seeing a further decline in their nutritional status during hospital admission. One of the causes identified is the ability to prepare food and eat independently. An older person who lives alone or has an informal carer, for example a loved one, may not be capable of consuming a balance of nutrients without support to eat. Healthcare assistants are generally responsible for monitoring a patient's capability to eat independently and reporting any concerns.

Eating aids (like those shown in Figure 4.1) allow independence when eating or drinking, so appropriate equipment must be provided to support individuals in these activities. Patients who request a hot drink will be served with a cup with a lid on if they are significantly at risk from spilling their drinks or they request a lid.

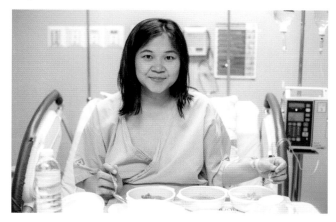

▲ Figure 4.1 Eating aids

In hospitals that are implementing a red tray initiative, patients who require support when feeding will have their food delivered on a red tray and their drinks in a red cup, for easy identification. Patients who have a red tray will:

▶ be given encouragement by nursing staff to eat at mealtimes
▶ be given help with eating if they need it
▶ be given plenty of time to eat
▶ be offered snacks throughout the day
▶ have what they eat recorded on a chart.

Similarly, patients with a red beaker or mug will be given encouragement and assistance, and offered a variety of hot and cold drinks throughout the day. Any food or drink intake will be recorded and monitored; food on average is made up of 20 per cent fluid.

Some items can be adapted to assist with eating and drinking (as shown in Figure 4.2). This might include:

▶ adaptations to the handles of cutlery, for example wide grip handles or a right-angled spoon/fork head for patients who have restricted hand and wrist movement or feel pain
▶ the use of a plate guard to ensure small foods are not pushed over the side of the plate; these are useful if a patient's peripheral vision is poor or they are using only one hand.

Appropriate equipment encourages independence and is empowering; however, providing hot drinks in a cup with a spout and handles is not always ideal as these may be associated with toddler cups.

A patient may need time to mentally adjust if their decline has been sudden, such as a stroke, but with rehabilitation and practice modified eating and drinking aids will perhaps no longer be needed.

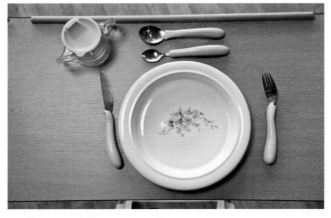

▲ Figure 4.2 Assistive aids

Adequate support

When giving support with eating and drinking you will use different levels and types of feeding technique.

▶ All patients must be in the upright position to avoid choking.
▶ Being seated, with their feet flat on the floor is preferable to the patient sitting in bed; the use of pillows to support their position is an adaption.
▶ Sitting at the same height as the patient you are assisting to eat will be more conducive to helping them to swallow; and you will need to be patient and give them only small amounts at a time.
▶ It may be appropriate to give a spoonful, say, and then carry out a different task while this is being eaten; this will reduce the pressure the patient might feel to eat with speed.
▶ For patients who may find it difficult to concentrate and are distracted it can be helpful to eat with the hospital dignity curtains pulled closed around them.
▶ A patient with a brain injury or a deterioration in cognition can be prompted to put food in their mouth, and may then need a prompt to chew this and swallow before the next mouthful.

Dignified care when dealing with any spillage and offering reassurance will make the mealtime experience positive and enjoyable.

Health and safety

When PEG tube feeding is not suitable, a 'feed at risk' approach is discussed with medical staff, the patient and their family, highlighting the potential consequences of this. For example, it may be the choice of a patient who is receiving end-of-life care to continue to eat and drink in the usual way, despite the risk of aspiration (food or liquid entering the airway).

In the Care Quality Commission's Adult inpatient survey 2022, around two-thirds of respondents who needed help from staff to eat their meals reported that they 'always' got this support (65 per cent), consistent with the 2021 results. However, this remains significantly lower than in 2020 where it was 69 per cent. Seventeen per cent of respondents said they 'never' received help to eat their meals, also consistent when compared to 2021.

Source: CQC (2022), 'Adult inpatient survey',
www.cqc.org.uk/publications/surveys/adult-inpatient-survey

According to the Malnutrition Task Force, an organisation established to raise awareness and offer guidance to help combat preventable under-nutrition and dehydration in later life, of the 11.6 million older people in the UK, more than 1 million are estimated to be malnourished or at risk of malnutrition. Clearly, then, the importance of routine clinical skills in relation to nutrition and hydration is underestimated.

Source: Malnutrition Task Force (2021), 'State of the Nation 2021: Older People and Malnutrition in the UK Today', www.malnutritiontaskforce.org.uk/sites/default/files/2021-10/State%20 of%20the%20Nation%202020%20F%20revise.pdf

Fluid balance is monitored and recorded

The patient's fluid intake and output may need to be recorded on a chart (like that in Figure 4.3) to prevent under- and over-hydration. This is especially the case for those who have a reduced ability to regulate their own fluid intake, such as: those who are Nil by Mouth before or following surgery; those who have a condition which causes them to lose their appetite; or people living with dementia who may have forgotten how or why to eat or drink.

An estimation of any fluids lost from vomiting is recorded, and the catheter bag measurement is added to the chart once it has been emptied. There should be an estimation of the volume of urine passed each time a patient visits the toilet: in adults this will vary from around 250 to 400 ml, about two cupfuls. Where a care and treatment plan requires accurate output measurements, urine is collected in a bedpan or through a catheter. To help with accuracy, the patient can be asked whether they feel they excreted a large or small amount of urine. Most people with normal bladder habits urinate every three to four hours.

Monitoring a patient who has chronic kidney disease (CKD) or cardiac failure requires close observation for signs of deterioration, which will show up in hydration levels. Information recorded over a 24-hour period will give a medical practitioner the information they need to start or adjust a treatment plan. If a patient develops oedema water retention there may be a need to restrict water intake, for example patients with heart failure.

A person living with dementia may no longer experience hunger or thirst and will need to be reminded to drink. Short-term memory problems may mean that, after each sip, they forget a drink has been delivered. In the end stages of dementia a patient may need to be prompted to put food in their mouth independently. A distraction can mean they do not chew the food so a second prompt may be required to encourage chewing. Without this intense support a patient may become malnourished or dehydrated.

Fluid balance chart

First name(s)	
Surname	

DOB			Date	
Patient weight	_____kg		24 hours from	
Record no.			To	

Intake (ml)		Enteral feeds	Output (ml)	
Time	Oral		Urine	Other
		NG/PEG/PEJ/NJ		

▲ Figure 4.3 A fluid balance chart

Food intake is monitored and recorded

A patient's food intake is monitored and recorded using a food diary or a nutrition care plan that documents their dietary needs, including information about allergies and intolerances, and assistance required. It records meals eaten, partly eaten or refused. It is particularly important to monitor the intake of food for patients who were found to be malnourished when admitted. Successful recovery in hospital and once discharged can be hampered by inadequate nutritional intake: muscle mass, for example, requires a good supply of protein, and bone repair a diet rich in calcium and vitamin D.

Individual's ability to swallow is monitored and assessed

A health condition that affects the nervous system, such as a brain injury or dementia, can impact on the co-ordination and muscle action used in swallowing. Mouth and throat cancers can also impact an individual's ability to swallow. A **barium swallow** investigates and identifies the extent of any damage, which will need close monitoring and assessment (Figure 4.4).

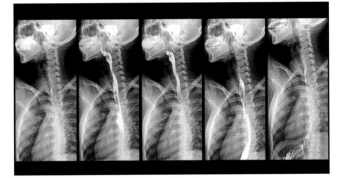

▲ Figure 4.4 An X-ray showing a barium swallow

Consider potential effects of medicines on eating and drinking

There are a number of considerations in relation to diet and fluids when administering medication.

> **Key terms**
>
> **Barium swallow:** a medical examination of the oesophagus and stomach. The patient drinks a liquid called barium while having an X-ray which records the position of the barium and identifies any blockages along the gastrointestinal (GI) tract.
>
> **Clostridium Difficile:** a bacterial infection of the colon, transmitted by poor hygiene when toileting, spread in faeces.

Certain foods can interact with medication and need to be avoided; for example warfarin is a blood thinner and the effect is more intense if grapefruit is consumed. A medicine may need to be taken in a specific time period before or after food. For example, medication for a thyroid condition needs to be taken 30 minutes before a meal, as food can block or slow down absorption. A patient who has been prescribed a medication that may harm the mucus lining of the stomach may be given lansoprazole to prevent stomach ulcers, which can form following damage caused by hydrochloric acid.

Prescribing professionals will consider all potential effects of medicines on eating and drinking in context. Monitoring stools using the Bristol stool chart or assessing levels of thirst will highlight the effect a drug can have on digestion or kidney efficiency. See K1.9 for more information on the Bristol stool chart.

K1.4 The range of clinical skills undertaken to promote and support wellbeing in relation to healthy bowel and bladder function in adult nursing

Dietary planning

Intervention may be required where the amount of food a patient consumes is not enough to provide the level of nutrition needed. Dietary supplements can be prescribed by a dietitian or other healthcare professional in the form of a drink or shake/nutritional bar. Medication can also be prescribed to soften or 'bulk up' a stool (faeces).

▶ A **diet plan** can be developed to address problems with managing faecal continence; eating more foods containing fibre and drinking more fluids improve constipation, and eating certain foods such as eggs can slow down bowel movement in diarrhoea. Foods with an acidic base, such as citrus fruits, pineapple and tomatoes, should be avoided for patients with an overactive bladder.

▶ In a postsurgical scenario, which limits a patient's movement for a period of time, attention is paid to protein in the diet. Protein supports healing, and following an extensive procedure muscle can atrophy (waste away) through lack of use, with protein needed to build muscle mass.

Collecting and analysing faecal samples

Faecal samples may be required for analysis – particularly if contamination or infection in the bowel such as **Clostridium Difficile** or norovirus is suspected. Stools are collected using a spatula and container system which is then tightly sealed and sent to the laboratory for analysis.

A microbiologist is the professional who will identify a specific form of infection after analysing a stool sample. Medication can then be prescribed if necessary and in some cases a further stool sample will be required in order to confirm that the infection is cleared.

It is important to prevent any sample from being contaminated with matter that is not related to the sample required.

Collecting and analysing urine samples

Urine samples are usually required when a urinary tract infection (UTI) is suspected. Urine can be collected in a urine pot at varying times of the day. For example, a standard urine test can be carried out at any time of day, whereas an early morning specimen will be required for glucose testing. The hormones secreted to waken an individual, including cortisol and growth hormone, act on the liver to boost the production of glucose to provide energy.

A GP may diagnose a UTI if protein and blood are detected in a routine dipstick test.

A urinalysis is a term given to a group of physical, chemical and **microscopical** tests on a sample of urine. If a UTI does not clear after advice and treatment, a urine culture analysis is more detailed and detects specific bacteria and yeast in a patient's urine so a more targeted treatment can be prescribed.

The test for gestational diabetes is a blood test, but an oral glucose tolerance test checks blood glucose levels after fasting then drinking a glucose solution, with a second test carried out two to three hours later which measures how a pregnant individual can process a large amount of sugar.

Key terms

Microscopical: using a microscope.

Digital rectal examination: an examination where a healthcare professional uses their finger (digit) to check for any problems inside a patient's bottom (rectum).

Endoscopy: a procedure where a tube camera, controlled by a doctor, is inserted in the anus for a lower bowel inspection. A tissue biopsy can be taken at the same time if necessary.

Colonoscopy: a procedure similar to an endoscopy, in which the flexible tube camera is used to inspect the colon and rectum.

Proctoscopy: an examination where a medical professional looks directly at the anal canal using a rigid inflexible proctoscope.

Rectal examination and administration of medicines

A **digital rectal examination** is usually carried out by a healthcare professional (doctor or nurse) as a routine prostate test in men aged 50-plus. The size of the prostate gland can be felt in males that are in the higher-risk age category for prostate cancer, using a gloved finger with lubricating gel applied. Patients who are experiencing bleeding from the bottom, bowel incontinence and long-term constipation will be referred to a consultant for further investigation.

Haemorrhoids are a common condition in people over the age of 50, or they may develop during pregnancy and childbirth. These are caused by pressure in the anus resulting in swollen veins which may become painful or will bleed when passing stools. Haemorrhoids can be treated with over-the-counter haemorrhoid cream or suppositories containing hydrocortisone. In more extreme cases a band is laced over the ballooning veins to cut off the blood supply to them so that the haemorrhoids drop off and clear.

Rectal medication is administered in the form of a suppository shaped for easy insertion, which melts at body temperature releasing medication that moves into the bloodstream as a result of diffusion through the wall of the bowel.

▶ Enemas can be self-administered, by means of a small bottle of fluid pushed into the anus using a small tube, which then stimulates the emptying of the rectum in cases of constipation or before an examination such as an **endoscopy** (Figure 4.5), **colonoscopy** or **protoscopy**. An enema can be given by a competent nurse if this is within their scope of practice.

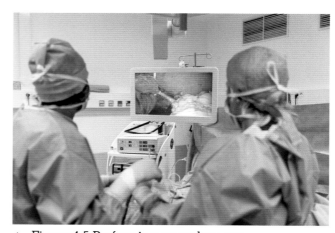
▲ Figure 4.5 Performing an endoscopy

▶ A suppository is given to a patient who vomits an oral medication or is being treated for constipation as it produces a gas, carbon dioxide, which stimulates the bowel, encouraging movement of faeces.

K1.5 The range of clinical skills undertaken to promote and support wellbeing in relation to mouth care in adult nursing

Mouth care is an essential aspect of personal hygiene clinical practice and impacts on a patient's emotional wellbeing, self-worth and dignity. Mouth Care Matters is a training initiative aimed at improving the oral health of inpatients.

Some patients will require more intensive oral care:
▶ Ventilated patients and those receiving oxygen therapy are at greater risk of experiencing dry mouth (xerostomia), causing discomfort and greater likelihood of developing oral health infections such as thrush.
▶ Patients living with dementia or who are experiencing delirium are unaware of personal hygiene, lose interest or resist intervention when confused.
▶ Adults living with a learning disability may need more support to understand the importance of, and co-operate with, good mouth care and oral hygiene generally.
▶ A terminally ill patient who is at end of life, an individual who has had a stroke or a frail older person perhaps lacks the ability to self-care.
▶ **Immunocompromised** patients are less resistant to oral infections, for example individuals with lupus are more prone to periodontal (gum) disease and jaw disorders.

Oral care assessment

On admission to a healthcare facility, an initial **oral care assessment is completed** using a mouth care assessment and patient record form.
▶ Using a pen torch, examination of lips, tongue, teeth and gums takes place, and checks on the palate and under the tongue are carried out.
▶ Dentures should be kept clean, and must be well-fitting and comfortable with a suitable storage container provided for patients while they are in hospital.

> ### Key term
>
> ***Immunocompromised***: it refers to individuals who have a weakened immune system, making them vulnerable to infections. The cause can be a medical condition, such as cancer, or immunosuppressive medication treatment, such as that for lupus.

▶ If any problems are identified during the examination, this should be recorded on the assessment form and a plan of care put in place with the patient's involvement. The recommended treatment must be documented and should also be included on the oral healthcare plan. In some circumstances, a dental specialist may be referred to and involved in the care if necessary.

Oral healthcare plan

An oral healthcare plan will be devised where additional support is needed to provide good mouth care. The equipment may include: a suitable toothbrush (which is usually a small head with soft bristles) and where applicable a sodium lauryl sulphate (SLS)-free toothpaste, as some patients have an allergic reaction to this ingredient.

A dry mouth care kit (such as that in Figure 4.6), which includes moisturiser gel, a soft cloth swab and an oral cavity cleanser, must be used regularly with patients who do not have enough saliva to lubricate their mouth and lips.

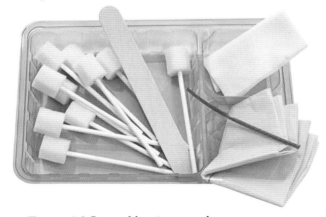

▲ Figure 4.6 An oral hygiene pack

Delivering daily mouth care

Daily mouth care is delivered based on a patient's needs and preferences. It does not have to be a health professional: visiting relatives may wish to carry out this care for the patient. As with all activities, a clear record of any actions taken must be made in the patient's records including the date, time and signature of the professional undertaking the role: see Figure 4.7 for an example.

K1.6 The range of clinical skills undertaken to promote and support wellbeing in relation to mental health in adult nursing

Promoting an individual's general health and wellbeing

A comprehensive care plan may include actions to **promote an individual's general health and wellbeing**, and this is especially important for those individuals who are admitted, treated and then discharged into the community mental health service.

In some cases, a patient will require a risk management plan, which will dictate the level of support required. A system of contact monitoring and easy communication channels is needed, checking on the suitability of medication and scheduling counselling appointments for outpatients.

Voluntary admissions and patients who are admitted under a court section will need to be monitored, for

---

{ **Mouth Care Matters**

NHS **Health Education England**

Mouth Care Assessment & Record

To be completed for every patient within **24 hours** of admission

Patient Name:	
D.O.B	
Hosp Number	
NHS Number	

1. Has the patient got:

Toothbrush	Y ☐	N ☐	Provided ☐
Toothpaste	Y ☐	N ☐	Provided ☐
Upper denture	Y ☐	N ☐	At home ☐
Lower denture	Y ☐	N ☐	At home ☐
Denture pot (named)	Y ☐	N ☐	At home ☐

2. Level of Support

Patient is fully dependent on others for mouth care	☐
Some assistance required e.g. unable to get to sink	☐
Patient is fully independent and can walk to sink	☐

Patients with **NO TEETH**, **NIL BY MOUTH** or **DYSPHAGIA** still require **REGULAR MOUTH CARE**

3. Does the patient have any pain or discomfort in the mouth? Y ☐ N ☐ Why? _____

Look in patient's mouth with a **LIGHT SOURCE**. Carry out **WEEKLY** assessment. Mark as **L, M** or **H** in the white box under today's date & sign.

	LOW RISK (L)	MEDIUM RISK (M)	HIGH RISK (H)*	Date	Date	Date
Lips	• Pink & moist	• Dry/cracked • Difficulty opening mouth	• Swollen • Ulcerated			
Action	None	Dry mouth care	Refer to DOCTOR			
Tongue	• Pink & moist	• Dry/fissured/shiny • Coated tongue • Secretions on tongue	• Looks abnormal • White coating • Very sore/ulcerated			
Action	None	Dry mouth care, brush tongue	Refer to DOCTOR			
Teeth/gums Advise the patient to visit dentist on d/c if problems with teeth not requiring urgent hospital treatment	• Clean • No broken/loose teeth	• Unclean • Broken teeth (no pain) • Bleeding/inflamed gums	• Severe pain • Facial swelling			
Action	2 x daily tooth-brushing	2 x daily tooth-brushing & clean the mouth	Refer to DOCTOR			
Cheeks/palate/under tongue An ulcer present for more than **2 weeks** must be referred to medics	• Clean • Saliva present • Looks healthy	• Mouth dry • Sticky secretions • Food debris • Ulcer <10 days	• Very dry/painful • Ulcer>10 days • Widespread ulceration • Looks abnormal			
Action	None	Clean the mouth/dry mouth care/ulcer care	Refer to DOCTOR			
Dentures Advise the patient to visit their dentist on discharge if the denture is loose	• Clean • Comfortable	• Unclean • Loose • Patient will not remove	• Lost • Broken and unable to wear			
Action	Clean daily	Denture cleaning, fixative, encourage daily removal to allow mouth to breathe	DATIX if lost or refer to dental team if broken			
For patients who are unable to communicate or cooperate with a mouth care assessment, signs of mouth related problems may include not eating/drinking, facial swelling & behavioural changes.			**Signature:**			

▲ Figure 4.7 An NHS mouth care assessment and recording form

example to observe them swallowing tablets during a medication round, and to check their appetite and any side effects of medication.

In general, physical exercise is to be encouraged as it releases endorphins, which can lift a mood. It is also useful if a patient keeps a diary that they can review with a psychiatric practitioner; this is useful and mindful practice. Everyone's mental health and illness journey is personal, which means that treatment needs to be tailored accordingly.

An individual's adherence to their mental healthcare plan

A patient's healthcare plan should be referred to, and its purpose reinforced if necessary, and they should be encouraged to ask questions.

Medication will initially be prescribed as a trial and a six-week period must pass before its suitability is reviewed, unless there are unmanageable side effects. Initial dosage is small, and this is increased weekly in some cases; patience is required and patients need to be reassured. For example, lamotrigine dosage starts as 25 mg orally and

side effects are monitored before increasing to a maximum dose of 400 mg.

Attendance and engagement with counselling sessions can identify a problem. If necessary, supportive measures such as changing to a new counsellor can help, as can a change of location to enable easier access.

Recognising key signs and symptoms of mental illness or distress

The diagram in Figure 4.8 shows the key signs and symptoms of mental illness.

A care plan can specifically include a requirement to monitor a patient for signs of an eating disorder, such as:

▶ an intense fear of weight gain
▶ concern with appearance or extreme mood changes, including uncontrollable 'highs' or feelings of euphoria, which can be an indication of bipolar or other mental illness.

Clear guidance will be included in a mental health care plan regarding the signs that need to be reported immediately, such as intensifying suicidal thoughts.

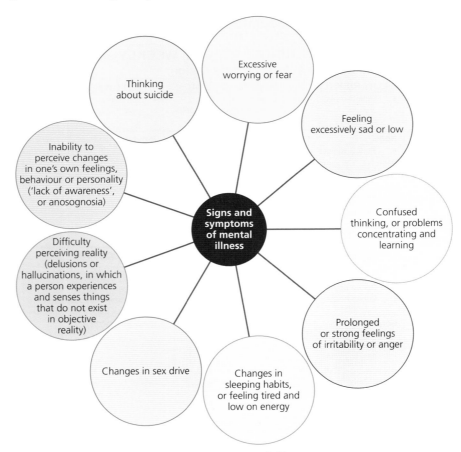

▲ Figure 4.8 Signs and symptoms of mental illness

Reporting safeguarding concerns

Clinical skills include **safeguarding patients** with high-risk behaviours, **escalating** concerns, **reporting** to the correct person and recording them for a review. For example, a patient with level 3 autism may have dangerous behaviours when distressed, such as banging their head on a wall. An informal carer can advise on any specific triggers and calming actions as part of risk assessment measures to minimise the likelihood of injury.

If a situation is not managed effectively there will be cause for immediate escalation by frontline nurses who witness any individual self-harm. For example, a relative or friend may be seen bringing alcohol to a patient at visiting times, and mixing alcohol with certain medications can have serious consequences.

K1.7 The range of clinical skills undertaken to promote and support wellbeing in relation to condition of skin, hair and nails in adult nursing

Skin integrity assessment

Skin integrity means skin health. A **skin integrity assessment** uses an assessment tool such as the Waterlow Scale and a **body mapping** form for initial and continuing monitoring, particularly with older patients and those with diabetes and limited movement, such as patients who are ventilated. Underweight patients may have less flesh over a pointy joint. Bony prominence will mean that they are at high risk of developing pressure damage. Rashes and dry skin/bruising is also something that will need to be monitored, as they may be indicators of a serious underlying condition such as sepsis or dehydration.

A frequent examination of skin-damaged areas and those that are vulnerable to damage can help prevent skin deterioration. Patients can have an impaired normal healing process condition for many reasons, such as frailty, diabetes and medical conditions which require steroids to be taken. Steroids can have a detrimental effect on the health of the skin. ANPO3 focuses on skin integrity and pressure injuries in more detail (see page 171).

Care plan devised to meet normal hygiene needs

It is good for the physical and mental health of the patient to be supported to maintain good levels of hygiene, such as having a shower or supported wash in bed. Consider the following points when working to a care plan:

▶ Independent washing should be encouraged wherever possible.

▶ Patients with full mobility and capacity can be encouraged to bathe without supervision and be instructed to use the emergency pull cord if there is a problem.

▶ Partial assistance may be required and/or the use of a shower stool for safety and comfort where a patient has limited mobility or lacks confidence to shower independently.

▶ Raising the arms above the head for some time while washing hair takes flexibility and strength.

▶ Pain around the spine area as a result of injury or arthritis may prevent the person bending down to undertake foot and nail care.

▶ The skin of older adults may be more frail as a result of medications that they take. It can become dry as a result of dehydration, and consideration should be given to the application of creams or moisturiser as directed for this.

▶ With age, skin loses its elasticity as collagen levels drop, and wrinkles appear. When assisting an older person to shave, take care to prevent small lacerations to the skin. It is important to identify the preference for shaving before embarking on a wet shave.

Some patients need support in cleaning areas of the body that are harder to reach, but as with all assistance, talking with the patient about what they would like help with is part of using a person-centred, empowering approach. Seeking a patient's consent and asking them to inform you when they are ready to start washing or drying an area is good practice. Observing the preferences of the individual and maintaining their dignity is essential as part of this care.

Maintenance through good nutrition and hydration

Nutrients, including vitamins, zinc and selenium, support the maintenance of healthy skin and hydration. A nutritional diet is the obvious source of these nutrients, so consider the existence of malnourishment in a patient and the dietary supplements they may need. Always refer to a dietitian where malnourishment is likely to have an impact on the healing process of skin.

In the first stage of healing the body has an inflammatory response, the purpose of which is to expel the initial cause of cell injury such as foreign body (splinter) or infection. Inflammation plays an important role in skin recovery, increasing the body's innate immune response. Too much inflammation, however, can lead to free radicals that cause damage. Zinc reduces inflammation, healing tissues and smoothing skin. It may be used as a dietary supplement for treating eczema and other skin conditions.

Applying dressings, ointments or simple wound dressings as prescribed/needed

Moderate skin damage will often require wound dressings to protect the surrounding skin structures while the wound heals.

The need for a simple wound dressing will be noted in the patient's care plan and applied as prescribed or needed. Attention needs to be paid to the type of dressing stated.

Referral to dermatologist or podiatrist if necessary

Toenail care

Cutting toenails involves skill, good strength and dexterity to safely cut and file nails. Although the growth rate of nails slows with age, they thicken, making nail care that bit more difficult. If a nurse is providing nail care, this offers the opportunity for an informal conversation about what the patient feels about their care, and allows the patient to be observed for signs of a deterioration in physical and mental wellbeing.

Nail coverings such as nail varnish, particularly if they are darker-coloured, significantly lower the oxygen saturation reading taken with a pulse oximeter clipped to the finger. One finger will need to have the covering removed to allow accurate readings; a clear explanation should be given to the patient so that they understand why this is necessary.

A podiatrist referral is needed in some cases of self-neglect and is not uncommon in older patients who find it difficult to look after their own feet.

Skin conditions

Skin rashes and moderate dry itchy skin can be painful and will need an assessment to ascertain the cause. A referral to a dermatologist (Figure 4.9) for expert advice and treatment will mean additional care plan responsibilities and monitoring.

Example of dermatology referral form

Referral date	
Referring physician	
Name of GP	
Address of practice	
Code of practice	
Telephone no.	
Patient details	
First name(s)	
Surname	
DOB	
Address	
Telephone no.	
NHS no.	
Reason for referral	
Affected body area	
Histology/Blood results (if available)	
Request for	Diagnosis ☐ Management ☐ Treatment ☐
Signature	

▲ Figure 4.9 Example of a dermatology referral form

▶ Psoriasis causes red, scaly skin; it is painful and will need creams or ointments and a discussion about any underlying cause, as it is associated with stress flare-ups.

▶ Atopic dermatitis is commonly known as eczema; it may also require bathing alongside daily treatment.

▶ A diagnosed skin condition will have named treatments, and monitoring these and the use of creams and ointments is an essential component of clinical practice.

K1.8 How effective communication skills, including ensuring the most appropriate communication techniques are adopted, support all routine clinical skills when assisting the adult nursing team

Effective communication skills are essential in healthcare. Research by Albert Mehrabian, who developed his Communication Model in the 1960s, broke down the types of communication as follows: 55 per cent visual/non-verbal, 38 per cent vocal and only 7 per cent verbal. Body language alone conveys a multitude of messages, and being self-aware and observing others are skills that contribute to the success of a patient–nurse interaction.

Source: Mehrabian, A. and Ferris, S.R. (1967), 'Inference of attitudes from nonverbal communication in two channels', *Journal of Consulting Psychology*, 31(3): 248–52.

doi: 10.1037/h0024648.

The formula for effective communication is to prevent or reduce barriers, focus, be aware of body language, appropriate delivery of verbal communication and check understanding so both parties fully understand at all times.

Some examples of communication barriers are:
▶ environmental factors, such as noise
▶ physical and sensory factors, such as deafness
▶ poor communication skills
▶ using jargon that is not easily understood, such as technical medical vocabulary.

Effective communication enhances the experience of the individual

There is a definite difference between a genuine smile and one that is forced: it's apparent in the eyes and tense/relaxed facial muscles – all signs that can be picked up by the receiver and can enhance or diminish the experience of the individual. Compassion can be shown in the smallest of gestures, such as:

▶ checking a patient who is on their own is feeling ok
▶ spending time with a patient to explain their condition to them
▶ offering a patient a drink as you are passing.

The value of compassion in the 6Cs of nursing supports a person-centred care approach and maintains the rights of service users, demonstrating respect and dignity.

Vulnerable people can feel threatened and behave out of character or act defensively, for example if a new diagnosis is unexpected. Observing these behaviours and addressing them can take just a few words and the time to listen. Anger can be diffused by taking a number of possible actions:

▶ acknowledge that the individual is angry and ask them if you can talk about why this is, perhaps arranging a later time to do this, if this is more appropriate

▶ avoid the term 'calm down', as this can inflame the situation

▶ sit down where possible

▶ lower your voice, use a soft tone and slow the pace slightly

▶ take care with body language, avoiding any sort of hand gestures

▶ make a judgement whether more or less eye contact is positive

▶ avoid being dismissive or judgemental as to whether they should feel anger in the situation

▶ slow the pace of conversation to aid understanding and clarify any misunderstandings; this could include paraphrasing or asking questions

▶ inform the person that you will be speaking to a manager about the issue to convey the importance of their feelings. It is important to record a significant outburst especially if the problem is unresolved.

If an interaction begins to give you cause for concern, such as disclosing a safeguarding issue, prompt a patient to expand on something they've said without asking them outright. Mirror what has been said at a slower pace, but lift your tone at the end as you would when asking a question. This avoids putting words in their mouth, which may be repeated in an abuse investigation, for example 'they made you feel dirty'. For example, a patient says a doctor makes them angry; repeat the sentence giving genuine eye contact and lifting your tone at the end; this cues the start of an expected response, encouraging the patient to continue and explain why the doctor makes them angry. It gives a moment to reflect, time to analyse what the doctor specifically does that they find annoying – is it frustration, misunderstanding, or is it the doctor's communication skills causing them to be upset?

117

Demonstrating empathy is an ongoing process. Basic empathy is the communication to another person of your understanding of their experience. It is useful to establish and develop relationships between nurse and patient. Listen and then, when the patient stops talking, allow a pause then follow with, 'You feel …', followed by the right category of emotion and the right intensity, then 'because …', followed by naming the experience and/or behaviours that give rise to those feelings. For example:

▶ 'You feel hurt because he left visiting until the last minute with no explanation and that is upsetting …'

▶ 'You feel annoyed with yourself because you didn't answer honestly …'

▶ 'You feel guilty because he put his pride aside and asked you directly for help and you didn't even answer him …'

The individual feels listened to

Acknowledgement and encouragement, being noticed and heard can be simply delivered as a visible action. Everyone wants to feel listened to, but this feeling is amplified when a person feels vulnerable, afraid or confused. If you take the time to listen when carrying out routine clinical tasks this will help you to gain an insight in to a patient's wellbeing and provide an opportunity to distract or reassure.

Active listening helps build a trusting relationship, which is essential for an enhanced patient experience. General rules for building a relationship using effective communication include:

▶ being honest – if you have not got the answer, say so and that you will find out; this builds up trust

▶ keeping a promise – if you say you will come back, then come back; if you say you will ask the doctor, ask the doctor.

You do not have to find a solution to fix everything. Some conversations are a way for a patient to work their way through an emotion, to understand why they felt or did something, and to find the solution themselves. There is no wrong or right feeling; if a person does not receive the message as you intended and becomes upset, take ownership of this and apologise for not being clear. For example:

▶ You bring an information leaflet to a patient to look at; they are offended as they feel the diagnosis is easy to understand.

▶ Apologise and say it is usual practice with all patients diagnosed with the illness and not personal, then collect the leaflet with a smile.

Active listening really means focusing on what and how something is said and acknowledging you have heard. This can mean gentle nodding or a single nod, good eye contact and saying 'yes' where appropriate or giving feedback to the patient. Asking permission to sit down next to the patient, so that your heads are at the same level, conveys equality; standing above them can suggest superiority or authority.

Gerald Egan, a communication theorist, developed the SOLER model for counselling, which is useful in a nursing context:

▶ Sit squarely, shoulder points in a rectangle so you are facing a person, sitting at the same height.

▶ Open posture, no folded arms or patient notes clipboard as a physical barrier.

▶ Lean forwards slightly, showing you are engaged in the interaction, with minimal movement.

▶ Eye contact at an appropriate level for the context; 70 per cent is average, more to show active listening and less at a time a patient is feeling threatened or getting undressed, for dignity.

▶ Relaxed, no tense muscles or conveying a state of alertness.

Source: Adapted from Egan, G. (2009), *The Skilled Helper*, Toronto: Nelson Education Ltd.

Body language actions to avoid include pointing, shrugging, slouching, looking at the ceiling, looking at your watch, eye-rolling and fidgeting.

The individual has a clear understanding of their treatment

Be clear and summarise key points in a complex conversation. For example, give an explanation for the need for three lots of tablets and then a summary: the blue and yellow capsules are to be taken after meals, the small white ones before you go to sleep and the pain relief tablets as required. If appropriate, you should name the medications and describe the expected outcome from taking the them along with a timescale on which improvements should occur. Be clear but also take steps to assess the patient's understanding (some points may need to be clarified). If a patient has a clear understanding of their treatment their stress levels will reduce.

A patient may want an explanation as to why they need to carry out physiotherapy exercises, have a change in diet or a referral to a second specialist due to a complex diagnosis. A patient's relative may want a more detailed explanation of a treatment plan, with the patient's permission. They may be more objective than the individual or vice versa.

Effective communication eases the individual's anxiety

Effective communication **eases an individual's anxiety** so they are confident and comfortable with treatments. In Egan's body language theory:

▶ a person who is nervous may display more finger movement, demonstrating a level of discomfort

▶ other signs of unease include rapid eye movement and speaking faster than appropriate.

A professional caring for an individual must show confidence through their body language, and what they say and how. Phrases such as 'I think', 'possibly' or 'I don't know' are not reassuring and can be replaced with, 'Some patients experience this and others do not' or 'I will double check with the nurse looking after you.'

The term 'emotional leakage' refers to a situation where verbal communication does not match non-verbal actions. For instance, a nurse tells a patient that they are important and says they have time to listen to them but looks at the clock on the wall and gives them no eye contact, showing that this is not a genuine message. Such mismatches are confusing and the patient can lose trust, their anxiety levels increase and they may stop asking questions, which would be a lost opportunity to allay their fears.

Effective communication enables the individual to continue to use the services provided

Once a patient has had a poor experience with one nurse there is a chance that a lasting memory will be formed and there will then be a mistrust of all nurses. A patient who is not included in decisions about their care, who has been ignored or not been treated with respect in terms of communication skills is less likely to attend a follow-up appointment.

Effective communication enables the individual's needs to be understood

Peplau's Interpersonal Relations Theory, as applied to the nurse–patient relationship, has different phases.

1 Orientation phase: The nurse introduces themselves as a professional, engages with the patient about the physiological measurements needed and the treatment. The patient is able to ask questions and get clear explanations, which they can talk over. A first impression of the nurse builds a rapport and the start of a trusting relationship.

2 Working phase, which has two subphases:
   ▶ Identification phase: The patient and nurse work together, in partnership, each with a role. These interactions more often than not are informal while the patient is monitored and treated. The interactions provide the basis for understanding, trust and acceptance, and enable the patient to be an active participant in their treatment.
   ▶ Exploitation phase: The patient is open to all that's on offer and takes advantage of all services, exploiting the patient–nurse relationship to address their needs and move towards recovery goals.

3 Resolution phase: A successful working relationship is achieved, with effective communication; the patient's needs are met and they move forwards for full independence. The patient no longer needs the care and is discharged, so the relationship ends.

Source: Hagerty, T.A., Samuels, W., Norcini-Pala, A. and Gigliotti, E. (2017), 'Peplau's Theory of Interpersonal Relations: An Alternate Factor Structure for Patient Experience Data?', *Nursing Science Quarterly*, 30(2):160-167. **doi: 10.1177/0894318417693286.**

The lasting effect of a patient's positive relationship with a nurse is that it will make things easier if there is a need for a nurse–patient relationship again. The trust will come quicker and, with reduced stress levels, recovery will be smoother.

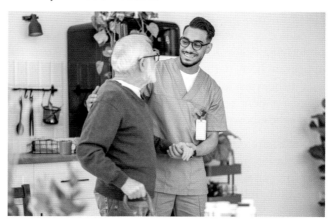

▲ Figure 4.10 Clear communication between nurse and patient helps understanding

Effective communication prevents the potential harm of a misunderstanding

Clear and effective communication (Figure 4.10) will prevent potential harm from misunderstandings, such as correct dosage of a medication prescribed on discharge. TTO is the acronym for medication to take out as a prescription on discharge, and the patient is responsible for taking this correctly and safely. Having a patient tell you when they should take medication and what the dose is confirms to you that they have understood and reassures them that they are right.

Trust and an approachable demeanour may convey safety for a patient who is experiencing cultural abuse. For instance, although female genital mutilation (FGM) is banned in the UK, it is known to take place, and hoodoo practices for removing bad spirits can present a safeguarding danger. In a hospital context, a patient disclosing to a person outside their culture can prevent further harm or protect others.

K1.9 How the collection of specimens and undertaking individual observations in adult nursing supports a range of risk assessments and clinical assessments undertaken by registered professionals

Braden Scale

Skin integrity assessment

Skin integrity assessment measures the likelihood of an individual developing a pressure injury. The **Braden Scale** is used to assess pressure injury risk during an assessment of skin condition (pressure ulcers are also known as pressure injuries). A pressure injury is damage that causes the skin to break down when the underlying tissue is damaged. Pressure injuries usually appear on bony parts of the body or where body weight is at its heaviest (and pressure is therefore the greatest) when a patient is lying or sitting down, for instance on the heels, elbows, sacral area and hips.

The pressure on the skin causes an element of vasodilation in surface capillaries so that blood flow to the skin surface and tissue is impaired (see ANPO3, page 180), cells die and skin breaks down as a result.

The Braden Scale was developed by Dr Barbara Braden and Dr Nancy Bergstrom in 1988 as a standardised evidence-based risk assessment tool to prevent injury and stop further deterioration following hospital admission. In 2021, Dr Amy Hester took their work even further by developing the Braden II Scale. The scale provides a means to record skin integrity and the risk of damage as part of skin monitoring recommendations in the care plan. The National Institute for Health and Care Excellence (NICE) recommends this tool as offering a uniform risk assessment and considers it to be valid and reliable.

The scale is made up of six subscales, with each score giving a measure of risk, for example in terms of sensory perception or mobility level, with a rating of 1 indicating no problem and 5 requiring immediate action. ANPO3 further details this aspect of care.

The six subscale categories are:
1. Sensory perception – can the person feel touch; the level of nerve stimuli impairment.
2. Moisture level – sweat or urine, for example skin that has a constantly moist surface breaks down.
3. Out of bed activity – exercise improves blood flow and muscle mass and reduces pressure time on vulnerable points.
4. In bed mobility – can adjust body position independently or requires assistance for comfort.
5. Nutrition – eats regular nutritious meals or rarely eats; use or non-use of dietary supplements.
6. Friction and shear – friction is repetitive damaging movement at location; shear involves gravity and weight.

For further details see Table 6.2 in ANPO3 (page 182).

Supports the observation of skin moisture levels and response to mild pressure being applied

In nursing clinical practice, use of the Braden Scale to assess skin integrity is supported by the observation of skin moisture levels and response to mild pressure being applied. Using the Braden Scale, interventions are detailed for all concerns. The levels of concern are recorded as:
▶ Very high risk: total score 9 or less
▶ High risk: total score 10–12
▶ Moderate risk: total score 13–14
▶ Mild risk: total score 15–18
▶ No risk: total score 19–23

Bristol stool chart

Assessing health in relation to stool type

The Bristol stool chart (Figure 4.11) was developed as a chart by Ken Heaton in 1977 to classify faeces into seven numbered and descriptive stool groups. The chart provides a standardised framework for stool monitoring. Type 1 is a very hard stool, and where appropriate the patient may require a laxative medication to relieve any symptoms. Type 7 is a very loose and watery stool, which may cause leakage at times. This can be caused by infection or other conditions relating to absorption of fluid in the bowel.

BRISTOL STOOL FORM SCALE

Type	Description	Image
TYPE 1	Separate hard lumps, like nuts	
TYPE 2	Lumpy and sausage-like	
TYPE 3	Sausage share with cracks	
TYPE 4	Like a smooth soft sausage or snake	
TYPE 5	Soft blobs with clear-cut edges	
TYPE 6	Mushy consistency with ragged edges	
TYPE 7	Liquid consistency with no solid pieces	

▲ Figure 4.11 NHS Bristol stool chart

Collecting faecal samples

A competent patient can self-assess and report back the level and type of stool they are experiencing. A qualified health professional may collect a stool sample if further investigations or treatment are required to manage symptoms.

Malnutrition Screening Tool (MST)

Using a MST to assess individuals experiencing malnutrition

A nutritional risk assessment tool commonly used in the healthcare setting is the **Malnutrition Screening Tool (MST)**, which can be used to make an **assessment of individuals who are malnourished** or at **risk of malnourishment** when they are admitted to the healthcare setting. **A body mass index (BMI) is calculated** as part of this assessment, and this gives an indication as to whether or not the patient is at the correct weight range (Figure 4.12a).

There are five steps to the MST:
1. Measure height and weight, calculate BMI score; if it is not possible to access these measurements, assess via observation to gain a clinical impression, for example very thin – underweight, very overweight – obese.
2. Note percentage unplanned weight loss, in the past three to six months, and score using the assessment table (Figure 4.12b).

Key term

National Patient Safety Agency: body responsible for identifying and reducing risks to patients receiving NHS care. The organisation leads national initiatives to improve patient safety.

3. Establish acute disease effect; no nutritional intake for five days or more scores highest.
4. Add together scores from steps 1, 2 and 3 to obtain overall risk of malnutrition.
5. Use referral guidelines and/or local policy to implement in an individual's care plan.

Adequate food and nutrition is an essential component of good healthcare and has been a focus of the regulators and the **National Patient Safety Agency** agenda since 2006.

Supporting the MST with height and weight measurements to calculate BMI

There are a number of methods to measure a BMI which use the height and weight measurement of an individual. Where it is not possible to measure the height and weight, the BMI can be estimated using the length of ulna measurement and mid upper arm circumference. However, because of the variation in weight distribution within an individual, this method is known to be an inaccurate method of assessment overall.

As part of a malnutrition risk assessment, a score of 0–1 indicates a low risk of malnutrition, 2 indicates a moderate risk of malnutrition and 3–5 indicates a high risk of malnutrition.

Waterlow Score

Assessing the risk of pressure injuries

The Waterlow Score (or Waterlow Scale) is a calculation of a patient's assessed risk of the development of a pressure injury.

As with the Braden Scale score, it is based on a number of calculations depending on current health of the individual and the existence of pre-existing skin damage. Age, medication, continence and mobility are also factors. The Waterlow score is measured at regular intervals depending on the risk to the individual. A score lower than 10 is minimal risk of damage occurring; 10–14 indicates 'At risk'; a score of 15–19 indicates 'High risk' and a score of 20 or above indicates 'Very high risk'.

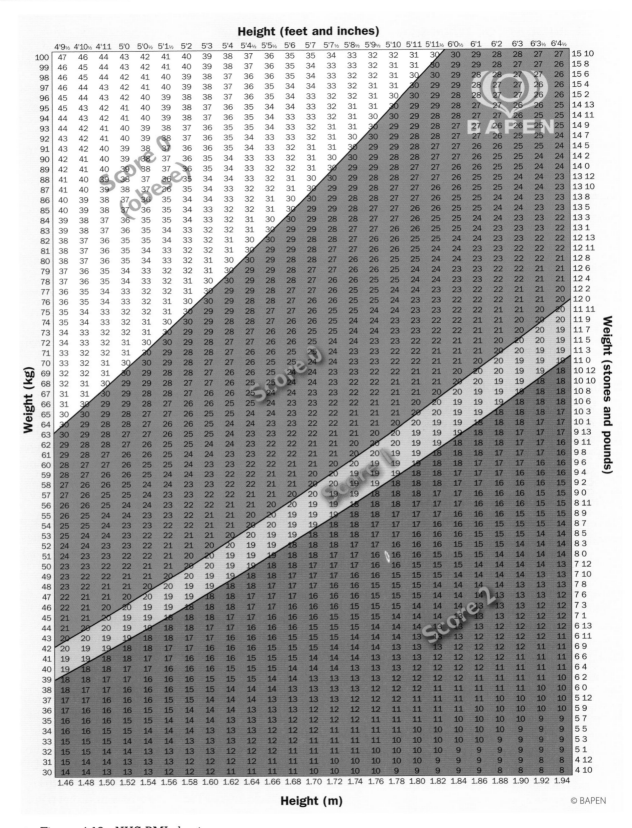

▲ Figure 4.12a NHS BMI chart

	Score 0 Wt loss < 5%	Score 1 Wt loss 5 - 10%	Score 2 Wt loss > 10%
	Weight loss in last 3 to 6 months		
kg	Less than (kg)	Between (kg)	More than (kg)
30	1.6	1.6 - 3.3	3.3
31	1.6	1.6 - 3.4	3.4
32	1.7	1.7 - 3.6	3.6
33	1.7	1.7 - 3.7	3.7
34	1.8	1.8 - 3.8	3.8
35	1.8	1.8 - 3.9	3.9
36	1.9	1.9 - 4.0	4.0
37	1.9	1.9 - 4.1	4.1
38	2.0	2.0 - 4.2	4.2
39	2.1	2.1 - 4.3	4.3
40	2.1	2.1 - 4.4	4.4
41	2.2	2.2 - 4.6	4.6
42	2.2	2.2 - 4.7	4.7
43	2.3	2.3 - 4.8	4.8
44	2.3	2.3 - 4.9	4.9
45	2.4	2.4 - 5.0	5.0
46	2.4	2.4 - 5.1	5.1
47	2.5	2.5 - 5.2	5.2
48	2.5	2.5 - 5.3	5.3
49	2.6	2.6 - 5.4	5.4
50	2.6	2.6 - 5.6	5.6
51	2.7	2.7 - 5.7	5.7
52	2.7	2.7 - 5.8	5.8
53	2.8	2.8 - 5.9	5.9
54	2.8	2.8 - 6.0	6.0
55	2.9	2.9 - 6.1	6.1
56	2.9	2.9 - 6.2	6.2
57	3.0	3.0 - 6.3	6.3
58	3.1	3.1 - 6.4	6.4
59	3.1	3.1 - 6.6	6.6
60	3.2	3.2 - 6.7	6.7
61	3.2	3.2 - 6.8	6.8
62	3.3	3.3 - 6.9	6.9
63	3.3	3.3 - 7.0	7.0
64	3.4	3.4 - 7.1	7.1

	Score 0 Wt loss < 5%	Score 1 Wt loss 5 - 10%	Score 2 Wt loss > 10%
	Weight loss in last 3 to 6 months		
kg	Less than (kg)	Between (kg)	More than (kg)
65	3.4	3.4 - 7.2	7.2
66	3.5	3.5 - 7.3	7.3
67	3.5	3.5 - 7.4	7.4
68	3.6	3.6 - 7.6	7.6
69	3.6	3.6 - 7.7	7.7
70	3.7	3.7 - 7.8	7.8
71	3.7	3.7 - 7.9	7.9
72	3.8	3.8 - 8.0	8.0
73	3.8	3.8 - 8.1	8.1
74	3.9	3.9 - 8.2	8.2
75	3.9	3.9 - 8.3	8.3
76	4.0	4.0 - 8.4	8.4
77	4.1	4.1 - 8.6	8.6
78	4.1	4.1 - 8.6	8.7
79	4.2	4.2 - 8.7	8.8
80	4.2	4.2 - 8.9	8.9
81	4.3	4.3 - 9.0	9.0
82	4.3	4.3 - 9.1	9.1
83	4.4	4.4 - 9.2	9.2
84	4.4	4.4 - 9.3	9.3
85	4.5	4.5 - 9.4	9.4
86	4.5	4.5 - 9.6	9.6
87	4.6	4.6 - 9.7	9.7
88	4.6	4.6 - 9.8	9.8
89	4.7	4.7 - 9.9	9.9
90	4.7	4.7 - 10.0	10.0
91	4.8	4.8 - 10.1	10.1
92	4.8	4.8 - 10.2	10.2
93	4.9	4.9 - 10.3	10.3
94	4.9	4.9 - 10.4	10.4
95	5.0	5.0 - 10.6	10.6
96	5.1	5.1 - 10.7	10.7
97	5.1	5.1 - 10.8	10.8
98	5.2	5.2 - 10.9	10.9
99	5.2	5.2 - 11.0	11.0

Current weight

© BAPEN

▲ Figure 4.12b NHS Malnutrition Universal Screening Tool (MUST) weight loss score table

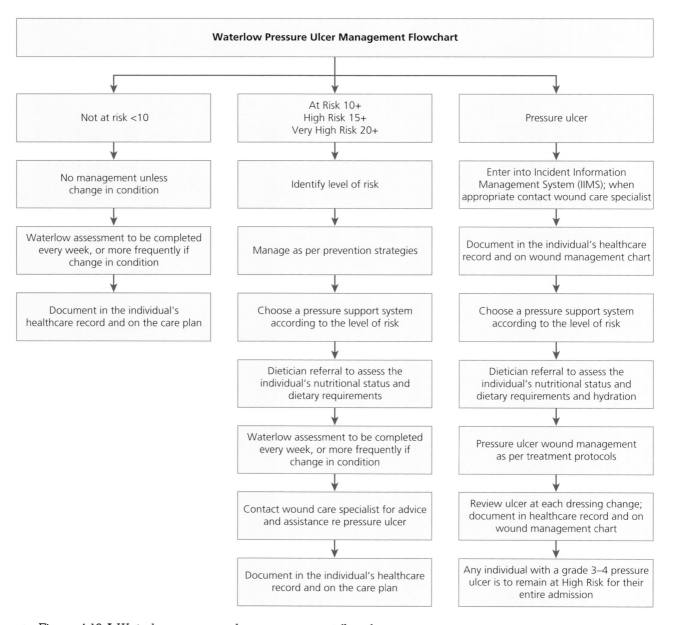

▲ Figure 4.13 A Waterlow pressure ulcer management flowchart

Supporting by observation of the skin, monitoring mobility and continence levels

Depending on the individual, the frequency of a Waterlow assessment is recorded in the care plan, for example four-hourly, daily, weekly or once every three months. This prompt ensures that changes are identified quickly and actions taken to reduce the risk of damage.

Oral health assessment

See section K1.5 for details of oral health assessment. This is an assessment to check whether an individual has oral health problems and needs to be referred for dental treatment. This risk assessment and monitoring tool is supported by observation of how an individual manages their daily mouth care routine.

Wound care

Assessing the state of a wound to prescribe appropriate treatment

Assessing the state of a wound is vital in order to prescribe the appropriate treatment. The stage a wound is at influences the treatment and care intervention response.

Haemostasis

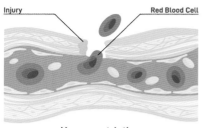
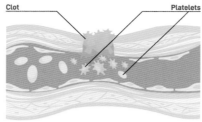
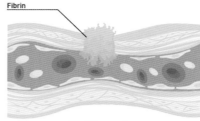

Vasoconstriction   Primary Haemostasis   Clot Formation

▲ Figure 4.14 Stages of wound healing

There are four important phases in the process of wound healing.

1 Haemostasis phase: starts at the onset of the injury, for example a deep cut, when the body initiates its emergency repair system starting with the blood's clotting process. The location, depth and size of the wound affect which blood vessels are damaged and the hole that needs to be plugged. Platelets, collagen and an enzyme called thrombin initiate the formation of a fibrin mesh, the clot. This will begin the tissue repair process. The injured vessel such as a vein will constrict to prevent any further blood loss. Blood loss which collects under the skin is known as a haematoma – or bruise. A patient's overall health, such as nutrition level, blood thinning medication and medical condition (for example haemophilia), can slow down the initial response, causing a greater amount of blood to be lost.

2 Inflammatory phase: this starts the defence mechanism to expel debris and destroy bacteria. Neutrophil cells peak between 24 and 48 hours after the injury occurs but are not always able to clear the site of pathogens. Macrophage cells are increased at the cut and secrete proteins to increase the immune reaction and facilitate skin and tissue repair. The characteristics of this phase are oedema, fluid swelling, erythema (visible redness), pain and generation of heat.

3 Proliferative phase: contraction of the wound's skin and tissue edges begin to come together following the formation of a scab, which protects the surface and prevents contamination. New blood cells are made to replace those lost, granulation tissue fills the wound bed from the bottom up; this prevents the formation of an abscess. Factors such as depth and location of the wound will have an impact on the length of time it takes to fully heal.

4 Remodelling (maturation) phase: new tissue progressively gains strength and flexibility, although scarred skin is thicker and less flexible. The skin's strength following repair may be limited and may not return to the pre-injury level.

Figure 4.15 shows the risk factors that influence the rate of the healing process.

Wound care and skin integrity

Wound care and assessment is commonly used in conjunction with a Braden Scale assessment for skin integrity (see page 120).

Continence

Assessing the causes of, and factors contributing to, urinary and faecal symptoms

There are many different causes of urinary and faecal symptoms. For example:

▶ Stress incontinence is where urine is leaked when the bladder is under pressure and the sphincters associated with this organ are unable to cope with controlling the passage of urine. Leaks may occur as a result of getting up from being seated, coughing or laughing suddenly.

▶ Pregnancy and a vaginal birth can cause permanent or temporary damage to the pelvic floor and bladder muscles.

▶ Obesity can cause excess weight in the abdominal area causing pressure on the bladder and pelvic floor muscles.

▶ Urge incontinence can be both a psychological and physical condition – a person is unable to get to the toilet in time as a result of mobility or proximity to the toilet facilities.

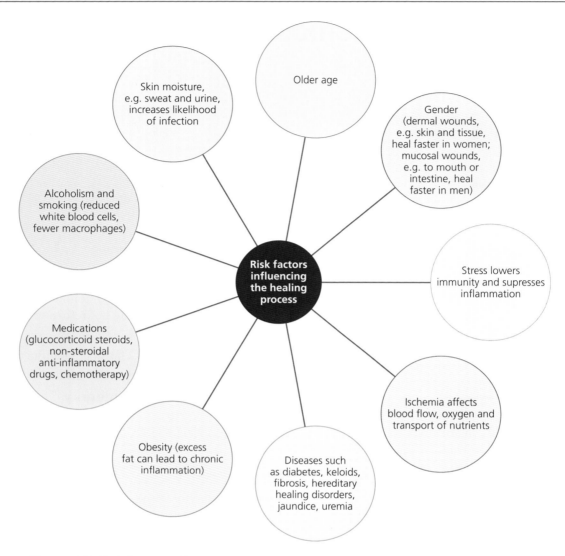

▲ Figure 4.15 Risk factors influencing the healing process

▶ Overflow incontinence happens as a result of being unable to control the emptying of the bladder, leading to an over-full bladder.

▶ Severe and chronic long-term constipation or diarrhoea contributes to faecal incontinence. Nerve damage to the area as a result of injury or surgery can be a causative factor.

▶ Certain health conditions, such as in a patient with irritable bowel syndrome (IBS), will lead to bouts of severe diarrhoea. Infections such as norovirus can cause profuse diarrhoea, which is frequently uncontrollable.

You would begin your assessment with a series of patient questions such as type of episode, which organ is affected (such as bladder or bowel), whether there is any pain associated with the episode and the duration of the flare-up.

Next comes a physical examination with regard to muscle action and control affecting faecal/urine retention and recording information such as the health and history of the individual.

The nursing role in maintaining personal hygiene for incontinence will include a skin assessment, as skin contact with urine can cause damage to the upper layers causing pain and excoriation. UTIs can be a causative factor for continence issues and should be ruled out before other treatments are considered.

Appropriate dietary planning can improve continence status

HCPO1 includes a detailed account of care plan responsibilities to reduce risks. See section K1.4 in this chapter for guidelines on dietary planning to manage incontinence.

Fluid balance

Assessing and interpreting fluid and electrolyte balance

Salts and minerals, such as sodium, potassium, chloride and bicarbonate, are important electrolytes which assist in maintaining a number of important body functions. Sodium and potassium are responsible for the generation of electrical impulses in the heart, and sodium also acts on the kidneys to regulate how much water is in the body. Blood tests are used to analyse levels of these essential elements in order to support a diagnosis and influence any diagnostic or treatment decisions.

Certain medications can cause an imbalance, such as the diuretics (water tablets) used as a common treatment for hypertension or heart failure. Electrolyte deficits can be addressed by using supplements such as zinc or potassium, usually in tablet form. In some cases electrolytes may need to be replaced through the introduction of intravenous fluids.

Supporting fluid balance with fluid intake and output monitoring

Dehydration is covered in HCPO1 K1.11, as is the importance of monitoring **fluid balance**.

Providing patients with opportunities to hydrate can aid the healing process and reduce the risk of a wide range of problems, for example UTIs, high blood pressure and, in more serious cases, kidney damage. Fluid balance monitoring is an essential role for the healthcare professional to prevent patients from becoming dehydrated or requiring additional fluids via an intravenous infusion. It is an important part of the practitioner's role to make sure fluid balance is documented accurately, including the input and output balance.

Nutrition assessment

Assessment to identify individuals who are at nutritional risk

Malnutrition hampers the body's healing process, reduces muscle mass, causing weakness, and adversely affects normal body function. Lack of individual nutrients causes specific health concerns.

Supporting assessment with food charts and physiological measurements

The clinical nursing skill of monitoring incorporates detailed recording of physiological measurements on a food chart and care plan; for example BMI assessment helps patients to be aware of their own intake and encourages them to be active in their own care. Recording information following daily consumption gives an opportunity for

you to have an informal conversation with a patient, highlighting any shortfalls, offering encouragement and involving the patient in their own care.

A patient may benefit from the introduction of the NHS Eatwell Guide (see ANPO2, pages 145–146) to inform them and prompt further interactions, including with regard to risk factors such as a BMI score that indicates an individual is underweight or obese. Referral to a dietitian may be relevant where more complex concerns exist, such as controlling diabetic intake or where other specialist diets may be required.

Pain assessment

Assessing pain levels to diagnose and determine suitable treatment

Patients with a health condition causing uncontrolled pain will benefit from a pain assessment and continual monitoring of levels to evaluate their responses to pain relief and inform approaches to their care.

Supporting pain assessment with a range of pain assessment tools

Pain assessment is different depending on the level of consciousness (NEWS2 records levels of consciousness).

Each pain assessment tool has a different purpose:

▶ The Abbey Pain Scale (Figure 4.16) is used with patients living with dementia, a cognitive disability or where a communication barrier exists.
▶ Numerical rating scales (NRS) are for competent adults who are capable of accurately associating a numerical score to a level of pain.
▶ Visual analogue scales (VAS) are a simplified technique where a patient selects a picture that best matches their pain level. These usually resemble simplified facial expressions.
▶ Categorical scales use words, possibly in conjunction with numbers, colours or location(s) on the body.
▶ The Face, Legs, Activity, Cry and Consolability (FLACC) scale is an observation chart used for signs of discomfort in the face or legs and to rate body movement, crying and **consolability** in relation to pain or discomfort. A score of 0–2 in each of the five key areas is totalled: 0 = Relaxed and comfortable; 1–3 = Mild discomfort; 4–6 = Moderate pain; 7–10 = Severe discomfort/pain.

> **Key term**
>
> ***Consolability:*** the rate/level to which an individual can be consoled, for instance feel less uncomfortable or respond to reassurance over a period of time, as a measurement.

▶ The Bolton Pain Assessment Tool (BPAT) scores patients' pain and includes a section to involve family and/or informal or paid carers as part of the assessment process. People close to the patient can give a timeline of pain intensity.

▶ The McGill Pain Index/Pain Scale for Complex Regional Pain Syndrome (CRPS) is a sensory assessment that focuses on three aspects:

– Sensory: sensitivity, skin colour or temperature changes
– Affective: how it affects you as a sufferer (for example fear, tension)
– Evaluative: finding where the pain is.

It consists of 78 words that describe pain, such as sharp, stabbing, sore, blinding or burning.

DATE AND TIME	DATE AND TIME	DATE AND TIME	DATE AND TIME	DATE AND TIME	DATE AND TIME	DATE AND TIME	DATE AND TIME	DATE AND TIME	DATE AND TIME	DATE AND TIME
VOCALISATION										
e.g. whimpering, groaning, crying										
Absent 0 Mild 1 Moderate 2 Severe 3										
FACIAL EXPRESSION										
e.g. looking tense, frowning, grimacing, looking frightened										
Absent 0 Mild 1 Moderate 2 Severe 3										
CHANGE IN BODY LANGUAGE										
e.g. fidgeting, rocking, guarding part of body, withdrawn										
Absent 0 Mild 1 Moderate 2 Severe 3										
BEHAVIOURAL CHANGE										
e.g. increased confusion, refusing to eat, alteration in usual patterns										
Absent 0 Mild 1 Moderate 2 Severe 3										
PHYSIOLOGICAL CHANGE										
e.g. temperature, pulse or blood pressure outside normal limits, perspiring, flushing or pallor										
Absent 0 Mild 1 Moderate 2 Severe 3										
PHYSICAL CHANGES										
e.g. skin tears, pressure areas, arthritis, contractures, previous injuries										
Absent 0 Mild 1 Moderate 2 Severe 3										
Total score =										
Signature of person completing score										
0–2 **NO PAIN**	**3–7** **MILD**			**8–13** **MODERATE**			**14 +** **SEVERE**			

Notes:

▲ Figure 4.16 The Abbey Pain Scale

Source: Adapted from Abbey, J., Piller, N., De Bellis, A., Esterman, A., Parker, D., Giles, L. and Lowcay, B. (2004), 'The Abbey pain scale: A 1-minute numerical indicator for people with end-stage dementia', *International Journal of Palliative Nursing*, 10(1):6–13.
doi: 10.12968/ijpn.2004.10.1.12013.

Mobility assessment

Assessing the individual's physical functions

Mobility assessments analyse patients' physical abilities so that the appropriate handling and mobility aids can be provided. A risk assessment for relevant ADLs is carried out independently.

▶ The Elderly Mobility Scale (EMS) is an assessment of mobility that considers locomotion, balance and key position changes, for example when lying in bed or seated.

▶ The Tinetti balance assessment tool is in two parts and has a 0–2 score rating. The first part assesses balance during tasks such as rising from a chair or when nudged. The second is about **gait**, such as foot clearance. This scale is used in the assessment of risk associated with falling.

Risk-assessing for trips and falls prevents injury or allows control measures to be put in place to reduce impact. A fractured hip (Figure 4.17) is a common fall injury in older people and is associated with high mortality.

The impact of a hip fracture may include loss of muscle mass, significant immobility and a higher risk of a repeated fall. Emotionally, an individual

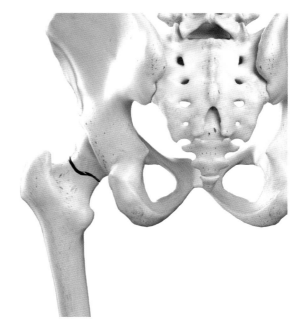

▲ Figure 4.17 A broken hip

may lack confidence as a result of the fall or develop depression influenced by pain and the effect of a loss of independence.

Supporting mobility by use of appropriate moving and handling techniques

Moving and handling techniques and equipment are required for the safety of both patient and nurse. See K1.10 and K1.11 later in this chapter for information on moving and handling techniques.

> **Key term**
>
> **Gait:** the way a person walks, or their pattern of walking.

> **Research**
>
> **S1.19 Support risk assessments for adults and escalate where appropriate**
>
> There is a variety of assessment tools used by healthcare practitioners in order to assess risk. Find out how these charts and assessment tool documents identify and evaluate risk, and how they trigger an escalation when deterioration or increased risk is identified:
>
> ▶ Braden Scale
> ▶ Bristol stool chart
> ▶ Malnutrition Screening Tool (MST)
> ▶ Waterlow Score
> ▶ Oral health assessment
> ▶ Wound assessment
> ▶ Continence assessment
>
> ▶ Fluid balance
> ▶ Nutrition assessment
> ▶ Pain assessment: Abbey Pain Scale, Bolton Pain Assessment Tool
> ▶ Mobility assessment
> ▶ Tinetti balance assessment tool.

Case study

S1.18 Demonstrate the ability to carry out clinical skills for individuals including clinical assessments and reporting findings

S1.19 Support risk assessments for adults and escalate where appropriate

Yezda is 78 years old and has been admitted to Rose Ward where you are on duty. You have been instructed to carry out a set of clinical assessments, recording outcomes on documentation. Yezda is an outpatient being treated for stage 5 breast cancer. She lives on her own and is fiercely independent. She had a fall and landed between the toilet and sink, cutting her head and elbow, and was not able to get up. She was discovered after two days.

She is feeling pain around the pelvis on one side: query fractured hip. She is dehydrated and says she has been losing her balance, was afraid to go out food shopping and her tinned food had run out. It is her first time in hospital and she will need a simple dressing on her wounds, reassurance and her questions answered. A test to check for a UTI will need you to assist Yezda with getting to the toilet using a walking frame. An observation of strength and balance is needed for a mobility risk assessment. An investigation into why she fell will follow when she is settled. The senior nurse would like you to report any concerns you have resulting from your clinical assessment, along with your suggested precautions.

Demonstrate how you would use the correct equipment to do each assessment and use effective communication skills when interacting with Yezda, keeping her informed of what you are doing and why. Cover the points below from the S1.18–19 criteria:

- weight (45 kg) height (5 ft 4 in); BMI calculation
- body temperature 37.9°C
- blood pressure and oxygen saturation 94 per cent
- respiration rate 19; heart rate 110 bpm
- instruct Yezda how you need to collect a urine sample
- assess her wounds, dress them and report no escalation needed
- Malnutrition Screening Tool (MST)
- Braden Scale; Yezda is underweight and has been lying on the floor for 48 hours
- Waterlow Score; include Yezda's treatment for cancer using a cytotoxic drug
- oral health assessment
- continence, stress bladder leaks getting up, pain
- Bristol stool, constipated
- nutrition assessment
- numerical pain assessment: vocalised – mild, face – moderate, guarded hip – severe, behavioural – mild confusion, physiological – moderate, physical changes – injured and specific to hip, McGill Pain Index assessment: communication barrier
- Elderly Mobility Scale (EMS) score: lying to sitting – independent, sitting to lying – independent; sitting to standing – stands but needs support; gait – uses walking frame, 6 metres in 17 seconds, reach approx. 15 cm
- Tinetti balance assessment tool: not hesitant, step through R, foot clearance foot drop R, symmetry unequal, step continuity stopping, path deviation, trunk uses arms, heels apart.

For Yezda's ongoing care, monitoring forms will need to be initiated:

- to monitor her fluid intake and output
- for dietary planning, requiring accurate physiological calculations for calorie intake; you will be promoting adequate nutrition and hydration while discussing what you are doing.

Evaluate your practical demonstration using Gibbs' reflective cycle to identify areas for improvement.

Moving and handling adults

In healthcare there are tasks that require the transfer, movement and positioning of an individual who is unable to do this independently. In 2020, research showed that 70 per cent of nurses had at least one episode of back pain every year, compared to 51–90 per cent of the general population in their whole lifetime.

Source: St John and St Elizabeth Hospital (2020), 'Back Care Awareness Week 2020: Back pain in nurses',
www.hje.org.uk/back-care-awareness-week-2020-back-pain-in-nurses/?fbclid=IwAR24B2QMFHmR-yOtTtSbnmh0J_2B-EXgt61EzOl33yLLoM5fCEkI77yCvJA

The spine vertebrae protect the nervous system's main highway from acute and chronic pain, but the back is also the number one location for injury, which can be down to repetitive movement and incidents that cause trauma. Shoulders, hips and knees are other common sites for injury as they are the weight-bearers when moving others, which is why, to prevent injury, there are regulations in place that specify steps and techniques to be used when working as a trainee nurse individually or in a pair.

K1.10 The fundamental principles of moving and handling individuals using evidence-based practice

As mentioned above, nurses are particularly susceptible to back pain. In the UK in 2022–2023 there were 473,000 workers with a work-related musculoskeletal disorder, and research in 2011 stated that, each year, more than 80,000 nurses injure their backs at work and 3,600 healthcare workers are forced to retire early.

Sources: HSE (2023), 'Health and safety statistics', www.hse.gov.uk/statistics

National Health Executive (2011), 'Huge cost of back injuries to the NHS', www.nationalhealthexecutive.com/News/huge-cost-of-back-injuries-to-the-nhs

Follow regulations and procedures

Incidents that cause muscle and skeletal (musculoskeletal) short- and long-term damage can be greatly reduced by following the regulations and procedures in:
► the Health and Safety at Work etc. Act 1974
► the Manual Handling Operations Regulations 1992, as amended by the Health and Safety (Miscellaneous Amendments) Regulations 2002.

Evidenced-based techniques have been developed to address this, and training for nurses is now mandatory. It is your responsibility to use the guidance when moving, handling and lifting patients: revise your knowledge from HCPO1 by reading the article at this link: **https://ojin.nursingworld.org/table-of-contents/volume-9-2004/number-3-september-2004/evidence-based-practices**

Establish whether the individual has a moving and handling risk assessment in place

A patient may have a mobility risk assessment that states the level of support needed for transfer, toileting and independence. It is your responsibility as a trainee nurse to:
► read the instructions and care plan guidance
► follow the instructions precisely, such as during a two-person slide-sheet turn
► report any incidences of concern, such as a decline in balance.

Maintain the individual's privacy and dignity

Before any actions take place, preparation is needed, such as ensuring ease of access to equipment, checking a patient knows what the plan is, and giving consideration to the **individual's privacy and dignity, for example closing the door or dignity curtains when using a hoist**.

Using a hoist sling with toileting means the patient's bottom is exposed during the lift, a move that is undignified. Effective communication skills, empathy and making sure any conversation you have with the patient before, during and after the move is not overheard will help the patient manage any feelings of distress.

The task

You will need to assess the moving and handling that is needed, such as:
► transferring a patient from a sitting position to standing
► transferring a patient from a wheelchair to the toilet.

A transfer or lift may need two people or appropriate equipment to perform it safely; adequate staffing must be in place as part of being prepared.

Assistive equipment, for example a hoist, must be available before a lift is executed and attention paid to the environment as changes can be necessary, so check the space in which the manoeuvre is planned. A 3.6 m^2 floor space is recommended, so furniture may need to be moved, including the hospital bed itself.

The individual's capabilities

Talking with the patient and reading their care plan will allow you to identify **the individual's capabilities** to assist with any move. Be mindful of preserving their dignity, and be respectful in terms of time and capability expectations, for example asking a patient to indicate they need the movement stopped if they feel pain, or allowing a minute for a patient to reposition themselves for comfort.

If the patient can move towards the edge of a chair or mattress, perhaps by shuffling, this will assist with weight-bearing, empowering them and making the experience less stressful in a sit-to-stand move. Narrating every step of using a hoist, from sliding the sling under the body to electronic movements, will keep a patient informed and reassured, and ensure they are ready and happy for the next step.

Being lifted up in a hoist increases a patient's feeling of vulnerability, so making slow movements with reassurance and using distraction techniques will make it a less anxious event, especially if the hoist is used several times a day for the same patient.

The capabilities of the handler

Only holders of a Moving and Handling Certificate, and with the necessary scope of practice, can move a patient, but consideration should still be given to the capabilities and confidence of your colleagues in terms of more complex moves. As a trainee nurse you will benefit from observing experienced staff carry out moves, how they complete the tasks, and their interaction with both the patient and their partner.

A certain type of move may require more height, a larger arm span or a higher level of strength, so the capabilities of the handler should be assessed with this in mind before transfer begins.

The needs of the individual

Moving and handling training focuses on learning and practising moves, but person-centred care is all about the patient's overall experience and the provision of compassionate care to maintain a high standard. A patient who is obese, bedbound or has chronic pain will need adapted lifts and encouragement to use open communication channels to make moving as comfortable and dignified as possible.

K1.11 How to safely move and handle individuals using specific moving and handling aids

Wheelchairs

A wheelchair should be positioned as close as possible to a transfer patient with the brakes applied.

▶ If the person is in a position to assist, lower their bed level with the wheelchair, removing the arm of the wheelchair and using a transfer board to allow them to move across independently while you monitor them for safety.

▶ Footplates need to be out the way when getting someone into a wheelchair and then their feet gently placed on them before moving.

▶ It may be necessary to use a seated-to-standing move onto a walking frame first and then support the patient's lowering into a wheelchair, which is moved in close behind them and the brakes applied.

▶ A transfer belt with loops to lift/guide upwards and steady a patient can be used as a safety precaution if necessary.

Walking aids/frames

A patient who needs the security of a walking aid/frame as they have a problem with balance or movement strength will usually be able to rise from seated to standing with mild or moderate support. Ensure the height of the aid is right and the patient has time to adjust to standing, as they may initially experience a moment of light-headedness.

Slide sheets

Slide sheets come in different sizes depending on the type of move: full body length for repositioning in bed for example, depending on the patient's height. The gentle sliding motion enables a patient to be manoeuvred on a flat surface without the need for lifting, such as in the case of ventilated, unconscious patients.

Hoists

A hoist comes with a set of instructions and must be maintained and checked to ensure that it is in safe working order before a move.

▶ A ceiling hoist can be used by one person; however, these are not common in hospitals and are more likely to be found in a nursing home, bathroom or changing facility.

▶ Mobile hoist lifting is a two-person task; sling hooks should be checked and brakes applied while positioning, and slow movement – supporting the patient to prevent any swinging – will make for a safe move.

Transfer board

A transfer board requires the patient to have a reasonable level of upper body strength. The board is put on a solid surface and acts as a bridge to allow the patient to move from one seated surface to another. For example, a lowered hospital bed to a wheelchair.

Transfer belt

Transfer belts assist with balance and movement of a patient from a sitting to a standing position or moving short distances. The transfer belt fits like a belt around the patient's waist and has a series of loops that act as handholds for the person assisting with upward movement and balance.

Sling

When a patient is unable to move themselves and is in a lying position, a sling is used to move them. The patient is rolled to one side and the sling, folded in half, is put on the surface next to the patient. The patient is then rolled on their other side and the second half of the sling is then flattened out. There are leg supports that are secured around the thigh so the head, torso and upper legs are supported when the sling is securely attached to a hoist. This move is used when changing bedding or repositioning and is only used for a short time.

K1.12 The importance of adhering to agreed ways of working when using appropriate techniques to safely move and handle individuals relevant to their condition

Avoiding any discomfort or injury to the individual

A **postoperative patient** will need moving from the surgical table to a trolley and then into bed. Care should be taken to avoid any rolling and a full body transfer board should be used, which requires four people for any move. The patient should be kept in a still position, avoiding any discomfort or injury, and observed for signs of pain; the move should take place on the count of three, co-ordinated by one person in the group. Correct positioning will avoid discomfort or injury to staff, who are responsible for following guidelines, checking equipment is in good working order and the correct use of equipment, following instructions.

Bariatric patients are classified as obese or morbidly obese. The Health Survey for England 2021 estimated that 25.9 per cent of adults in England were obese and a further 37.9 per cent overweight but not obese. Obesity is usually defined as having a body mass index (BMI) of 30 or above. A BMI between 25 and 30 is classified as overweight. Scotland's rate is higher, and in Northern Ireland and Wales the rate is slightly less. Patients who have a BMI above 30 are at higher risk of health complications and have a higher likelihood of needing medical intervention compared to those in the healthy BMI range.

Source: UK Parliament, House of Commons Library (2023), 'Obesity statistics', **https://researchbriefings.files.parliament.uk/documents/SN03336/ SN03336.pdf**

Rising rates of obesity (Figure 4.18) mean increasing hospital admissions for patients who need specialist care and adapted forms of moving, handling and lifting. Hospitals have specialised wheelchairs, beds and hoists for safe lifting and transfer, and a higher number of staff will be needed to carry out adapted techniques.

- A transfer belt is not used, as the belt length and distribution of handle spacing is not supportive enough for a safe lift.
- The larger-sized slide sheets are made of stronger material and have reinforced additional handles to accommodate a three- or four-person move compared to the average two-person move.
- The average maximum lift weight for a mobile hoist is 150 kg (24 stone), whereas a track hoist can lift 240 kg (32 stone). Hospital policy will state whether

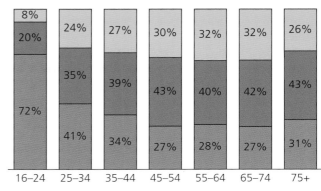

Key
- Obese
- Overweight
- Neither overweight or obese

▲ Figure 4.18 Almost three-quarters of people aged 45–74 in England are overweight or obese

Source: NHS Digital (2022), 'Health Survey for England 2021: Data tables', Overweight and obesity tables, Table 1,

https://digital.nhs.uk/data-and-information/publications/statistical/health-survey-for-england/2021/health-survey-for-england-2021-data-tables

a heavy lift requires three or four people to assist the mechanical lift.

Avoiding any discomfort or injury to yourself

Following moving and handling regulations can cause a dilemma when a patient starts to lose balance or fall. Stepping in to support them may lessen the injury to the patient, minimising damage; however, the instruction is to stand back and not attempt to intervene as this is more likely to cause injury to both the patient and health professional.

A large proportion of workplace musculoskeletal injuries are caused by sudden strain or poor positioning when attempting to stop a full-fall patient incident.

Maintaining an individual's privacy and dignity

Respecting an individual's privacy and dignity is an essential aspect of all moves.

- Particular attention is required when moving a bariatric patient. Locating specialised equipment and ensuring there are enough staff available prior to undertaking the move is good preparation and will prevent the patient from waiting longer than necessary.
- Privacy at a time when the patient is feeling vulnerable and sensitive to judgement will support their emotional security and reduce anxiety. It will also increase trust in the healthcare team carrying out the manoeuvre.

Practice points

S1.20 Demonstrate safe practice when moving and/or positioning the individual for treatment or to complete clinical skills using appropriate moving and handling aids

S1.21 Monitor and maintain the environment, equipment and resources when assisting with clinical skills for individuals

You are a trainee nurse. You need to revise and practise your moving, handling and lifting skills, adhering to regulations and procedures within the Health and Safety at Work etc. Act 1974 and the Manual Handling Operations Regulations 1992, as amended by the Health and Safety (Miscellaneous Amendments) Regulations 2002. Check equipment is in good working order and is clean.

Working with a manikin (and a partner in a two-person move), you are to produce a training video, narrating your demonstration of each of the below:

1 Your manikin is a 35-year-old rehabilitation patient who has paraplegia. You must:
   ▶ assist with movement, from bed to standing using a transfer belt on to a stationary walking frame
   ▶ assist from stationary walking frame to seated in a wheelchair
   ▶ assist with transfer from wheelchair to comfortable seat using transfer board.

2 Your manikin is a 42-year-old with advanced motor neurone disease (MND) who is an inpatient with minimal control over their movement. You must:
   ▶ reposition them – roll from lying on right-hand side to left on their request, using a slide sheet
   ▶ hoist from the bed to sitting in a hospital chair by the bed.

3 Evaluate your practical demonstrations using Gibbs' reflective cycle to identify areas for improvement.

Making effective use of all equipment

Older people are more likely to lose muscle mass and become frail as they reach their eighties and nineties. This requires extra vigilance regarding pressure and pain management, which must be noted. A move technique may take longer and require adaptations; for example cushioning in a hoist sling or repositioning in bed are important in preparing for the move to happen. Using the equipment effectively and selecting the most suitable equipment for the task is important from a safety perspective. Following guidelines and a person-centred approach are clinical tasks in everyday nursing.

Equipment, resources and environment used in clinical skills for adults

Equipment used in support of clinical skills, and the immediate environment where tasks are carried out, must meet safety regulations. When equipment is used or moved around frequently, its actions can be affected, so safety checks will be required before use. Medical equipment is required to go through regular checks to enable safe use. Some items will have an initial check by the manufacturer, and where needed there will be routine visits and **calibration** inspections by specialists. Other equipment, for example a hoist, must have timely routine checks or be checked before use.

The Provision and Use of Work Equipment Regulations (PUWER) 1998 require that equipment provided for use at work is suitable for the intended use; for example specialist equipment could include a 250 kg bariatric patient hoist for the movement of a bariatric patient.

The Lifting Operations and Lifting Equipment Regulations 1998 (LOLER) state that there should be health and safety organisation leads who oversee employees' safety while using lifting equipment.

K1.13 When monitoring, recording and supporting the overall care and wellbeing of individuals, the range of equipment and resources used, where to source and how to check them

Equipment and resources used

In HCPO3 you learned about the equipment used to assess and monitor a patient's vital signs. You have practised using equipment and resources for medical and personal care.

Key term

Calibration: a procedure for detecting and fixing uncertainties in equipment used to take measurements.

Medical devices

You need to know how to use the following medical devices:

▶ manual and automatic blood pressure monitors (blood pressure)
▶ tympanic thermometer (temperature)
▶ pulse oximeter (oxygen saturation)
▶ glucometer (blood sugar levels)
▶ scales and tape measure (weight and height).

See HCPO3 K3.4 for details of how to use the first four items listed above. Scales and tape measure are to be used as follows:

▶ With portable floor scales, a freestanding column scale or a chair scale can be used to weigh a patient, to assist with calculating their BMI. Some hospital beds are also weighing scales.
▶ A stadiometer measures height on a stand or attached to the wall; patients who are unable to stand for any period of time will have their height calculated. This measurement from the base of the heel to knee height, using a broad calliper device or tape measure, can be used to calculate an estimated height.

Personal care equipment

Hospital ward care and community care offer different personal care equipment where possible, depending on the patient's needs. Examples are specialised mechanical beds, commodes and pressure-relieving mattresses.

Specialised mechanical beds

Curative care (or acute) beds, rehabilitative care beds and long-term care beds can be manual, semi-electric or fully electric. Each type will have its own manufacturer's instructions.

If you observe experienced staff using different types of beds and ask for detailed training on their usage, this will benefit both the patient and your colleagues (in terms of your being able to act swiftly).

Most hospitals have electrical beds with functions that move the whole main body of the bed up and down, a top part that can be moved up and down, and a part that bends and extends the legs, or lifts the legs up and down, along with side rails which can be raised for safety. You can adjust the bed using a mechanical controller, which allows slow, smooth movement.

Acute hospital beds have a red emergency button on their controls that, if pressed, drops the height of the bed to allow instant access for staff to get on to carry out CPR. A patient who is in pain will require you to use your skills to avoid a wrong move, such as raising their legs instead of lowering them.

Manual beds have the same range of movement but have levers that need to be cranked by hand. Applying a brake to the wheels is done using a foot lever. Minor movement requires one member of staff, while more advanced moves need two.

Commodes

A commode is a seated frame, on wheels for ease of movement, with a concealed commode pot to contain urine and faeces. This pot has a lid, which is removed for emptying and cleaned after use.

A patient with a mobility concern requiring the toilet can be offered a commode, particularly at night, and assisted to use it safely. Commodes should never be used as transfer aids.

Pressure-relieving mattresses

All hospital beds have waterproof surfaces, and **pressure-relieving mattresses** as a standard. However, in cases where the patient is at very high risk of developing pressure injury, inflatable air mattresses can be used to ensure that there is consistent automated pressure relief.

Practice points

S1.21 Monitor and maintain the environment, equipment and resources when assisting with clinical skills for individuals

S1.33 Assist with individuals' overall comfort and wellbeing including bed comfort

The manikin is in an electric hospital bed. Demonstrate effective controller use and hospital bed calibration:

1 A flat bed at the highest point for a patient bed bath
2 Raise back to comfortable upright position at patient visiting time
3 Lower back for comfort for patient who is using an oxygen mark and is tired
4 Elevate legs by approx. 20 cm to improve comfort and circulation for patient
5 Emergency low flat bed for patient CPR access

Test yourself

S1.20 Demonstrate safe practice when moving and/or positioning the individual for treatment or to complete clinical skills using appropriate moving and handling aids

1   Why should footrests be folded out of the way when a patient is being seated in a wheelchair?
2   Why should the height of a walking frame be checked after the patient's first step?
3   When would a tetrapod walking stick be used instead of a regular Coopers walking stick?
4   Why are hoist slings and slide sheets different colours?

Sensor pads

For patients living with dementia, and in caring for older people and individuals with a mental illness, there may be a need for a sensor pad. These sense a change in pressure as a patient gets out of bed, sending an alarm to the nurses' station and alerting staff to monitor the movement of the patient who gets up in the night. Patients are unaware of the presence of the discreet device, meaning a dignified, quick response can be actioned.

Individual personal care equipment

Walking aids

These are useful for independent movement for a patient once it is established they can be used safely; sometimes a patient will need support in using a walking aid to stand and sit, before and after use. A mobility risk assessment, detailing specifics, will be recorded in a care plan so that usage and support is clear.

Hearing aids

Hearing aids are essential for communication and should be treated with care, being kept clean and in good working order. Hearing aids can be easily lost if patients are being transferred between wards and departments. It is important to ensure that the hearing aids are transferred with the patient and kept safely in a hearing aid case or within the patient's belongings.

A hearing aid might be uncomfortable when a patient puts pressure on it while lying in bed. If hearing aids are removed at this point, you should be aware that this causes a communication barrier, and adapt your skills to ensure the patient can hear. This may include putting the hearing aid back in position, ensuring you are facing the patient for lip-reading or using written communication as an alternative. Consider the patient's choice.

Glasses

As with hearing aids, glasses can be removed for sleeping and resting in bed for comfort, if this is the patient's choice. It is essential that glasses are available for use when the patient needs to read, at either a long or short distance. Having orientation to an unfamiliar environment is more difficult if glasses are not available when needed, such as reading the mealtime menu or signing a consent form. An individual who is unable to see distance may not see the ward clock or toilet signage, and as such may easily become disorientated.

Dentures

Dentures may comprise a complete top and bottom set or separate denture plates which contain false teeth that fill a gap to enable eating and talking. These may come loose, and if so become a potential choke hazard. Assisting with denture removal requires gloves and gently loosening the denture by putting the finger and thumb in the mouth in a pincer grip. Patients should be gently encouraged to undertake this practice independently, although assistance might need to be given to clean the dentures once removed. A patient's preparation for surgery will include the removal of any dental fixtures.

Like glasses, dentures may easily get misplaced if removed. Agree a place and system with a patient for where they will be stored, such as a bedside cabinet. Care should be taken to make sure these are transferred with the patient if they move between wards or departments.

Where to source equipment and resources

The location of stored equipment and resource access will be explained as part of a ward induction. In bank nursing, familiarising yourself at the start of a shift with the help of a supervisor is good practice, as some equipment such as resuscitation equipment may be needed in a hurry.

Storerooms

Storerooms, medical and laundry utility spaces, and the **sluice room** will be located in different spaces depending on the ward. Surgical and medicine trolleys are usually stored in the same place as items such as wound dressing kits, which remains locked for staff entry only. Stock checks and audits are carried out to ensure equipment is monitored and reordered as necessary before items run out.

Key term

Sluice room: a specialist infection prevention room for storing bed/bedside toileting equipment, and for the safe and effective disposal of human waste.

Medical equipment libraries

A medical equipment library (MEL) has stock that is checked out and returned, for example bariatric equipment or suction machines, which are not stored on each ward. Staff who stock-control items of equipment are responsible for maintaining them in good working order but will need feedback from ward staff if there is a concern.

External agencies

Outsourcing equipment using external agencies may happen if waiting times exceed the government-set targets or specialised equipment is not used often enough to justify a purchase.

Private hospitals can ease the pressure of meeting treatment waiting times at a cost to hospital trusts, and out-of-hours care may be sourced in certain locations. The equipment can be borrowed and returned, and a loan cost will be charged. The cost may also include hiring staff with the relevant expertise in using this high-tech equipment.

Procurement of equipment from other areas

Purchasing and acquiring equipment is a decision made at management level. A requisition will be completed by a department or ward and considered by the hospital trust's financial and resourcing team. A trainee nurse may be part of the department audit and assist in determining what should be in the requisition, for example calculating predicted use, cost savings and enhanced patient care. Ward managers and departmental leads may be required to write a business case for the purchase of expensive non-standard equipment.

How to check equipment and resources

The responsibility for maintaining equipment that is safe for use in clinical skills assessment and monitoring lies with the staff using the equipment and the protocols in place for maintenance. Standard safe practice means doing the following:

▶ Following **standard operating procedures** (SOPs), which state preparation needed before use, level of staffing and training needed, following instructions clearly during and after use. For example, there may be a need for equipment calibration, infection prevention steps, safety PPE or risk assessment control measures to prevent harm.

▶ Completing **calibration of equipment when required (for example weekly, monthly or annually)**, for example defibrillators, weighing scales and **spirometers**. Medical equipment calibration is the process of ensuring the equipment is functioning as it should be and to the industry standard. The calibration of equipment is necessary to ensure readings are accurate and the equipment is functioning as it should and can be used safely. Records are kept and review dates set on some items of equipment, whereas others are checked before each use. First line calibration of smaller electrical devices means they are often automatically checked at start-up when switched on. There may be a need to change flat batteries, such as in a tympanic thermometer or blood pressure monitor. Measuring temperature with one thermometer and then another will confirm accurate functioning if both readings are exactly the same. This is recorded and frequency of changes monitored.

▶ Adhering to guidance on **checking equipment and resources for damage**. If equipment – such as mechanical hoist, weighing scales with limited capacity and medical equipment such as spare defibrillators – is used or stored incorrectly it can get damaged.

▶ Completing equipment check records. The Health and Safety at Work etc. Act 1974 states that equipment must be maintained to prevent dangerous occurrences, the specifics of which are not stated. Hospital policy will have uniform processes in place, for instance portable appliance testing (PAT) carried out by a qualified outsourced company for smaller devices. Manufacturers of larger equipment will provide timely maintenance checks as part of a lifetime purchase. Manufacturers often provide post-market vigilance instructions and reports for the Medicines and Healthcare products Regulatory Agency (MHRA). Many manufacturers will be expected to deliver training before and after equipment purchase to ensure correct use.

Key term

Spirometer: assessment equipment to assist with diagnosing and monitoring of certain lung conditions by measuring how much air is inhaled and exhaled in one forced breath.

Practice points

S1.21 Monitor and maintain the environment, equipment and resources when assisting with clinical skills for individuals

S1.22 Demonstrate the ability to perform first line calibration on clinical equipment

You are a trainee nurse. You need to perform infection prevention measures and first line calibration on the equipment listed below.

1 Using correct documentation you must report and record checks to the following equipment:
   ▶ automatic and manual blood pressure monitors
   ▶ tympanic thermometer
   ▶ pulse oximeter
   ▶ non-electronic weighing scales
   ▶ glucometer.
2 You discover the following:
   ▶ the thermometer is displaying 2°C lower than it should be
   ▶ the battery for the pulse oximeter is flat.

Explain what action you should now take.

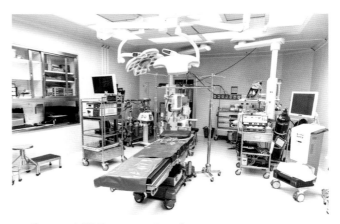

▲ Figure 4.19 An operating theatre

blade. A stainless-steel operating trolley (OT) carries sealed sterilised equipment that is needed in surgery and is subject to recorded checks each time there is new planned or emergency surgery.

Monthly checking requirements

Examples of **monthly inspections** include:
▶ theatre lighting
▶ video feedback endoscopy equipment
▶ operating theatre bed.

A hospital theatre manager is the lead on risk-managing the equipment in a particular operating theatre (Figure 4.19) or all the theatres in the hospital. They will be responsible for staff training, allocation of staff to complete checks and managing timely manufacturer's checks on larger equipment, such as the operating theatre bed. Mobile equipment units such as endoscopy or ECG equipment will be examined and their functioning checked on a schedule overseen by the manager.

Documentation to be completed

Records of usage, checks and replacement of equipment must be recorded, signed and dated. Each type of check will have its own checklist which forms part of regulatory safety activity.

K1.14 The procedures of how to check emergency equipment

Checking by a registered professional

Equipment is checked by a registered professional, such as a registered nurse, and not by a trainee nurse.
▶ In theatre, anaesthesia equipment will be checked by a qualified anaesthetist.
▶ Surgical lights, table and monitors will be checked by authorised staff, such as a theatre nurse.

Daily checking requirements

▶ Portable oxygen cylinders should be checked on a daily basis, and empty or near empty oxygen cylinders replaced immediately.
▶ Defibrillators are checked daily and should not be used unless the green light is on.
▶ Suction units or lines will also need checking for correct functioning.
▶ Equipment that is disposable, such as kidney bowls, dressings and sutra kits, will be subject to an inventory checking system and an order will be needed to replace depleting stock.
▶ Sterilised surgical equipment stocktaking will take place before and after surgery, to ensure that nothing is left in the patient after surgery, such as a swab or a small piece from a damaged surgical

K1.15 The different environments in which clinical skills in adult nursing are undertaken

NHS hospital wards, outpatient units or specialist departments

Adult nursing with competent clinical skills is used in different locations, such as NHS hospital wards, outpatient units and specialist departments such as an oncology chemotherapy treatment room.

NHS hospital wards

NHS hospital general wards will have non-specialist medical and nursing practitioners; specialist wards such as a stroke ward will have expert qualified staff. Specialist rehabilitation and mobility equipment, and frequent visits by physio and speech and language therapists, aim to meet the needs of the specific service users in wards.

Outpatient units

Outpatients is an area with clinics where patients are seen by appointment only. An appointment could involve the use of larger equipment, such as an MRI scanner or a second appointment with a consultant to go through the findings from a scan.

Outpatient nurses assist medical practitioners and may be involved in an examination or minor procedures. Some clinics are nurse-led, such as in the case of pre-op assessments, and nurses are often responsible for correct information delivery before consent forms are signed.

Specialist departments

Nurses who are specialised in supporting patients who are attending an appointment for a measured dose of intravenous chemotherapy will be proficient in maintaining infection prevention of peripherally inserted central catheter (PICC) lines and safety measures when setting up chemotherapy and other drug treatment fluids for patients, for example those admitted as day cases.

The community

Care can take place in an individual's home, such as palliative care, in a GP surgery, such as mental health care, and in a nursing or residential home.

Individual's home

The majority of patients with life-limiting conditions and at the end stage of a terminal illness choose to stay at home if possible. Their treatment is likely to be focused on pain management and reducing side effects. Macmillan nurses support palliative community nurses and are also specialists in patient welfare.

GP surgery

A patient who is experiencing episodes of poor mental health can benefit from remaining in the community, in their own home or a relative's home. Specialist community mental health nurses hold clinics in local GP surgeries or can home visit to monitor the progress of treatments and escalate any concerns.

Nursing home

A nursing home provides residential accommodation for a variety of individuals who require daily treatment and hospital-type facilities but not enough intervention to require inpatient care in hospital. Nurses and other health professionals are employed by nursing homes to work closely with the residents. A GP is usually responsible for the provision of medical care to the residents unless an emergency occurs.

The regulators monitor standards in all locations and seek feedback from service users, their families and healthcare professionals who support the home.

Prison hospitals

Prisoners often have poorer health than do the general population. Prison hospitals provide a healthcare service and mental health support. Specialist services to deal with dental care and addiction and to support survivors of abuse meet the needs of the prison population and require expert nursing staff who are trained in working with offenders.

Other types of nursing environment

Voluntary or private-sector hospitals

Health professionals are required to work in the private healthcare sector such as hospitals and clinics. The private sector now supports the NHS with work relating to waiting list targets and general decision making around diagnostics. The clinical skills for these nurses and other health professionals are the same as any hospital, but patient care is often provided in individual rooms rather than wards, and more time may be allocated to spend with individuals as the staff to patient ratio is higher.

Hospices

Hospice care is provided by healthcare professionals who are specialists in care for patients at the end of life. These staff are often experts in pain and symptom management and the provision of support to friends and family of the patient. Palliative nursing is primarily about making patients comfortable, meeting their needs and providing symptom management. Excellent communication skills to support the patient and their family are of paramount importance, and this type of nursing helps people find their way through a difficult time.

A Macmillan nurse is a registered nurse with specialist skills in the management of the end of life.

Clinics

Nursing also takes place in outreach clinics such as sexual health and hospital outpatients, covering the whole spectrum of care. Each clinic is a specialist area with nurses whose clinical skills and knowledge support the patient's needs such as diabetic reviews, undertaking cervical cytology clinics and reviewing wounds following surgery.

K1.16 The range of checks to emergency equipment and why these checks are carried out

Full range of checks to emergency equipment

In K1.14 you learned about who carries out checks on emergency equipment and the required frequency of these checks, depending on the type of equipment and its use. Table 4.2 lists the full range of checks to emergency equipment, along with explanations.

Why checks are carried out

▶ The purpose of having an audit system of checking **is to ensure that equipment is working effectively** and fit for purpose.

▶ Checks are carried out to **ensure everything is available, in good working order and located correctly**.

▶ Decontamination of medical equipment will **ensure infection prevention compliance**, and is usually carried out in the hospital sterile services department. In many cases, medical equipment such as scopes and resuscitation equipment is single-use only. Correct sterilisation processes reduce the risk of cross-contamination and support infection prevention policy.

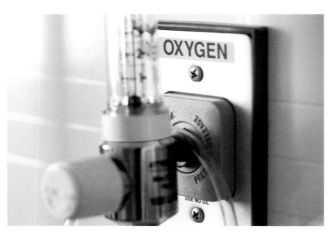

▲ Figure 4.20 Oxygen regulator

▼ Table 4.2 Checks to emergency equipment

Checks to emergency equipment	Explanation
Resuscitation checklist	All resuscitation equipment must be checked on a daily basis by a registered nurse who, using a standardised form, will check and sign that: • all equipment is present and in the right location; for example there must be a new sharps bin on a resuscitation trolley, and a PPE dispenser • suction equipment is clean, functioning (calibrated) and has been left with tubing attached; this is standard practice among professionals, for example a portable suction machine will have the correct size tubes in place but not the Yankauer suction tip for oral and airway clearance – this is attached later and the most appropriate size connected; there are additional sizes of other airway equipment that must be present and available. Most equipment, such as an endotracheal tube, is single-use and disposable. A rigid bronchoscope opens up the oral cavity and trachea; it is a hollow metal tube and helps with inserting ventilation tubes. This is sterilised, and checks for the presence of different sizes of sterile equipment are needed before and after resuscitation trolley use. Sterilised equipment should have an unbroken seal. Expiry dates should be checked on perishable equipment as appropriate, such as antiseptic fluids and disposable resuscitation trolley sized tubing. The tube materials degrade over time; expiry dates are clearly visible and must be checked.
Calibration of equipment	Equipment must be calibrated in accordance with the manufacturer's instructions, for example vaccine fridge temperature checks. Testing may indicate a deviation from what is expected, such as an oxygen regulator not delivering the correct level to a mask worn by a patient (Figure 4.20).
Defibrillator charge	Defibrillators do an automatic self-check when switched on, indicated by a flashing 'egg timer' until it becomes a solid green light. This quickly ensures it is charged and working correctly. This piece of equipment has a life expectancy of ten years. The defibrillation electrodes must be present and not expired.
Oxygen cylinder full	There is a gauge that shows whether an oxygen cylinder is full; manufacturers calibrate these, sending them to a laboratory that uses precise equipment. If the cylinder has been used and is only partially full it is exchanged for a full one daily.

Assessment practice

Your task is to demonstrate the correct procedures in delivering a total support care package to meet physical and mental wellbeing needs, maintain standards and health and safety, and report any concerns you may have. You will need a manikin and a partner for the moving and handling tasks.

You are to demonstrate your understanding of the HCPO1 and ANPO1 knowledge and skills, completing the case study tasks below.

Patient A

You are a nurse receiving a new admission. You must carry out initial assessments and complete monitoring documentation for the patient's notes.

▶ The patient is 83 years old. She is living with dementia and has been knocked over by an electric scooter in the park and is very muddy.

▶ An X-ray shows a broken hip and she has grazes on her hand and chin; she shows discomfort in her face and has two noticeable broken teeth.

▶ Her husband is with her and has brought her medication: warfarin blood thinner and statins for high blood cholesterol. She has now been given morphine as pain relief and antibiotics.

▶ A urine catheter is in place and her wounds need re-dressing after you have given her a bed bath. You can use a slide sheet to carry out a skin integrity assessment and reposition her for comfort.

▶ The patient's husband needs to be kept informed of every action you take; she lacks capacity and he is her advocate.

▶ You can see that the patient is underweight and dehydrated, and her husband says she has had diarrhoea for two days; she is double incontinent and he has used an incontinence pad that is too big; the skin on her bottom is sore.

Your assessment will include the patient's husband, who is her next of kin.

Using the advice and guidance given in this chapter, your assessment and monitoring must cover:
▶ nutrition and hydration
▶ bowel, bladder and skin assessments to gather maximum accurate information
▶ investigating oral health
▶ providing well-fitting incontinence wear
▶ obtaining a stool sample
▶ obtaining an Abbey Pain Scale score an hour after the patient arrives on the ward.

Include her husband in your assessment: he can be asked to carry out dry mouth care and monitor her pain levels.

Patient B

You have built a good working relationship with a patient on your ward over the past 12 weeks. Their discharge is imminent, and a mobility assessment will influence a suitable care package for when they go home.

▶ Following a car accident, the patient had two femur breaks and an L2 spinal cord injury, which has caused paralysis from the knee downwards.

▶ In the accident, his brother was killed instantly and observations have noted he refuses to acknowledge this.

▶ He has a BMI of 30 and you will need to discuss a food diary and calorie intake information.

▶ A mobility risk assessment is carried out and the patient has been cleared to demonstrate their safe skills to move from bed to chair and chair to bariatric wheelchair. He will need a bed controller, a walking frame and a transfer board.

During these tasks you will need to ensure dignity is maintained. Use the opportunity to communicate and to look for any signs of mental ill health.

Adult Nursing PO2: Supporting individuals to meet activities of daily living

Support for inpatients and patients in the community should meet their medical and physical needs as recorded in a care plan. Activities to maintain good nutrition and hydration, and a good standard of personal hygiene require effective communication skills to explain the purpose of your clinical duties and encourage patients to participate in their own care.

Informal carers need to work in partnership with medical and social care professionals to provide the most appropriate level of tailored care.

Learning outcomes

The core knowledge outcomes that you must understand and learn:

K2.1 the purpose and importance of supporting the individual with a range of activities of daily living

K2.2 the different types of long-term conditions and their impact on activities of daily living

K2.3 how to support or enable individuals to complete activities of daily living in line with their care plan, using a person-centred and enabling approach

K2.4 the different types of carers and their role in meeting the needs of individuals

K2.5 the concept of informal carers and the general rights of carers when supporting individuals to meet activities of daily living

K2.6 the possible roles of informal carers and the importance of working in partnership with them when supporting individuals to meet activities of daily living

K2.7 the symptoms and implications associated with frailty

K2.8 the importance of early diagnosis in relation to dementia and other cognitive issues, why depression, delirium and the normal ageing process may be mistaken for dementia and how other conditions may contribute to early onset dementia

K2.9 the factors that impact on the care of the dying and the deceased to ensure most appropriate care is provided.

Skills outcomes

The skills you will need to demonstrate:

S2.10 support or enable individuals to maintain good nutrition and hydration and record details

S2.11 support or enable individuals to maintain continence

S2.12 support or enable individuals to maintain good personal hygiene

S2.13 support or enable individuals to dress and undress

S2.14 support or enable individuals to be mobile

S2.15 support or enable individuals to rest, sleep and keep safe

S2.16 support or enable individuals to express their sexuality

S2.17 appropriately manage situations in which individuals cannot do things for themselves

S2.18 support individuals to manage own health and wellbeing, offering appropriate guidance within the scope of role, knowledge and responsibilities

S2.19 advise carers on supporting an individual to manage their own condition within scope of role, knowledge and responsibilities

S2.20 provide appropriate care that helps individuals with advanced, progressive and life-limiting conditions to live as well as possible.

Activities of daily living

There are many nursing theories connected with supporting people with their everyday needs, but the Roper–Logan–Tierney Model is the one most commonly used in the UK. This model acts as a guide for assessing a patient's capabilities to carry out day-to-day tasks, taking into account their environmental, physical and mental wellbeing as factors.

The level of care necessary will depend on a patient's capacity and capabilities, and it should aim to maintain a safe environment for the patient while they are carrying out basic daily living tasks. Some individuals may require assistance only for certain types of task, while others will need complete care; however, this is reviewed since care needs change in terms of improvement or deterioration of physical or mental health conditions.

K2.1 The purpose and importance of supporting the individual with a range of activities of daily living

Nutrition and hydration

On a cellular level, the human body needs **nutrients, fluid** and oxygen to function. These three elements are the foundation of tissues, organs and body systems. There are many types of cells and each type of cell will carry out a different function within the body.

For the body to function and maintain optimal health, adequate nourishment at a cellular level is required. This is even more important when a person is recovering from surgery or illness, or has a health condition that hospitalises them. Speed of recovery and management of physical or mental illness can be hindered by the insufficient consumption of hydration or nutrients. Malnutrition is responsible for an increase in hospital admissions and an increase in the length of stay for many patients.

Principles of good nutrition and hydration

A balanced diet, adequate portion sizes and a sufficient intake of fluids are the principles of good nutrition and hydration. A core role for the healthcare professional is to ensure that as part of the recovery process and care planning principles, the patient is encouraged to maintain a good diet and fluid intake in order to support the body to heal and repair.

Different types of diet

Many health conditions can be improved by the intake of a modified diet. For example:

- a fall in levels of oestrogen in perimenopause or testosterone in prostate cancer treatment; this will affect bone density, requiring more vitamin D-rich foods and a dietary supplement
- the pancreas and liver are organs that play a role in converting food nutrients into a useable format for cells; health conditions affecting these will have a significant impact
- health conditions that affect appetite directly or as a consequence of wanting to avoid symptoms, such as inflammatory bowel disease diarrhoea and painful gut spasms, can be addressed by changing foods and using suitable treatments.

Diets can be modified. For instance, in the form of:
- an increased level of protein for cell repair
- lower-cholesterol foods as a treatment for heart disease.

Alternative forms of nutrition and hydration

Table 5.1 shows how patients who are unable to eat and/or drink in the usual way may receive fluids and nutrients in an alternative form.

▼ Table 5.1 Alternative forms of nutrition and hydration

Form	Explanation
Percutaneous endoscopic gastrostomy (PEG)	This is a type of feeding tube: ▶ percutaneous means 'through the skin' ▶ endoscopy refers to equipment used to examine the digestive tract ▶ gastrostomy refers to the opening into the stomach. PEG tubes allow nutrients to be carried directly into the stomach bypassing the mouth and oesophagus. This type of **enteral** feeding requires a procedure in which the PEG tube is inserted through the wall of the abdomen straight to the stomach (Figure 5.1). Patients might be fitted with a PEG tube because they have difficulty with swallowing, problems with appetite or an inability to take adequate nutrition through the mouth, for instance as a result of cancer of the oesophagus or stomach, or dysphagia (difficulty swallowing).

Form	Explanation
	The tube must be carefully monitored and cleaned. It may need to be replaced periodically. A PEG tube which is infected or blocked will need an immediate review and may require replacing.
	Patients with a PEG tube can be fed manually: the external clamp is unscrewed and a feeding syringe attached, and approx. 50–60 ml of liquid, called a food bolus, pushed down the tube every 20 seconds in a slow and methodically way. **Pump feeding is set up as part of an automatic system: a feed bag is attached to the tube and will run for several hours via a controlled insertion pump.**
	The tube needs to be flushed before and after the administration of food, as occasionally there are blockages. Flushing may not clear a blockage so there is the option of massaging the tube or using a feeding syringe to withdraw the formula fluid. The health professional must be trained and competent to use the tube for the administration of medication or feed.
	PEG feeding requires a thorough cleaning routine to prevent infection.
Percutaneous endoscopic jejunostomy (PEJ) feeding	This is similar to PEG feeding but the tube goes directly into the jejunum section of the small intestine. This method is for patients who are unable to tolerate food in their stomach, for example if they have stomach cancer, or are at risk of getting food in their lungs due to **reflux**.
	As with PEG feeding, PEJ feeding requires a thorough cleaning routine to prevent infection, and the use of pre-prepared sterile food tube bags.
Nasogastric (NG) feeding	A tube is passed through the nose or mouth into the stomach. The tube enters the stomach via the oesophagus sphincter. PEG/PEJ feeding is more suitable for long-term use compared to NG feeding.
Total parenteral nutrition (TPN)	This is a type of patient feeding that bypasses the gastrointestinal tract entirely. Parenteral means 'outside the digestive tract' and is the only option for some patients who have had abdominal surgery, certain chemotherapy treatments or have a bowel obstruction. A special formula is given through a vein, which provides all the nutrients the body needs.
Intravenous (IV) infusion fluids	These are solutions administered directly into a vein via a cannula (a small plastic tube inserted into a large vein). IV fluids are used to prevent or treat dehydration, replenishing the body with nutrients and fluids. This method is used for patients who are injured, dehydrated from illness, malnourished or undergoing surgery.

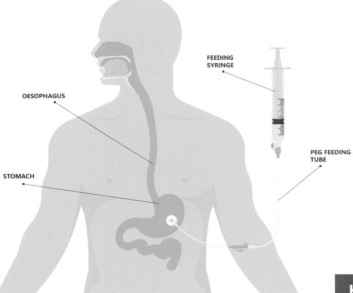

▲ Figure 5.1 PEG tube feeding

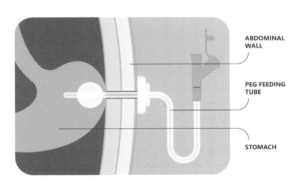

PEG TUBE FEEDING
PERCUTANEOUS ENDOSCOPIC GASTROSTOMY

Key terms

Enteral: passing through the intestine, either naturally via the mouth and oesophagus, or through an artificial means such as a nasogastric tube.

Reflux: when stomach acid repeatedly backflows through the oesophagus sphincter.

Methods of monitoring and recording nutrition and hydration intake

You have already learned about documentation and observation methods used in **monitoring and recording patients' nutrition and hydration intake**, in HCPO3 K3.5 and ANPO1 K1.3.

▶ A food and drink chart records and reports a patient's consumption over a time period.

▶ Information can be gained directly from the patient or a relative, to ascertain intake and output prior to medical treatment.

▶ Blood tests specifically looking at the level of cholesterol, vitamins or minerals will give an indication of current levels, but other tests will be used to investigate why there is a deficiency and its effect.

Signs and symptoms of poor nutrition and inadequate hydration

Dehydration and malnutrition can be easy to identify under certain circumstances. However, a low BMI is not a good indicator of nutritional status (see Table 5.2).

▼ Table 5.2 Signs and symptoms of poor nutrition and inadequate hydration

Signs and symptoms of poor nutrition	Signs and symptoms of inadequate hydration
Signs of undernourishment may include: ▶ weight loss ▶ weight gain (obesity is also a type of malnourishment) ▶ poorly controlled diabetes ▶ confusion ▶ bone density reduction ▶ vitamin deficiency ▶ poor wound healing ▶ infection risk ▶ constipation/diarrhoea.	Symptoms of dehydration are: ▶ thirst ▶ reduced urine output ▶ confusion ▶ falls ▶ dry skin ▶ dry mucosal membranes ▶ low blood pressure ▶ increased heart rate.

Promoting good nutrition and hydration

It is important to offer dietary education and promote adequate nutrition and hydration when working with people experiencing ill health. This is particularly important if the person is being discharged from hospital and has a history of dehydration or malnourishment.

Health promotion campaigns

Examples of health promotion campaigns relating to dietary intake are:

▶ The 5 A Day health promotion campaign encourages a higher intake of different fruits and vegetables, according to their size and what is classed as a portion, aiming to raise people's vitamin and mineral intake.

▶ Consensus Action on Salt Health is an education campaign to explain the health dangers of excess salt in the diet and the importance of checking food labels. A high salt intake is a contributing factor to health risks such as hypertension, kidney disease and heart disease. Takeaway food and ready meals can have a high salt content; adding salt to boiling vegetables has been usual practice, to reduce the amount of water entering the vegetables and add seasoning.

▶ Give Up Loving Pop (GULP) is aimed at children but is also useful for adults in raising awareness of calorie intake and replacing carbonated drinks with alternatives. Sugary drinks interact with bacteria in the mouth and increase its acidity, a cause of damage to teeth.

A casual conversation with the patient while you are taking observation measurements offers a good opportunity for you to reinforce the importance of change for good health.

Current government guidelines

The current government guidelines for the recommended proportion of food groups in a meal is visually represented in the Eatwell Guide (Figure 5.2). This is a simple representation that does not include more scientific information about particular macronutrients and micronutrients.

Using the Eatwell Guide, patients outside the healthy category range on a BMI scale, for example, can see clearly the types of foods and guided amounts they need to eat per day; and it will help them to discuss their current and future diet with a better understanding. Patients who recognise calorie intake and food labelling can be given suggestions about how to increase or decrease their intake, such as sugary snack swaps and modifying the amount of fried or takeaway foods that they eat.

The Eatwell Guide recommends fluid consumption of six to eight glasses a day; this can be in the form of water, lower-fat milk and sugar-free drinks including tea and coffee. This amount assumes that around 20 per cent of foods contribute to the daily fluid intake too.

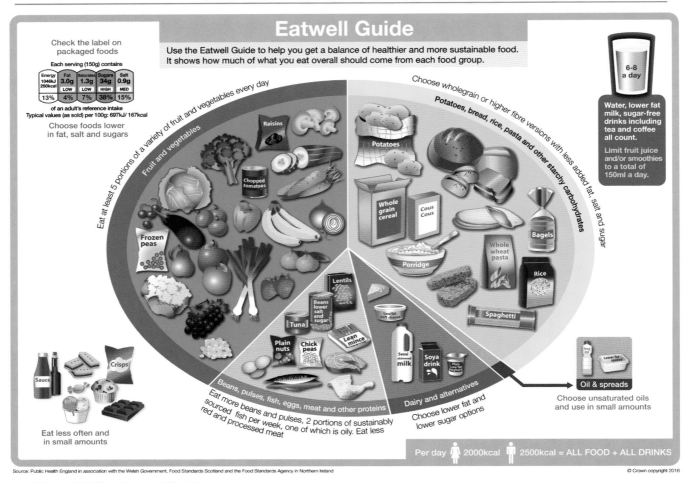

▲ Figure 5.2 The Eatwell Guide

Individual healthy options within a clinical or community setting

A dietician working as part of a multidisciplinary team is tasked with personalising advice and guidance for an individual, designing a food diary plan that will gradually change their habits to more healthy options and choices.

Dieticians work across all sectors of the healthcare system, including within an acute care clinical environment, outpatients departments or community setting based at a GP surgery. In some cases, morbidly obese patients will need a home visit. Current diet is considered and new diet routines planned to effect a gradual change, and factors like cooking ability and food preferences are considered.

Discussing improvements to diet with a patient must consider their values, for example according to religious practice, or choices such as vegetarianism or veganism. Suggesting a food that is outside the principles a person lives by can be offensive and demonstrates a lack of understanding and poor person-centred

Test yourself

S2.10 Support or enable individuals to maintain good nutrition and hydration and record details

You are a nurse on a ward. You have been tasked with maintaining and recording nutrition and hydration for patients.

A speech and language therapist has carried out a bedside swallow (dysphagia) assessment, which indicated a significant choke risk for a patient in your care. The individual is Jewish, has an obese BMI, and needs lower-energy foods and changes to their diet to address their type 2 diabetes diagnosis.

Would you be able to talk with the patient/a relative to explain the points below?

1 Alternative methods of eating
2 How cultural needs will be met
3 Changes needed to support weight loss and blood sugar levels
4 Where, why and how nutrition and hydration are recorded

care. Talking with a patient and their relatives about the individual's preferences when analysing dietary changes is respectful.

Maintaining continence

Offering reminders and prompts to use the toilet

Individuals with bowel or bladder retention problems should be offered dignified advice regarding maintaining continence.

▶ Inpatients can be reminded, a prompt to use the toilet can be given, and relatives directed to continue when a nurse is not present.

▶ Pelvic floor exercises can be explained, and a patient can be prompted to carry them out to help with better control by strengthening the pelvic floor muscle (Figure 5.3).

▶ A patient living with dementia or a brain injury may not feel the urge to go to the toilet or may forget to go. This could be overcome by the use of a toilet schedule.

▶ You should observe any verbal or visual cues which indicate that a patient may need the toilet, such as pacing, pulling trousers down or pulling back the bed covers when lying down.

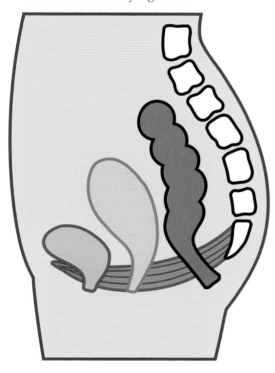

▲ Figure 5.3 The pelvic floor muscle (shown in the image as a red 'crescent') can be strengthened through exercise to improve continence

Ensuring an appropriate environment for the individual

Toilet anxiety, or shy bladder syndrome, needs to be addressed by ensuring an appropriate environment for the individual – as far as this is possible in a hospital and other environments such as care homes in social care.

You may need to **support the mobility of a patient** who needs to go to the toilet; ensuring the availability of facilities and responding in a timely manner will reassure them. An awareness that a patient may suddenly need to go to the toilet in the middle of a medical consultation avoids stress and anxiety surrounding toileting.

When a patient is in the toilet cubicle or facility, their dignity can be maintained by you first ensuring they are confident in using the call alarm cord if they need any support, before you step away to allow them their privacy. This will mean that any noises occurring while toileting are not overheard, if possible. Undisturbed time and not feeling rushed will make the toileting experience less stressful for the patient.

Aids and adaptations

Individuals have the option of a catheter or **penile sheath** while remaining an inpatient.

▶ A penile sheath is a soft, flexible silicone sheath that fits over the penis and has medical adhesive on the inside. It has an outlet tube at the tip, which drains into a catheter bag. There is a low risk of infection but there is always the risk of some leakage.

▶ A catheter is more invasive, with less chance of leakage, and is sometimes a patient's preference. When the catheter tube is inserted through the urethra an aqueous lubricant reduces the risk of pain and discomfort. Once the tube reaches the bladder a balloon at the tip of the tube is inflated so it remains in place and is not ejected with bladder contractions. When removing the tube, the balloon is deflated to allow it to be removed with ease.

Key term

Penile sheath: silicone tube condom attached to a urine collection bag.

Maintaining the individual's privacy and dignity

Maintaining the individual's privacy and dignity during their personal toileting time is more difficult with patients who are bedbound. Consideration for the safety of a patient while toileting independently will form part of a mobility risk assessment and safety measures may need to be put in place. For example, a patient who is at risk of a fall going to and using the toilet must be informed not to attempt this on their own.

▶ Pulling the curtains around a bed visually protects a person, but those with a condition causing Type 7 Bristol stool chart **defecation** will be conscious of noise heard by other patients and visitors.

▶ Moving a patient bed nearer the toilet facility can benefit others, as can the use of the call alarm.

▶ A patient may be able to be offered choices such as having support to use a commode rather than using a bed pan or using the toilet with support rather than the commode.

▶ Hygiene support after toileting may be all that is needed for some patients, perineal care for hygiene must include the patient washing their hands afterwards; this may require a prompt.

▶ Incontinence pads in various sizes should be readily available and patients informed about the correct size for them.

Mental and/or physical ability to use the toilet

Toileting takes a level of mental ability, and certain patients will need support with this.

Physically being able to get to the toilet on time, the ability to lower down to seated and wipe all require different levels of support. Personal hygiene and infection prevention are important factors every time the toilet is used. Toileting requires reasonable control of movement and for some aspects the ability to twist.

A patient with cognitive impairment affecting memory, such as dementia, may not recognise a toilet and can transiently forget where it is located. In some instances putting up the seat is forgotten and the toilet is used with the lid down. Incidents like this are undignified and can be distressing.

Key term

Defecation: discharging faeces from the digestive system.

In cases of spinal cord damage and paralysis, an injury above level T11/T12 vertebrae means muscles around the sphincters and pelvic floor may be tight, leading to constipation and no or slow excretion of urine. An injury of these vertebrae and below can affect muscles, meaning they may be loose and more relaxed, which leads to stool incontinence. Incontinence is a physical condition; it restricts what a person can do and how they feel.

Nerve and muscle actions work together for bladder and bowel control, and brain degeneration, such as in the case of motor neurone disease (MND), or a cognitive decline, such as in dementia, mean limitations in the control of the sphincters that control the outflow of urine and faeces.

Research

S2.11 Support or enable individuals to maintain continence

Continence issues are often related to weakened muscles around the bladder and anus. Causes can include damage to the perineum during childbirth, a neurological condition or obesity.

There are a number of different types of continence issues such as urge incontinence, which is the sudden, unexpected and frequent need to urinate. There can be a problem with the bladder's detrusor muscles, which ordinarily relax as the bladder fills, spontaneously contracting and causing leakage.

What exercises can improve the level of incontinence a patient is experiencing?

Personal hygiene

An important aspect of adequate personal hygiene is the physical and mental effect of feeling fresh and clean, such as clean teeth and fresh breath or clean hair washed with a pleasant smelling shampoo. Some people need to wash their hair every day but it is more common to be two or three times a week. For Afro hair, recommendations are washing hair every 7–10 days. It is important to cleanse the scalp to ensure optimum health and hair growth.

Daily personal hygiene tasks can become a cause of anxiety for patients who under usual circumstances take pride in their appearance. For example, being restricted to hospital facilities and without their usual toiletries, a patient may be unable to maintain their usual appearance which can affect an individual's overall wellbeing.

Food spillage by a patient who drips food while eating a meal in bed, which would be addressed immediately at home, may need to wait while other tasks take priority in a hospital ward, such as other patients being given support to eat, or a medication round for tablets required right after eating has taken place.

Infection prevention

Patients' lack of hand and nail hygiene can lead to a transference of bacteria, viruses and fungus, leading to infections and diseases, like gastroenteritis, flu, hepatitis A, athletes foot and a mite transfer causing a scabies spread. Bathing, washing and wearing clean clothing all help to prevent infection. Additionally, feeling clean can lift a patient's mood. Intimate care – the cleaning of the breasts, genital area and, to some extent, washing the hair – is very personal.

You have already learned about the physical steps for a bed bath and cleansing of the vaginal and penile areas. These are physical actions and, during such tasks, you must use effective communication to prepare and reassure patients who already feel vulnerable.

Dignity and privacy

By using a modesty blanket, covering exposed parts of the body that have been washed or are next on the list, you will preserve a patient's dignity at a sensitive time. Privacy encompasses a patient's preferences, such as their own nickname for the genital area and making sure conversations are not overheard, as well as actions such as shaving pubic areas.

You can reassure patients by distracting them from the cause of their distress; use appropriate humour or talk about what is going on outside the ward, such as the weather.

Personal clothing from home is comforting, allowing a patient to feel at ease with an item when almost everything else feels out of their control.

Promoting independence

A patient who has been cared for for a long time can start to relinquish (give up) their role in personal care and dressing, moving towards dependency. If you ask a patient like this what they would like to wear and their reply is 'You choose, I don't care', this signals a need for greater inclusion.

Techniques to encourage a person to choose clothing can be more covert so that this is not disempowering. Describing two or three items, holding them up and giving good eye contact, with a smile and slight nod, inviting the patient to choose, is preferable to telling them they must choose.

Where possible, promote independence in how personal care is executed; patients who either do not or partially self-care can be encouraged to do more through empowering communication practices and working at the pace of the patient. For example, you could hold a rolled-up sock in front of a person's feet and encourage them to choose which one goes on first; for example, their right foot might be the one they have started with all their lives.

Intimate care

Personal hygiene tasks that include the vagina, penis and anus require direct contact and exposure of the sexual parts of the body. Faecal incontinence in particular can reach or cover these parts, and regular cleaning will prevent soreness and infection.

There is a high risk of urinary tract infection and cleanliness must be carefully maintained. A female patient has a shorter urethra than a male and the vaginal entrance is in close proximity to the anus and faecal output. Wiping should be from front to back to avoid the transfer of faeces in the vaginal area.

This process requires sensitivity and steps need to be taken to maintain a patient's privacy and dignity, for example during hygiene tasks, as well as recognising it is undignified for them to be left wet or soiled. Reassurance is essential throughout, and communication that distracts may benefit a patient's emotional comfort.

Checking skin integrity

This is a really important role – skin integrity must be checked on a regular basis, particularly for those at a high risk of developing pressure injury. Supporting a person to bathe and dress gives the health professional an ideal opportunity to review the skin and identify any marks or bruising that need treatment or assessing.

Personal appearance

Supporting a patient to maintain their personal appearance is part of overall holistic care, as it can benefit their mental health.

Upholding and supporting personal choice and supporting independence

Complementing a patient's choice and supporting their independence help with forming positive self-esteem and interpersonal relationships.

A ward's temperature will usually be between 23°C and 27°C. This is comfortably warm, meaning lighter clothes should be worn by most patients. An older patient may feel the cold if they are underweight and have less insulating fat. There are certain medical conditions with the symptom pyrexia, a temperature above 37°C, where a patient will feel warmer and may decide on minimal clothing for the duration. A new inpatient may need to be informed about average ward temperature before making their own decision as to what to wear.

The use of foot coverings avoids having bare feet on the floor as part of infection prevention, and non-slip items are suggested to avoid incidents of injury through slipping. Although a hospital gown, disposable underwear and foot coverings can be provided, patients are encouraged to bring clothing from home, to support their individuality, empowerment and comfort.

A menu choice may need a more detailed verbal description to help a patient decide what they want to eat. Influencing a patient's choice by personal input which is leading is not person-centred and should be avoided.

Recognising altered body image

For individuals who have had an accident with life-changing consequences or had a limb removed, such as in the removal of damaged tissue in bacterial meningitis to stop the spread of the infection, the change is sudden and the patient will need time and support with recognising their altered appearance and functioning.

The impact of such changes will differ from patient to patient, for a number of reasons. Some may be very sensitive while others are willing to joke. It is a period of grieving a loss, which is a personal journey. The wound will need care, during which you can encourage communication, answer patients' questions honestly and communicate that there will be good and bad days ahead. You should give clear instructions to the patient to ask for assistance when needed; this is empowering and avoids over-caring.

A patient who has had a mastectomy will have had one or both breasts removed as part of breast cancer treatment. Not everyone can have reconstructive surgery and for those that can there is a significant period for healing. Psychological support such as counselling can be offered and in some cases a referral for mental health care may be appropriate.

Dressing and undressing

While some elements of dressing and undressing can be completed by the patient, others – such as putting on socks or getting an item of clothing over the head – will be challenging for some.

Putting on a cardigan requires an element of spinal and shoulder flexibility, so assistance may be required. The patient can then choose if they have

buttons done up or the garment left open. Effective communication, when giving the individual control over what level of assistance they want, can be achieved using empowering language. Hovering while a person dresses themselves at a slow pace can make the individual feel pressured. They may feel more comfortable if a task such as straightening the bed or refreshing a water jug is carried out as they take their time to complete dressing independently. This means you are available but not standing over the individual.

A patient may be required to wear compression socks due to a medical condition or post-surgery. These are designed to apply pressure to the lower legs, helping to maintain blood flow and reduce discomfort and swelling. They may be used to help prevent health problems like blood clots and deep vein thrombosis (DVT), for example. Compression socks are tight and support to put these on may be required before the patient dresses themselves independently.

Oral care

Correct care and fit of dentures

Dentures are made to fit an individual, but even so they may initially cause discomfort. Dental plaque can build up on dentures as it does on natural teeth; plaque contains pathogens and may cause odour. Most patients will be able to remove and replace their dentures.

Dentures are removed at night and stored in a denture cup, which should be clearly labelled. Cleaning the dentures after removal using a cleaning paste and toothpaste will ensure they are ready at whatever time the patient wakes. The cleaning process should use warm water to rinse and not hot, as this can damage them.

The denture cup should be put in reach of the patient where possible. They will then be able to choose when to put the dentures in. Offering to assist with dentures is good practice.

Promoting dental hygiene

Oral care and promoting dental hygiene twice a day can mean providing a toothbrush and toothpaste for emergency patients. In ANP01 there is more about good mouth care practice.

▶ An individual can need total mouth care support, for example a ventilated patient.
▶ Others may need to be advised on an effective brushing technique and given the means to floss.

If you are working with a patient who may not have a good dental routine as their norm, you could support them to clean their teeth while you are assisting them, and a toothbrush can be provided in the short term.

A patient with a learning disability, cognitive deterioration or poor personal hygiene may need you to demonstrate how they can clean their teeth effectively.

Regular visits to the dentist

It is important to recommend regular visits to the dentist. Medication side effects, such as a dry mouth, increase the risk of gum disease, as do autoimmune illnesses like lupus. Dental checks will need to be more frequent, for example every three months in patients who are at high risk of teeth and gum problems.

Oral health assessment

Without encouragement, a patient who is feeling low may neglect self-care tasks. An oral assessment (Figure 5.4) can form part of an overall assessment for a new admission, if appropriate. If a concern is raised the assessment should be repeated weekly and recorded in the care plan by a medical professional. An oral health assessment offers an opportunity to talk with and listen to the individual.

This assessment covers a risk rating of low, medium or high and covers lips, tongue, teeth and gums as well as inside cheeks and under the tongue. A dry mouth, ulcers and loose or sore dentures may be observed and appropriate actions recorded in the care plan for trainee nurses to give support with. In certain cases it may be necessary for the patient to be referred for specialist care.

In 2016 NICE guideline NG48 was introduced to maintain and improve oral care in nursing homes. The CQC checks that this element of personal care is satisfactory, in both nursing home and hospital inspections.

Mobility
Encourage and support independence

A patient may feel that some aspects of their life are out of their control due to the effects of their illness, and you may need to encourage them to carry out self-care independently as much as they can. Others who are in hospital for the first time may make assumptions, for example believing they can hand over their care to nursing staff while they are on the ward. Talking with a patient about what they feel they can and cannot do will enable conversations between the patient and health professional about what their limitations are and how the health professional can support them.

Appropriate risk assessment

Being independently mobile enables a patient to move freely and independently around the healthcare environment. Despite this, however, a mobility risk assessment must be carried out to assess the potential for falls, which may occur as a result of the illness or other existing conditions.

A mobility assessment, such as the Elderly Mobility Scale (EMS), analyses the capability and safety of a patient carrying out tasks. For the EMS there are seven ADLs; a score of above 14 is seen as being independently safe, 10 to 14 is seen as requiring some assistance and below 10 is high risk and seen as needing an increasing level of support.

In some cases, the internationally recognised Morse Fall Scale assessment tool is used to identify risk factors for falls in hospitalised patients. The total score may be used to predict future falls, but it is more important to identify risk factors using the scale and then plan care to address those risk factors. Not all NHS hospitals use this and you may come across the Falls Risk Assessment Tool (FRAT) or the observation system, Avoiding Falls Level of Observation Assessment Tool (AFLOAT), which aims to reduce risk and improve patient safety and patient outcomes and experience.

Before any movement takes place, ensuring a patient has enough room to manoeuvre, a walking frame within easy reach and instructions to use the nurse call bell will be an outcome of an assessment of this kind. A physiotherapist is involved in the assessment and an occupational therapist will suggest appropriate mobility aids where required. A mobility assessment may also be used in conjunction with or instead of a Tinetti balance assessment, where appropriate.

Aids and adaptations

There are medical conditions which affect balance, such as benign paroxysmal positional vertigo (BPPV); others cause muscle weakness and tremors, such as Parkinson's Disease or Multiple Sclerosis. Supporting mobility aids can be precautionary and need to be identified in an assessment.

Deterioration of progressive conditions needs monitoring so more supportive equipment is provided when needed. Some medical conditions such as a hip fracture will mean a mobility aid such as a walking frame is needed temporarily. Improvements during the healing process could mean the frame is no longer needed and the patient will move to using one or two walking sticks.

▶ A patient can be given an assistive aid for the first time, given instruction and checked to see it is used safely; a question and answer opportunity will lower the risk of an injury caused by a fall.

{Mouth Care Matters

NHS
Health Education England

Patient Name:	
D.O.B	
MRN Number	
NHS Number	

Mouth care assessment
Complete **WEEKLY** if the patient has a red box ticked
on the front page/or if their condition deteriorates

Look in the patient's mouth using a LIGHT SOURCE and carry out a WEEKLY mouth care assessment. Mark as L, M or H in the white box under today's date and sign.

DATE: DATE: DATE: DATE: DATE:

	LOW RISK (L)	MEDIUM RISK (M)	HIGH RISK (H)*					
Lips	• Pink & moist	• Dry/cracked • Difficulty opening the mouth	• Swollen • Ulcerated					
Action	None	Dry mouth care	Refer to DOCTOR					
Tongue	• Pink & moist	• Dry/fissured/shiny	• Looks abnormal • White coating • Very sore/ulcerated					
Action	None	Dry mouth care	Refer to DOCTOR					
Teeth & gums	• Clean • Teeth not broken • Teeth not loose	• Unclean • Broken teeth (no pain) • Bleeding/inflamed gums	• Severe pain • Facial swelling					
Action	2 x daily toothbrushing	Daily toothbrushing and clean the mouth	Refer to DOCTOR or dental team	Advise the patient to visit their dentist on discharge if there any problems with their teeth that do not require urgent treatment in hospital				
Cheeks/ palate & under tongue	• Clean • Saliva present • Looks healthy	• Mouth dry • Sticky secretions • Food debris • Ulcer <10 days	• Very dry/painful • Ulcer >10 days • Widespread ulceration • Looks abnormal					
Action	None	Clean the mouth/dry mouth care/ulcer care	Refer to DOCTOR	An ulcer present for more than **2 weeks** must be referred to the doctor				
Dentures	• Clean • Comfortable	• Unclean • Loose • Patient will not remove	• Lost • Broken and unable to wear					
Action	Clean daily	• Denture care • Dental fixative • Encourage removal	DATIX if lost or refer to dental team if broken	Remember to place the denture sunflower at the patient's bedside. Advise the patient to visit their dentist on discharge if the denture is loose				

*For patients who are unable to communicate or cooperate with a mouth care assessment, signs of mouth related problems may include not eating/drinking, facial swelling & behavioural changes

Signature:

Dry mouth care	Ulcer care	Denture care
Frequent sips of water unless nil by mouth	Rinse mouth with saline	Advise the patient to leave denture out at night in a named denture pot with a lid
Moisturise dry mouth gel onto the tongue, cheeks and palate	Anti-inflammatory mouth spray – discuss with doctor	If the patient has oral thrush, soak in chlorhexidine (0.2%) mouthwash for 15 minutes twice a day, rinse thoroughly and encourage the patient to leave the denture out whilst the mouth heals
Hydrate with a moist toothbrush	ULCER PRESENT FOR MORE THAN 2 WEEKS; REFER TO DOCTOR	
Apply lip balm to dry lips		
Keep mouth clean		

Figure 5.4 A mouth care assessment form

Case study

S2.14 Support or enable individuals to be mobile

Using the Elderly Mobility Scale (EMS) form or online calculator, assess the scale for this patient and interpret his support needs.

Viraj is 93 and has suffered a minor heart attack. His discharge is being planned, and you have been asked to complete an EMS. You have been caring for Viraj for five days and have supported him with using a walking frame to go to the toilet, speaking to a relative on the nursing station phone and taking him to a quiet space for him to carry out puja worship by himself.

You have supported and observed the following:
▶ Viraj has used the hospital bed rails to sit up and lower himself back down.
▶ He can make his way to the edge of the bed sitting; he needs support to stand but this is minimal and can be carried out with only yourself to support him for safety.
▶ He can then stand after a short spell of dizziness lasting about four or five seconds, and he needs the walking frame to be passed to him as reaching can upset his balance.
▶ Once supported by the walking frame, Viraj can walk for approximately 12 m to the toilet, which takes him roughly a minute.
▶ He is able to transfer from the walking frame to the toilet frame, a reach of 20 cm, and has the call bell at his side if he needs support to get off the toilet and back onto the walking frame.
▶ As he gets stronger this need has become less frequent, which you have recorded.

▶ A stabilising walking frame can be enough to enable an individual to move from bed to hospital chair and back.
▶ Raising the height of a chair is an adaptation for people who need a hand to sit and stand, reducing the drop and demand for leg muscle strength.

Repositioning

The importance of helping with **repositioning** for a patient who has reduced mobility cannot be underestimated. Repositioning ensures that blood flow to the tissues is maintained and the risk of developing pressure injuries is reduced. There is a variety of recommendations around the timing of repositioning, but with the addition of pressure-relieving equipment such as airflow mattresses, the usual schedule of repositioning is around every four hours.

▶ Pressure injuries occur when the blood flow to the tissue is reduced. This most commonly occurs over the bony prominences such as the hip, shoulders, heels and elbows.
▶ A patient who is unwell but able to reposition themselves may need prompting to change their position. In some cases, pain medication can increase drowsiness and reduce the patient's natural desire to move and reposition themselves. Close monitoring of patients for this reason is essential.

Explaining the purpose of repositioning and agreeing the timing of actions with the patient is best practice where possible. Talking to the patient before, during and after any supportive movements keeps them informed and is a common courtesy.

Environmental factors

Environmental factors are responsible for patient slips, trips and falls, whether this is on the hospital ward or in their own home in the community. Hazards such as floor rugs, a change in height or pattern of the floor surfaces, poor lighting or steps in and out of the property should be noted on a risk assessment and where possible adaptations made to reduce the risk.

Being vigilant during home visits and reporting any other concerns form part of a risk management review for improvements.

Sleep and rest

How sleep and rest enhance recovery and improve physical and mental wellbeing

The importance of sleep, as a restorative function, should not be underestimated (Figure 5.5). Research shows that sleep deficit has been linked to obesity, type 2 diabetes and cardiovascular disease; it also slows the healing process.

Source: Knutson, K.L. and Van Cauter, E. (2008), 'Associations between sleep loss and increased risk of obesity and diabetes', *Annals of the New York Academy of Sciences*, 1129:287-304. **doi: 10.1196/annals.1417.033.**

Practice points

S2.11 Support or enable individuals to maintain continence

S2.12 Support or enable individuals to maintain good personal hygiene

S2.13 Support or enable individuals to dress and undress

S2.14 Support or enable individuals to be mobile

You will need a manikin or partner for this demonstration. Your task is to produce a training video where you narrate what you are doing and the purpose of each action, covering all points in the skills criteria S2.11–14.

You are nurse on a ward. Your patient rings the call bell as they require support with toileting; their incontinence pad is uncomfortable. They are recovering after surgery and they are able to walk with the support of a walking frame. After talking with the patient you decide to get them to the hospital toilet and shower room safely. You will be on hand to assist with toileting, bathing, oral care and dressing.

▶ What do you need to do to prepare before the patient makes their way to the bathing area using a walking frame?

▶ Explain what steps you would go through in order to make a training video for new trainee nurses. There is a toilet frame, shower rail and shower chair available for safe use.

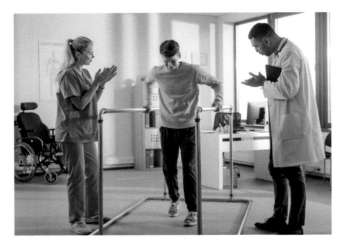

▲ Figure 5.5 Sufficient sleep and rest will produce better results in physiotherapy sessions

Some suggestions for promoting rest and sleep might include:

▶ Delay carrying out physiological measurement observations on a sleeping patient if they are not essential. Always check this with a senior member of staff.

▶ Keep noise to a minimum and handle the patient gently so as not to disturb them unnecessarily.

▶ Encouraging a patient to sit in a chair during the day or to sit up in bed with mental stimulation may help to orientate their body to the natural day and night rhythms. This includes being dressed in clothes during the day rather than staying in nightwear all day.

▶ Using earplugs and blocking disturbances caused by light using a face mask may be the choice of some patients.

▶ Appropriate lighting, natural light and darkness on the ward will help to orientate patients, particularly if they are living with dementia.

How sleep and rest increase productivity

A well-rested patient will be more **productive** in a physiotherapy or counselling session, for example, and will have an increased chance of a positive outlook.

Expressing sexuality

There is a lot of one-to-one contact time during activities for daily living, occasions when a patient can ask questions, be reassured and express themselves. Communicating acceptance and compassion for all supports an individual to be themselves. Expressing sexuality is hugely personal but an important part of who we are.

It is a basic human right for people to express their sexuality. Sometimes a patient may need reassurance and encouragement to empower them to do so. This could include explaining how they are protected by law and that all service providers will provide care which shows fairness and equality.

The CQC published 'Promoting sexual safety through empowerment' in February 2020, which guides providers on how to support people's sexuality in adult social care. The same can be applied to healthcare as trainee nurses use a person-centred approach to care, considering people's holistic needs. Understanding of a person's sexual identity should help with knowing how to support a patient appropriately to express their sexuality in a way that supports, empowers and protects them from harm.

Some patients with a cognitive deficit or who are victims of long-term sexual abuse may overtly display sexuality, creating a risk which will need to be closely monitored. It is important that healthcare workers build up a good professional relationship and trust with a patient of another gender to themselves. The use of effective interpersonal communication skills is important and provides reassurance.

Source: CQC (2020), 'Promoting sexual safety through empowerment', www.cqc.org.uk/sites/default/files/20200225_sexual_safety_sexuality.pdf

Gender expression

It is good practice to ask individuals about gender pronouns as part of a hospital ward admission process. Patients who attend outpatients or are cared for in the community should be given an opportunity to openly discuss gender expression. In both cases, effective communication skills require sensitivity, as this can be a deeply personal issue for some individuals.

Learning from patients who have experienced discrimination will provide you with a deeper understanding of the challenges faced by a diverse population. Engaging a person to talk about their life, what is important to them and their future aspirations can be an opportunity to build trust between the patient and healthcare giver, and demonstrates good interpersonal skills. For example:

- ▶ respecting an individual's style preferences, for example hairstyle, style of dress or make-up, and admiring individuality support healthy self-esteem
- ▶ make-up can be used by some as a camouflage and protective layer for a person who feels vulnerable and anxious
- ▶ a particular item of clothing may hold sentimental value or have meaning, making a patient feel stronger or less exposed
- ▶ ignoring an obvious statement of individuality, such as noticeable multiple hair colours, comes across as avoidance; taking a naturally occurring opportunity to make a positive comment about their expression of uniqueness is preferable.

Cultural preferences

Sexuality and identity are an important part of a patient's life. Some may believe this is private information and may be reluctant to discuss this with someone who is unknown to them. Others may welcome the opportunity to discuss their thoughts.

A patient may overtly display signs of sexuality, in their appearance or in open conversation for example. Being guided by the individual themselves as to the level of confidentiality they prefer means they have ownership;

a patient may want this part of their life acknowledged publicly, for example talking about Pride celebrations.

Females may require a health worker of the same gender to provide care, and if there is CCTV in a bedroom area they might not want to be observed by a male.

The impact of certain conditions

Patients will have limitations and specific physical needs depending on their personal situation and health status. For example, some illnesses, such as anal cancer, have a higher likelihood of occurrence in people who are gay and a patient's fear of this being overheard adds to a distressing diagnosis.

Most patients will have anxieties around being in hospital, emotional needs such as that for reassurance, and fears that require distraction techniques. Research has shown that lesbian, gay and bisexual patients have an elevated risk of an anxiety or depression diagnosis.

Sources: Bostwick, W.B., Boyd, C.J., Hughes, T.L. and McCabe, S.E. (2010), 'Dimensions of sexual orientation and the prevalence of mood and anxiety disorders in the United States', *American Journal of Public Health*, 100(3):468–475. doi: **10.2105/AJPH.2008.152942.**

Bos, H.M., Boschloo, L., Schoevers, R.A. and Sandfort, T.G. (2015), 'Depression and anxiety in patients with and without same-sex attraction: differences in clinical expression, lifestyle factors, and vulnerability indicators', *Brain and Behaviour*, 5(9): e00363. doi: **10.1002/brb3.363.**

Certain conditions, such as dementia, can cause a person to forget their religious or cultural preferences, for instance the desire to eat certain foods or attend a place of worship on a specific day.

Professional boundaries

Boundaries refer to what is acceptable and unacceptable at work or outside of work relating to patients and other members of staff. Standards protect a nurse and their patients' safety; clinical daily activities are always in the best interest of an individual, and supporting communication should remain positive and uphold the professional reputation of the NMC. Any evidence of sexually inappropriate behaviour or unprofessional language or activity may result in disciplinary action. This includes accepting gifts or money for care.

A hospital will have a Professional Boundaries and Relationship Policy, giving clarity for all. This can be referred to if someone is unsure. Certain terms and actions should be avoided, such as keeping a secret, vocally taking sides against other professionals or relatives, or being flirtatious, even in jest. In a professional relationship there should be no hint of any kind of romance or sexual attraction. Having unprofessional relationships with vulnerable patients and acting in such a way as to bring the hospital or community trust into disrepute will result in an immediate suspension while this is investigated and dealt with swiftly as an attempt to regain trust in the organisation and provision. A report will also be sent to both the CQC and NMC. Innocent suggestions can be misconstrued, such as saying you will 'have a word' with a late visitor; something that was intended as humour can, when repeated, lead to a complaint.

A patient who has been sexually abused as a child may not fully understand appropriate behaviours, linking trying to please with a person who is dominating, in authority, displaying provocative behaviour.

Confusion over gender and sexuality may be displayed in inappropriate behaviour. Talking honestly and signposting the patient for support by experts in this area is good practice and a supportive measure.

Politely making the professional boundaries clear may not improve some situations. In cases where this is a problem, swapping patients with another professional to minimise contact is advisable, or you may need to have another professional attend while you are carrying out a one-to-one consultation.

There needs to be a space between the nurse's authority and the patient's vulnerability: respect the imbalance, safeguard and avoid over-involvement, at the same time as delivering therapeutic care. Empathising as a human builds a bridge but crossing that bridge by being overfamiliar is misconduct. Spending more time than is necessary with a patient once is acceptable but doing so repeatedly is not. Seeking advice from a supervisor about a particular patient's behaviour is good practice when you have concerns, such as being offered an expensive gift.

K2.2 The different types of long-term conditions and their impact on activities of daily living

Physical conditions

Chronic long-term physical conditions, for example chronic fatigue, can take time to be diagnosed and there will be a period of acceptance. Medications to manage symptoms and improve quality of life involve a trial period that can end in the need for a different prescription due to the side effects experienced. The period of time during which a medication that will have the desired effect is sought is frustrating for both prescribing physician and patient. The individual can feel demoralised, defeated and reluctant to continue trialling drugs. Couple this with their new physical limitations and being unable to complete activities of daily living without support and, for the majority of patients, the emotional impact of the long-term condition can often outweigh the physical effects.

A musculoskeletal injury, such as a fractured limb, may result in a period of restrictive activity and movement during the healing process. Depending on the severity or location of the damage, it may significantly impact the patient's ability to carry out self-care tasks. Their speed of getting out of bed and walking to the shower, for example, will be slower, and the patient may need a

---

Key term

Appendectomy: surgery under general anaesthetic to remove the appendix.

Practice points

S2.15 Support or enable individuals to rest, sleep and keep safe
S2.16 Support or enable individuals to express their sexuality

You will need a partner for this demonstration. Your task is to produce a training video to promote communication in a clinical setting.

You are a nurse on a ward. You check on a patient who looks upset. It is their first time in hospital and away from home. They have had an emergency **appendectomy** and share their concerns about feeling vulnerable. Their home environment is living with a supportive family who accept that they will complete their transgender surgery soon. In the hospital setting the patient feels scared and alone, and tells you they will not be able to sleep.

▶ Explain the importance of sleep and rest; suggest ideas of how to get quality sleep while in hospital.
▶ Using effective communication skills, reassure the patient and encourage them to be themselves for positive emotional wellbeing.

Evaluate your training video performance using Gibbs' reflective cycle to identify areas for improvement.

waterproof covering for broken skin or a plaster cast if appropriate.

A patient who has no or limited ability to reposition themselves independently will be at greater risk of developing pressure injuries. This risk will increase if the person has a very high or very low BMI, or if they are living with continence issues. There is specific learning for this in ANPO3, which focuses on skin integrity.

As with many long-term conditions, it is important to consider the patient's mental health and provide support for them to come to terms with and manage the ongoing restrictions that may occur as a result. Personal characteristics such as having a positive outlook can help with patient resilience, so being able to offer support and encouragement is therefore a key part of the health professional's role.

Obesity

In 2018, the Royal College of Physicians stated that obesity should be recognised as a chronic progressive disease that has biological, pathological and genetic factors as contributors. The World Health Organization (WHO) had previously declared obesity a disease in 1997.

Bariatric patients may experience problems managing their skin hygiene as obesity puts a strain on lymphatic vessels, resulting in swelling to the affected limb or body part. **Oedema** (Figures 5.6 and 5.7), and **cellulitis** are common in the lower legs of patients living with obesity, and they may require frequent antibiotics to manage these conditions. Excessive **adipose tissue**, which ordinarily insulates the body, has a poor blood supply; lack of oxygenated blood to a wound will slow down the healing process.

Bariatric specialised hospital equipment is strengthened for a larger weight capacity and wider than standard for comfort. A BMI calculation can be obtained using a specially calibrated digital chair weighing scale, which records higher weights than an average domestic bathroom weighing scale. Furthermore, modified moving, handling and lifting

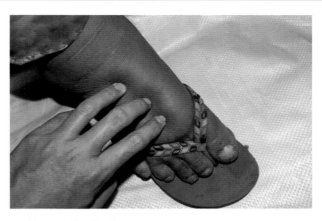

▲ Figure 5.6 Oedema

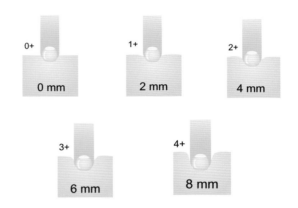

0+ No pitting edema
1+ Mild pitting edema. 2 mm depression that disappears rapidly.
2+ Moderate pitting edema. 4 mm depression that disappears in 10-15 seconds.
3+ Moderately severe pitting edema. 6mm depression that may last more than 1 minute.
4+ Severe pitting edema. 8 mm depression that can last more than 2 minutes.

▲ Figure 5.7 Pitting Oedema grading

techniques are often required to prevent injury to the health professional and patient during transportation. Seeking advice from bariatric experts or moving and handling experts is essential where this process is required.

Mental health conditions

Specialist communication skills are necessary when supporting a patient who has a cognitive impairment. In conditions such as Down's syndrome or moderate dementia, it is common that the person will have a lower level of understanding and comprehension. They may also have difficulty retaining and recalling information. The level of difficulty will be personal to that individual.

Talking with a patient's advocate who accompanies them will assist you in pitching their care at the right level. The patient may have a trigger that will cause them instant distress, or a term or item that gives them comfort. For the health professional, ascertaining the

> ### Key terms
>
> **Oedema:** a fluid build-up, often in ankles and hands, causing swelling and puffiness.
>
> **Cellulitis:** painful bacterial infection of the dermis layer of the skin.
>
> **Adipose tissue:** a type of connective tissue that specialises in the storage of fat.

individual's communication level becomes a priority in order to ensure they are involved in the decision making where possible.

If a patient lacks capacity to understand the importance of undertaking daily living activities

The Mental Capacity Act 2005 (amended 2019) describes daily living activities, and in situations where a person does not have capacity to understand or undertake them, personalised care is of paramount importance. Each patient's needs are unique, and consulting the patient themselves, their carers and relatives can help you to build a picture that enables you to support them with the activities of daily living (ADLs) in the most appropriate manner. Learning disability nurses are professionals who have expertise in the care of individuals living with neurodiversity. They have the expertise to advise other care professionals about the most appropriate support for a patient who has a cognitive impairment on a non-specialist ward.

If a patient lacks motivation

A common symptom of a mental health condition is a lack of desire or motivation to undertake ADLs, or not recognising their importance. For example:

▶ A patient with depression may not see the point or worth of good personal hygiene, nutrition or appearance.

▶ People living with severe obsessive-compulsive disorder (OCD) may have a germ-related obsession and compulsions around excessive cleaning.

▶ In many cases of mental illness, intrusive thoughts replace normal thinking; the frustration and anger that result could be directed at the nurse who is in charge of their care. In these circumstances, a risk assessment will identify that it is safer for staff to work in pairs to provide the support the individual needs. This can also be a requirement to ensure staff safety.

▶ A person with mild OCD can find themselves in a position of heightened fear, associating hospitals with infections and death.

Encouraging open communication, recording and reporting concerns will enable actions to be taken to better support a patient who is not coping in a ward environment. Registered mental health nurses can share their experience and techniques as good practice, which will help other health professionals to care for patients who require more specialist support, in addition to being an opportunity for learning.

If a patient lacks cognition around personal safety

In some cases, a patient may lack cognition around personal safety when undertaking ADLs. For example:

▶ slippery, wet floors in walk-in showers

▶ rinsing off soap

▶ drinking hot drinks.

A risk assessment for the individual in this situation will assess the level of care and support needed to prevent harm. Assistance with prompts may be needed when the patient is bathing, eating and drinking.

Health and safety

All hospital walk-in showers have control measures in place to prevent/reduce the incidence of slips and falls. Heat and humidity can cause dizziness, so it is advisable for a patient to use a shower stool/chair to remain seated while they are showering. A walking frame can be used to transfer to seated and balance assisted by using the shower grab rails. Patients should be encouraged to take their time.

Sensory impairment

The term sensory impairment covers all the senses. When a patient with a visual or hearing impairment is hospitalised they may be unable to complete activities of daily living without support. An initial communication assessment will give an outline of the patient's abilities as a starting point, but the finer points will require further discussion with the patient, a family member or an informal carer as appropriate. Some examples may be:

▶ A ward can be noisy, with unfamiliar noises due to the hard flooring and lack of soft furnishings. A side room may be more suitable if this is an option or being mindful of the patient's experience.

▶ A patient who has a sight impairment could find the environment detrimental to their mental wellbeing and be more dependent than they would ordinarily be. Extra consideration and time should be given for orientation and communication.

▶ Talking with the patient to find out their specific needs may require a wheelchair move, finding a quieter space and investigating what they are capable of and where full or partial support is needed.

▶ Minimal support, for example passing a flannel when they are washing and being able to describe mobility equipment, may be all that is requested.

▶ A patient who has a hearing impairment can write down what support they feel they need; a British Sign Language interpreter is an option for an individual whose hearing has been impaired for some time.

▶ An older person with a progressive deterioration in hearing and who requires a high level of support can use a picture exchange communication system (PECS) to indicate, for example, their level of pain, their thirst or their urge to toilet.

▶ Alternatively, a document listing daily living tasks, broken down into smaller tasks, can be used. With this approach a patient takes their time in ticking what they can do and identifying tasks they need support with. This method is empowering and allows for slow processing, as the document is given to the patient to complete at their own pace.

K2.3 How to support or enable individuals to complete activities of daily living in line with their care plan, using a person-centred and enabling approach

A patient's care plan is a document that includes their medical history, personal details, a course of action with expected outcomes, a review and monitoring plan, and details of who is doing what and when. This is the basis of a personalised holistic plan of care which enables a patient to have autonomy and tailored support.

When working with a patient there are different factors to consider outside the plan, as described below, recognising their uniqueness, adapting or modifying care practices and listening to an individual's perspectives.

Age groups

A care plan will document a patient's date of birth and age; the finer details, such as maturity, how a patient feels about their age or ageing, is not recorded. **Age group** characteristics tend to be generic, not personal:

▶ There are sprightly **octogenarians** who might be willing to try a suggested treatment plan and have a positive outlook on their treatment.

▶ In contrast there are patients of the same age who feel withdrawing from society is part of the ageing process and may demonstrate reluctance to take part in planning their care in conjunction with the health professionals.

It should not be assumed that a person in their early twenties will be more conscious about their appearance than someone in their nineties. Without

talking with the patient to understand their views on treatment, their perception and reality is not known.

Environment

The hospital environment first thing in the morning compared to during late afternoon visiting time is very different, and can impact on a patient's confidence, concentration and outlook. Depending on the patient's relationship with their visitors, this may affect their behaviours, for example they might become more self-conscious and not drink from a spouted cup or they may like to demonstrate their coping skills to prove their acceptance of care support.

When the ward is quiet and one-to-one support for mobility is carried out, one person may feel motivated to utilise the time to improve, while another may reject the attention due to feeling pressured to perform.

Coming to terms with a sudden reduction in independence, due to a stroke, for instance, or change in body image after surgery may take a period of time to adjust, impacting on a person's willingness to engage in therapies on a ward. When a person is discharged and has accepted such changes they may be more willing to participate as an outpatient.

A healthcare environment can cause white coat syndrome when blood pressure is taken, or give rise to feelings of helplessness and anxieties about treatment and unfamiliar surroundings. For others there is an element of security; being surrounded by experts reduces their worries, making them feel positive about recovery and their return home.

For most, having care delivered within their own home is preferable where possible. Home comforts can make an individual happier to attempt ADLs with support. Empathising with an individual patient, listening, offering methods that enable and empower them, reflecting and being open to further modification, support the provision of individualised care.

Religion

Article 9 of the Human Rights Act 1998 states that a person has protected rights to hold both religious and non-religious beliefs. The cultural needs of patients must be addressed without prejudice. A religion is personal to an individual, and levels of devoutness and commitment will vary: assuming one person who is Catholic requires the same provision as another is a mistake. Religious texts can be interpreted differently by people of the same religion, and originating from a specific regional location can slightly alter practice.

Key term

Octogenarian: a person aged from 80 to 89.

Meeting patients' individual and specific cultural needs, for example foods that can/cannot be eaten, requires confirmation. A quick conversation, giving opportunities for a particular practice to be discussed, avoids misunderstandings and supports person-centred care. For example:

▶ Judaism and Islam prohibit the eating of pork and pig products such as gelatine.

▶ Muslim and Hindu females can observe purdah; the restrictions on social practices and expected behaviours in connection with this can be at various levels – purdah was not traditionally observed by women of a lower class, for instance.

▶ A seriously ill patient may not be dressed in religious clothing during their treatment and will have areas of the body exposed at times, such as wound checks, that causes distress.

▶ The CQC has guidance on the support of religious or spiritual beliefs practices, for example encouraging people to keep religious or spiritual items with them, such as the Bible or Quran, and for these to be stored safely.

▶ In terms of specific methods or times of worship, some events – such as communal worship – are streamed online when they cannot be attended in person; it is good practice to provide access.

▶ Some Muslim people may want to fast during Ramadan. Adjustment to the timing of their medication is needed, as this should be taken with food where possible.

Research

S2.17 Appropriately manage situations in which individuals cannot do things for themselves

Patients facing a communication barrier may not be able to discuss their cultural/religious needs openly. An individual's beliefs are very important to them, and actions to maintain their right to dignity, equality and inclusion are supported by the Equality Act 2010. Dietary requirements, prayer, religious texts and important traditions should be respected where possible and the patient supported to carry out religious practice as required. Consulting a family member is good practice and a patient's notes will usually identify their religion.

Click on this link to read about fasting and religion: **www.britannica.com/topic/fasting** then create your own resource with relevant points pertaining to caring for a patient.

Individual needs and preferences

Needs

Monitoring health through observations to source measurement data, ensuring needs are met through personal care, toileting, and adequate fluid and nutrition are all clinical tasks that meet individual needs.

For example, a patient's motivation to self-care could be that they are working towards a goal such as returning to work or walking their daughter down the aisle at her wedding.

Finding out about a patient's preferred way of doing a particular care task will build a better working relationship; attention to detail and keeping an open mind are delivering compassionate care as described in the 6Cs of nursing. Reminding a patient of their goal can be helpful if appropriate: when their sense of purpose is diminishing, for example, revisiting their intended target could reinvigorate them.

A setback in treatment is demoralising, and adapting communication and the delivery of care plan tasks can positively reframe and encourage forward thinking, looking past the temporary disappointment. A positive patient experience enables medical and nursing staff to build a good working relationship with them. Future medical needs such as further treatments will feel less daunting, and the patient is likely to be more co-operative and compliant.

Preferences

Some patients may prefer to be fully dressed during the day, whereas others are happy to remain in their nightwear. An individual may want support in getting into a chair for visiting times or to have the bed back lifted upright, while others would prefer to remain slightly elevated.

Preferences around the desire to have lights on or off at night or having tea or coffee in the morning, for example, will be documented in the care plan.

Social interaction and positive relationships

A patient can be naturally sociable and easy to interact with, making it easy to gauge how well they are doing. However, social interaction can feel threatening for some, for example a patient admitted following a domestic violence injury. Personality traits are not written in a care plan: for example an introvert is a person who likes their own company and is selective about who they talk to, while an extrovert is talkative and enjoys socialising.

Enabling a patient who is reserved to ask questions is not something that will see immediate results; you will need to build a relationship with them and talk with colleagues in a shift handover to discuss progress and tips on supporting them to ask questions and share their preferences.

A patient who has had a bad experience while being cared for previously may find it difficult to form a positive relationship. Encouraging an exchange about this is a step forward and reservations can be addressed. Building a positive trust-based relationship between patient and professional will require good interpersonal skills. The impact of poor communication or negative experiences in healthcare situations in the past can have a lasting impact.

Health and Care Act 2022

The Health and Care Act 2022 states that a provider must ensure that appropriate person-centred care and treatment is provided. This must be enabling, empowering and personalised. Every effort must be made to provide care that takes into account diversities. This legislation removes barriers to integration of services across different parts of the NHS, enabling care providers to work better together than with previous Acts. For example, support for independence may need surgical intervention and physiotherapy to enable a person to carry out all ADLs.

The role of carers in meeting the needs of adults

Care comes from a variety of sources, and some of the most personal care is delivered by people who volunteer their time, usually to support a loved one. The Family Resources Survey estimated that, in 2020/21, around 7 per cent of the UK population (4.9 million people) were providing informal care, and in England there were an estimated 334,300 carers aged 24 or younger carrying out adult caring tasks daily.

Source: Department for Work and Pensions (2010), 'Family Resources Survey', www.gov.uk/government/collections/family-resources-survey--2 (last update March 2024)

Caring for someone often takes priority over working and earning money; in addition this role can be socially isolating due to its nature. Ongoing daily care for a loved one is a continuous job which is varied and diverse – from supporting with daily care needs to caring for a person at the end of their life.

K2.4 The different types of carers and their role in meeting the needs of individuals

Types of carer

There are two types of carer outside the hospital environment:

1   **Informal carers:** provide unpaid care in a voluntary capacity to family, friends or neighbours as required. Volunteers and befrienders who offer care and support on a more ad hoc basis all contribute significantly to a person's wellbeing and quality of life.
2   Formal carers: paid **healthcare workers** who carry out daily tasks for the patient, who may be living in their own home with the additional support. Examples of formal care givers are usually referred to as domiciliary home care givers but may include meals-on-wheels services, chaplaincy services and dog walkers.

During a hospital stay, a patient may prefer to receive assistance from a family member when washing and dressing rather than support from nursing staff. This can be carried out at visiting times. Family members will often bring in clean clothing and nightwear, removing soiled clothing to take home to launder where appropriate.

Family members may also bring in reading material or activities for the patient to do for entertainment and stimulation while they are in hospital.

Depending on the financial situation, some patients are entitled to financial support to meet their care needs once they return home. This may include full care packages, support from the local authority to pay heating bills and other types of support. It is important to advise a patient and their family that financial help may be available for care giving on discharge from hospital.

Types of support

Friends and relatives may be in a position to offer **financial support**, such as paying for private care, paying for care at home or supporting a person with transport and escorting to appointments.

They may be in a position to **practically support**, for example caring for a pet at home while the person is in hospital or offering to provide meals for the patient once they have been discharged home.

Where there are no living relatives or appropriate friends, a patient may be entitled to an **advocate**, which is a person specially appointed to speak up for the patient

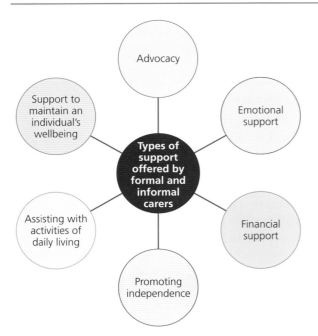

▲ Figure 5.8 Types of support offered by formal and informal carers

There may be a number of informal carers working as a unit, with specific times and dates when they spend time with the person who needs assistance and will be returning home. These people will have relevant information that is helpful when assessing needs and noting history. Often, they will know the person best and can share information about their usual behaviour as a baseline assessment for changes that have occurred through injury or ill health.

For example, a neighbour can shop for the person and drop round a meal, keeping an individual company at times, while a family helps with financial support, such as paying for a meals-on-wheels delivery.

A neighbour's location is an advantage over an individual's family who may be further away. Contact between family and neighbours will ensure support to meet the person's needs is provided in one way or another. Innovative technology allows a monitoring system to be set up, with contact via video calls offering a check-in and an opportunity to catch up, and enabling long-distance emotional support.

Amount of informal care and activities undertaken

The amount and type of informal care varies depending on need, availability and resources. A relative with a car may offer to visit on days when there is an outpatients appointment, transporting the patient and acting as an advocate.

Community nurses are specialists in this field of nursing: they provide end of life care, administer medications, manage complex dressings, diagnose deterioration, assess wound management and identify care needs that have become apparent. In some circumstances, they can offer training for informal carers who are willing to carry out these tasks themselves, depending on the patient's preferences and the informal carer's confidence.

and support them in their best interests. There are charities, such as Mencap, that specialise in providing advocates who are experienced in this support.

Visiting time can be **emotionally supportive** to a patient. The need to feel connected to others and the world outside the ward is an important part of emotional wellbeing. Having the opportunity to socialise, share anxieties and feel secure with people can reduce the stress of being in hospital and feelings of isolation that may occur.

Visiting is also essential for the person living at home, particularly if they live alone.

Figure 5.8 presents some of the types of support that can be offered by formal and informal carers.

K2.5 The concept of informal carers and the general rights of carers when supporting individuals to meet activities of daily living

The concept of informal carers

Any person who provides care on an unpaid basis (often close friends or family)

An informal carer is any person who provides care on an unpaid basis. This type of carer is often a family member, close friend or neighbour of the individual, who offers help and support simply because they care about the person.

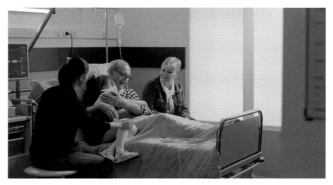

▲ Figure 5.9 Informal care can take place at home or in hospital

Rights of informal carers

Informal carers are entitled to:
- an assessment of their needs as a care giver, such as planned respite care
- financial support through benefits if eligible
- flexible working arrangements from an employer
- take unpaid leave to provide support in emergencies.

Carers' rights provision falls under the Equality Act 2010 and, as such, employers must allow flexible working hours for informal carers, and unpaid leave should they need to take time out in an emergency. They cannot lose their job and may be entitled to more financial support on an individual basis.

Financial support through benefits if eligible

Informal care givers may have a right to access financial aid from the government. To be eligible, the following criteria must be met: the care needs to be delivered for more than 35 hours per week, the person must earn less than £139 per week in an additional job and they cannot be studying for more than 21 hours per week. Carer's Allowance is £81.90 per week (current amount as of July 2024).

A carer's assessment is usually carried out face to face and conducted by a health and social care worker. It considers areas such as:
- the role requirements of that person as a care giver
- how that person feels about providing care support
- whether they are able or willing to carry on as a carer
- their own health
- any additional employment or work
- other care-giving responsibilities that might exist
- what the carer enjoys doing in their free time
- whether they have plans for emergencies when they may not be able to provide their usual care.

Depending on the situation, there may also be financial support for transport and respite care. This gives the main informal carer time each week or at a weekend when paid local authority carers can be appointed to look after their loved one while they are able to have a break, say to go out shopping or meet with a friend. Some care givers choose not to have respite care in place even though they are entitled to it.

General carers' rights

An employer must respect an informal carer's rights, and they must abide by the Equality Act 2010's stipulation that ensures carers are not disadvantaged or discriminated against, such as being denied a promotion or pay rise in line with other employees.

In general, informal carers' rights are:
- to be respected and not be abused, safeguarded
- to not be discriminated against
- to be treated in alignment with the Equality Act 2010.

With some health conditions, such as advanced dementia or a brain injury, the person an informal carer is providing care for may have outbursts of aggression and even violence. In cases such as these a risk assessment will be carried out and actions suggested if their loved one's behaviour causes a risk to the care giver. This can be a very sensitive situation, and care givers are often afraid to ask for support as it may seem like they are unable to cope, and their care-giving role may cease as a result.

Informal care giving is a very rewarding role, and it is often the last thing a family member can do for their loved one at the end of their life.

K2.6 The possible roles of informal carers and the importance of working in partnership with them when supporting individuals to meet activities of daily living

What might be included in an informal carer's role?

Providing personal care

A long-term partner or spouse may confidently and competently provide personal care. However, moving and handling regulations still apply, and training should be offered particularly in relation to complex movements requiring more than one person.

Where there is conflict between the care giver and the patient, sensitive communication is required to identify the best approach to care giving. This might be that the informal care giver provides less structured support and paid care givers are appointed to carry out the main support for the patient.

Monitoring medication

Medication that needs to be taken throughout the day can be monitored by an informal carer, using prompts where necessary, and recorded on the medications chart as required.

Undertaking practical care tasks

Commitment to providing practical care, such as shopping or doing laundry, needs to be co-ordinated, so as to avoid omissions and duplications. Checking that informal care is in place for certain tasks needs to be recorded in a care plan and reviewed from time to time. For example, a son or daughter may initially feel they have the time to support their parent to wash and dress before they go to work but then become overwhelmed; in such cases alternative arrangements will need to be put in place once the concerns have been raised.

Working in partnership with carers is beneficial in terms of reducing dependency on services and personalising care for a patient. However, this needs to be organised and co-ordinated in a systematic way, with regular reviews to maintain a good standard of care provision tailored to the needs of the patient.

Providing company and emotional support

Relatives and close or long-time friends may have a wealth of knowledge of and history with the individual who requires care; they are best suited to provide them with company and emotional support. They will know the person well enough to use appropriate humour, tried and tested techniques to distract them or encourage communication, and when to escalate a concern. This is a key component of providing social support to another individual.

Acting as a power of attorney in property and financial affairs

A patient who has sudden or progressive cognitive impairment will benefit from a trusted relative or friend to make decisions on their behalf in their best interest. Legally this will be a person who holds power of attorney, overseeing an individual's health and welfare, as well as their property and financial affairs.

To hold a lasting power of attorney (LPA), a person must first be registered with the Office of the Public Guardian (OPG). Checking who holds a patient's LPA requires a secure access code to use on the OPG's online service in cases where paperwork has been lost.

It is good practice to involve informal carers in care plan meetings as a matter of course. Someone who holds a LPA must also be consulted, whether present or not. LPAs should be made when the person involved is fully cognitive with no impairment of mind.

Working in partnership with informal carers

Recognising and valuing the support provided by informal carers

The combined efforts of integrated care, working in partnership with informal carers, means the team behind a patient's care has immeasurable value. As noted earlier, the Family Resources Survey estimated that, in 2021/22, around 7 per cent of the UK population (4.9 million people) were providing informal care. The survey defines informal caring as care that is not a paid job, and that can occur for many, or only a few, hours per week. (The Family Resources Survey is a continuous household survey implemented by the government. It collects information from a representative sample of private households in the UK.)

Source: Department for Work and Pensions (2010), 'Family Resources Survey', www.gov.uk/government/collections/family-resources-survey--2 (last update March 2024)

According to Professor Matt Bennett and Dr Maria Petrillo of the ESRC Centre for Care at the University of Sheffield, unpaid carers in England and Wales contribute a staggering £445 million to the economy every day – that's £162 billion per year.

Source: University of Sheffield (2023), 'Cost of unpaid care in England and Wales now exceeds that of NHS budget', www.sheffield.ac.uk/news/cost-unpaid-care-england-and-wales-now-exceeds-nhs-budget

The financial savings to the country provided by informal carers is just one benefit: a person being cared for at home will reduce hospital admissions, and informal carers will provide convenient transport and give the individual being cared for a better quality of life.

Ensuring carers are involved in discussions about the care being provided to an individual

Including carers in discussions about an individual's care has many benefits: the valuable insights contributed and flexible support offered can be combined with expert knowledge of how a treatment plan will work in practice.

Developing a working relationship with carers

Having a good working relationship with carers will enhance the experience of the patient.

An informal carer can be shown how to dress a minor wound, such as a pressure injury, how to carry out personal care and assist their loved one to safely use mobility aids. They are in a position to quickly observe any decline in health status and make a decision about the need for further medical intervention.

An informal carer is a valuable asset and should be included in any care planning meetings with the permission of the patient.

Reflect

S2.18 Support individuals to manage own health and wellbeing, offering appropriate guidance within the scope of role, knowledge and responsibilities

Advance care planning is for people whose mental capacity may decline, for example due to progressive illness.

Someone to hold a lasting power of attorney (LPA) can be chosen by a patient; they are registered and will be legally in control of a patient's health and welfare and/or property and finances when the person is unable to manage these independently.

Advance decisions are documented choices, such as refusal of a specific medical treatment. These are legally binding.

Advance statements are recorded information about how the patient feels about their health and care, such as what is important to them. These are not legal, but every effort should be made to honour and respect them.

Consider the following situation.

One person is sociable, articulate and has good self-esteem. Another person is reserved, has no close family or friends, is a victim of long-term abuse and does not feel valued in life. Both have an inoperable brain tumour, which is a progressive illness. They have been told that there will be a period of time where they will lack capacity before dying and the idea of advance care planning has been suggested.

▶ What factors might affect how each person responds to an opportunity to document an advanced care plan?
▶ What support is there to ensure their true feelings are recorded and wishes carried out?

Case study

S2.19 Advise carers on supporting an individual to manage their own condition within scope of role, knowledge and responsibilities

Working with a partner, role-play effective use of verbal, non-verbal and written communication skills. Your partner should play the role of the informal carer and you the trainee nurse. Video-record this task and reflect on your demonstration, analysing points in S2.19, then use your reflective journal to analyse areas that can be improved.

Lewie, who is 61, is admitted to hospital and is on the stroke ward following a moderate brain injury caused by a blood clot. He has weakness on his right side, some confusion and is more confident in speaking his first language, German, than English as he finds this easier.

His wife, Adelinde, is managing her anxiety following Lewie's sudden stroke by being practical and keeping busy. She wishes to carry out his personal hygiene and toileting support while he is in hospital, as well as any assistance he needs at mealtimes. Doctors are carrying out a thorough examination in the afternoon, reviewing scans and blood-clotting status, along with other investigations.

Adelinde has questions that you need to answer in an unambiguous way using appropriate language and terminology. Like Lewie, her first language is German. She has a good understanding of spoken English but less so of written text.

You need to answer Adelinde's questions:
1 How long will her husband be in hospital and when can he go home?
2 Will he get better and return to his full functioning soon?
3 Can she support him to toilet and shower and dress him, instead of nursing staff?
4 Are there clean towels for him when showering or does she need to bring some from home?
5 Is she able to borrow a walking frame to help him get from the bed to the bathroom facilities?
6 Is she able to have some written information, which she can translate on her smartphone into German, to help them both to understand about symptoms, diagnosis and treatment for a stroke?
7 Is there anything else she can do?

K2.7 The symptoms and implications associated with frailty

The World Health Organization (WHO) defines frailty as a recognisable state in which the ability of older people to cope with everyday or acute stressors is compromised by an increased vulnerability brought about by age-associated declines in physiological reserve and function across multiple organ systems. The NHS medical definition is the group of older people who are at highest risk of adverse outcomes such as falls, disability, admission to hospital or the need for long-term care.

Deconditioning

▶ The process of becoming frail is deconditioning caused by reduction in mobility. Chronic pain caused by arthritis or other health conditions, coupled with the decrease in activity, contributes to frailty.

▶ Muscle wastage in the pelvic area directly impacts on the control of bowel and urine continence. Limited mobility and speed of movement adds to problems with getting to the toilet in time for people in later life.

▶ There is an increased falls risk: a fall from standing is a forceful impact on the wrists and pelvic area, which land first. More than 85 per cent of hip fractures occur in people who are over 65 years.

Loss of bone density and muscle mass

Inactivity and hormone changes are responsible for a decline in muscle mass and strength, and a decrease in bone density. Adequate and quality sleep can be hampered by joint pain. Both men and women produce less growth hormone, which regulates body fat, meaning bones can protrude. Balance requires co-ordination of leg muscles and core strength; losing balance is more common in the older population, caused by a multitude of age-related conditions.

Dementia/cognitive decline

The slowing down of thought processes can be mistaken for forgetfulness; cognitive decline means a longer length of time is needed to recall a previous solution, to reason and keep up with a conversation, for example. It does not mean the person is incapable of thinking, having opinions or participating in everyday activities. Requiring longer to remember a person's name can be frustrating, but the more upset an individual becomes the less likely they are to recall it.

Dementia chiefly affects older people, after the age of 65; the likelihood of developing dementia almost doubles every five years. The Office for National Statistics

(ONS) recorded that the number of people living in England and Wales aged 65 years and over increased from 9.2 million in 2011 to more than 11 million in 2021. The demand on healthcare services will rise with the continuing growth of the ageing population.

Early detection of illness, preventing ill health associated with ageing and promoting healthier choices like more active lifestyles can improve people's quality of life and lessen the strain on medical and social care services. Hypertension, particularly midlife high blood pressure, has been related to a higher risk of cognitive decline and dementia, including Alzheimer's disease.

Sources: Office for National Statistics (2023), 'Profile of the older population living in England and Wales in 2021 and changes since 2011', www.ons.gov.uk/peoplepopulationandcommunity/ birthsdeathsandmarriages/ageing/articles/ profileoftheolderpopulationlivinginenglandandwalesin2021and changessince2011/2023-04-03

Sierra, C. (2020), 'Hypertension and the risk of dementia', *Frontiers in Cardiovascular Medicine*, 7:5. doi: 10.3389/fcvm.2020.00005.

Mental health illnesses

Constant pain, incontinence and the gradual or sudden loss of independence are cited as the main causes of depression and other mental health conditions in older age.

Supporting a spouse or sibling who is living with dementia can mean that an increase in fundamental care is needed, such as personal hygiene, managing toileting or help with eating and drinking. The person may not recognise them, get upset or agitated and restrict the carer's opportunity to rest and carry out their own tasks without risk to the other person. The resulting responsibility and strain can cause the onset of depression in the person caring, which they do not recognise in themselves as they put the needs of the person needing care above their own.

Loneliness after the passing of a long-term partner or friend leaves a big void and can be isolating. An older person living in the community may not see anyone to talk to unless they go out. If their mobility is poor and there has been a decline in their sight and hearing, socialising and getting out may be too much of a challenge for them. Being aware that their actions are slower, and that other people might get frustrated or annoyed at their speed of movement and processing, can mean a withdrawal of contact. A key feature of social disengagement theory is that social withdrawal in later adulthood is a natural progression as we age – resulting in social disengagement and preferring our own company. Depression and anxiety may go unnoticed by others and an older person may be reluctant to seek help.

Higher risk of developing infections

The risk of developing cancer significantly increases as we age, and a weakening immune system puts older people at higher risk of developing infections.

A lack of appetite as a result of reduced movement is often a reason for a person eating less. Mental ill health and infection also play their parts in reducing appetite.

K2.8 The importance of early diagnosis in relation to dementia and other cognitive issues, why depression, delirium and the normal ageing process may be mistaken for dementia and how other conditions may contribute to early onset dementia

Similarities between the symptoms of depression and delirium

There are multiple types of dementia and Alzheimer's disease is the most common.

▶ Dementia is not a specific disease; it is a general term for impaired cognitive functioning affecting memory recall, problem solving, perception and decision making, interfering with everyday life.

▶ Delirium is a mental state characterised by confusion, disorientation and not being in the present reality; for example a person is unaware that they are in a hospital ward.

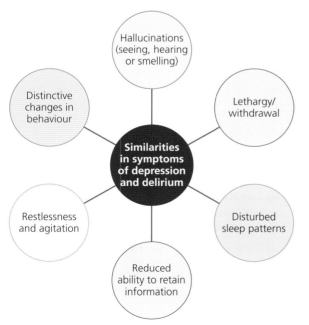

▲ Figure 5.10 Similarities in symptoms of depression and delirium

Dementia and delirium are alike, and they can be experienced at the same time. There are similarities between the symptoms of depression and delirium (Figure 5.10), but generally the onset of dementia is seen in symptoms that occur over time, moving from minor signs to those that become more noticeable. Delirium occurs over a shorter time span, sometimes appearing suddenly. Patients living with dementia can have good and bad times of day where symptoms become more obvious; for instance, they may be more alert in the morning, but their memory recall and thinking stay roughly at the same level. In comparison, delirium can present several times a day with no obvious trigger, coming and going.

Similarities between the symptoms of the normal ageing process and dementia

There are some similarities between just getting older and developing dementia:

▶ There are, for example, **disturbed sleeping patterns**. An older person who has painful joints, has not been active during the day and has catnapped will not have a full night's quality sleep.

▶ Overthinking means out-of-control dissection and analysis of a situation, resulting in anxiety, agitation and the **reduced ability to retain information**, being preoccupied with hyperfocused thoughts.

▶ For some people, the normal ageing process causes a **reduction in mobility** and **reduced appetite**, resulting in them appearing uninterested and withdrawn.

▶ **Reduced sensory capacity**, such as hearing and sight impairment, impacts on a person's confidence when socialising, especially in a group. A conscious effort to interact at a quieter time and slower pace can identify the reason for withdrawal and tiredness in an open conversation.

Why early diagnosis of dementia and other cognitive issues is important

An early diagnosis of dementia will improve the **quality of life of both the person living with dementia and their loved ones**. The difficulty for a person caring for a loved one is that sometimes being in a state of denial or wanting to protect the person from other people's judgement means they do not seek medical assessment.

Trying to avoid the label of a dementia diagnosis is common, but **appropriate medication may slow down the progress of the disease**; therefore the earlier dementia is diagnosed the better.

Medication aims to prevent an enzyme from breaking down a substance called acetylcholine in the brain, which plays a role in neurons' communication in the synaptic gap. Memory recall and function deteriorate as the passage of nerve messages in the brain slows and ceases to communicate effectively.

Planning and having **early access to support services** improves support for the main person caring for the individual who is living with dementia and enables them to stay together living at home. As their short-term memory declines the importance of remaining in surroundings that are familiar becomes more apparent, resulting in less confusion and distress.

Legal documentation

In the early stages of dementia, **legal documentation** can be discussed and arrangements made. For example:
▶ **lasting power of attorney (LPA)** (as explained above)
▶ an **advanced directive** – legal and clinical instructions about future treatment choices, recorded before there is a lack of capacity.

How other factors may contribute to early onset dementia

Early onset dementia is the diagnosis when symptoms are present before the age of 65; it can occur any time after the age of 30 and represents 5–6 per cent of all dementia cases in the UK. Factors that contribute to early onset dementia could be:
▶ a **stroke**
▶ **lifestyle factors**, including **alcoholism**
▶ an **acquired brain injury**
▶ an **existing genetic condition** such as Huntington's disease.

A University of Cambridge study showed that the damage to the brain caused by dementia can begin nine years before a diagnosis. Denial and dismissing symptoms as due to old age contribute to this statistic.

Source: University of Cambridge (2022), 'Scientists detect dementia signs as early as nine years ahead of diagnosis', www.cam.ac.uk/research/news/scientists-detect-dementia-signs-as-early-as-nine-years-ahead-of-diagnosis

K2.9 The factors that impact on the care of the dying and the deceased to ensure most appropriate care is provided

The NHS Palliative and End of Life Care (PEoLC) Statutory Guidance for Integrated Care Boards (2022) document sets out the legal duties and an Integrated Care System (ICS) approach. There are six key areas, referred to as 'Ambitions', in the delivery of PEoLC and principles for advance care planning (see Table 5.3).

▼ Table 5.3 Six key areas for end of life care

Key areas	These areas as reflected in K2.9	What this means in practice
Ambition 1: Each person is seen as an individual	Recognition of religious and cultural beliefs	Different religions have different spiritual practices before death and immediately after, and including the timescale before the next stage and what that is. For example, in the Hindu religion, cremation takes place within 24 hours of death.
Ambition 2: Each person gets fair access to care	Providing care and support to the carer and family, including emotional and practical bereavement support	A leaflet is given to the family before the death of a loved one at the end stage of life or after a sudden death, which guides them through NHS processes, options and their rights.
Ambition 3: Maximising comfort and wellbeing	Pain management to relieve distress and discomfort	Many palliative care patients have more than one pain. A comprehensive assessment and regular reviews identify intensity and location before the most appropriate pain relief is prescribed.
Ambition 4: Care is co-ordinated	Medical healthcare, social care, informal carers and community	A patient in the end stages of life may move from hospital as treatment stops and return home for pain-management medication. At home or in a hospice there is still medical intervention, such as from a community palliative nurse. Working alongside social carers supporting the family unit may be a charity-funded Macmillan nurse, for example.

Key areas	These areas as reflected in K2.9	What this means in practice
Ambition 5: All staff are prepared to care	Following agreed care plan, with regular reviews; recognition of policies and procedures around death	Hospital policy states that personal care after death needs to be carried out within two to four hours of the person dying, to preserve their appearance, condition and dignity. The body temperature needs time to lower and refrigeration in a mortuary should take place within four hours. Trainee nurses will be aware of policies and can discuss coping strategies with their supervisor.
Ambition 6: Each community is prepared to help	Local councils' voluntary and charity organisations	If the deceased's family does not have the money for funeral expenses, they may be eligible for local council means-tested financial support. Charities run helplines for the bereaved and offer guidance with practical matters such as access to a loved one's bank account and cancelling a phone contract. NHS-funded counselling support can be offered in the short term and specialist charities can offer counselling, such as those supporting a family which has experienced an MND patient's death. Bereavement support groups – local or specialist – are an option some people find beneficial while they are on the grieving journey.

Recognition of wishes regarding resuscitation and organ donation

Advance care planning is a voluntary discussion that offers an opportunity for the individual to plan their future care, support and treatments before they experience deterioration and lack of capacity. A document states and records a patient's wishes regarding resuscitation and organ donation.

Recognition that care does not stop at point of death

The care given by nurses following a hospital death was traditionally referred to as 'last offices'. This term has since been replaced with 'care after death', which is more respectful in a multicultural society. This updated terminology better reflects the clinical tasks involved in nursing after a patient has died, including the support offered to family and informal carers. The term 'next of kin' is now referred to as family; the concept of family does not mean simply genetics but encompasses those that are not blood relatives, representing modern living arrangements.

Most people have a 'good death' in their preferred place, most commonly at home or in a care home. On occasions where a patient has been brought to hospital, care should follow an agreed care plan, with reference to wishes as set out in an advance care plan. After death, the deceased patient's eyes should be closed, applying light pressure for 30 seconds, and their body

repositioned so they are lying on their back, to preserve their appearance, condition and dignity. The personal care after death must be carried out within two to four hours of the person dying and after the patient has been certified as deceased.

Figure 5.10 presents the different aspects of care after death. The deceased person's family may have questions that need to be answered honestly, as well as signposting to bereavement services.

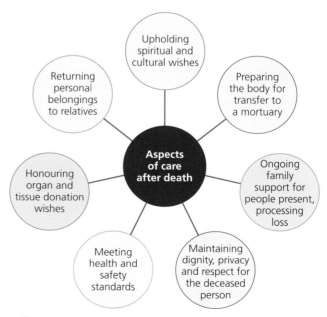

▲ Figure 5.11 Aspects of care after death

Case study

S2.20 Provide appropriate care that helps individuals with advanced, progressive and life limiting conditions to live as well as possible

Working with a partner, role-play effective use of verbal, non-verbal and written communication skills. Cover all points in S2.20. You may wish to refer to the list as you go through points discussed with the informal carer.

Your partner should play the role of the informal carer, Mal, and you will play the trainee nurse. Video-record this task, reflect on your demonstration and use your reflective journal to analyse areas that can be improved. You must record significant information.

Karol has been offered a place at the local hospice and her husband, Mal, has asked how the hospice works. He would like reassurance that the care plan he has been involved in will be implemented, and he wants to know how the hospice will ensure she is comfortable, and ensure her emotional wellbeing and Catholic spiritual needs will be maintained.

Karol is unable to communicate. She relaxes when gentle music is heard, and Mal has information to discuss on her behalf. He would like to know if there is a prayer room, that there will be no withdrawal of life support care before her time and that the priest can visit when Mal feels she needs to see him.

Assessment practice

S2.17 Appropriately manage situations in which individuals cannot do things for themselves
S2.18 Support individuals to manage own health and wellbeing, offering appropriate guidance within the scope of role, knowledge and responsibilities

Your task is to demonstrate correct clinical skills, following all relevant regulations and delivering consistent good practice. You will need a partner in a simulated ward situation, who will play the role of a recovering stroke patient.

You are to demonstrate your understanding of HCPO1, HCPO2, ANPO1 and ANPO2 knowledge and skills, completing a number of tasks.

During your demonstration you must narrate what you are doing using the correct terminology and explain why you are taking each action.

It would be an enhanced learning experience if you have your demonstration recorded so you can evaluate your practical demonstration using Gibbs' reflective cycle to identify any areas for improvement.

Bibek is 70 and, without prior warning, had a life-changing ischemic stroke. He is usually a physically active, sociable man, who takes part in physical outdoor activities and plays an active role in grandparenting. He was brought in to hospital by ambulance and was given tissue plasminogen activator (tPA) medication to break up the clot and get blood flowing to his brain while in A&E. After 24 hours an assessment identifies significant weakness to the right side of his body, aphasia and incontinence. He is mentally alert, but his speech is fragmented and he is hard to understand. His wife is in shock and cries. He has communicated he wants her to go home.

Bibek is left-handed. He has good muscle tone for his age and appears to understand basic instructions at his own pace. A mobility assessment has been completed: he can move to the edge of the bed and, with minor support, stand up, sit in a wheelchair, and get on and off a toilet. The doctors are confident that physiotherapy rehabilitation will have Bibek functioning independently. Adaptations needed at home and outpatient rehabilitation appointments are noted in his care plan. Bibek refuses to eat or drink; he is not interested in his personal appearance and has stopped any written communication he initially used.

Your role is to encourage Bibek to participate in his own care, educate him in eating, care and mobility aids, and participate in rehabilitation activities. Refer to points in the skills criteria for S2.17–18.

Adult Nursing PO3: Assisting with skin integrity assessments, and with the care and treatment of skin conditions

The skin is the largest organ of the body and is the body's main protection from external factors such as bacteria and ultraviolet (UV) rays. It is made of several layers and one of the main functions is to maintain hydration within the body. Hydration is maintained as the skin preserves water in conjunction with other bodily systems and provides us with a waterproof layer.

However, the skin can be vulnerable to damage caused by irritants, injury and prolonged pressure, and any physical damage to the upper layers of the skin can cause us to be vulnerable to infections such as bacteria and viruses which can enter the body through the damaged layers.

Skin integrity is the name given to the monitoring of skin health including assessments on admission and at regular intervals throughout a treatment programme. The purpose of skin monitoring in hospital or care home settings is to prevent tissue damage and monitor other bodily systems such as the heart and the lungs.

Actions to prevent and support the recovery of the skin are within the scope of practice of trainee and registered nurses.

Learning outcomes

The core knowledge outcomes that you must understand and learn:

K3.1 the function and structure of the skin

K3.2 the pathophysiology of the skin ageing process and the factors affecting skin integrity

K3.3 common skin conditions seen in individuals and the possible causes of skin conditions

K3.4 how pressure injuries develop, the common sites, early symptoms and the preventative measures to avoid the development of a pressure injury

K3.5 how to carry out assessments of skin integrity and why it is important to do so

K3.6 the types of treatment that can be used to care for skin and prevent or treat skin conditions.

Skills outcomes

The skills you will need to demonstrate:

S3.7 assist with skin integrity assessments, treatment and care of skin conditions, working within scope of role, knowledge and responsibilities

S3.8 check skin integrity using appropriate assessment documentation and inform others

S3.9 demonstrate the ability to provide the appropriate care to reduce the risk of pressure ulcers developing or deteriorating and record interventions

S3.10 undertake and record interventions to treat and prevent skin conditions (for example repositioning of the individual) in line with your roles and responsibilities

S3.11 demonstrate the ability to advise and discuss with both individuals and carers about how to prevent pressure injuries.

Skin physiology and pathophysiology

Skin is the largest organ in the body and has many functions, such as playing a vital role in the homeostasis mechanism, thermoregulation. The skin has three main layers – the **epidermis**, dermis and hypodermis – each of which has a different role and composition.

If the skin becomes damaged by an injury, penetration or burn, for example, the process of healing has four stages which will often result in the formation of scar tissue at the end stage.

> **Key term**
>
> **Epidermis:** outer layer of skin, which acts as a protective barrier.

In later adulthood the skin will often change, becoming thinner and paler. It may become semi-translucent and frequently pigment spots will appear, especially in skin that has been regularly exposed to sunlight. These changes are not as visible in dark skin tones.

Ageing skin deteriorates, losing its firmness and the loss of collagen means it loses its elasticity. Over time the skin produces less secretions, leaving the skin drier, so extra care is required when caring for an older person as dry, frail skin is very prone to damage.

With darker skin, monitoring for pressure damage, rashes and bruising can be more difficult so extra vigilance is required to prevent skin damage from being missed.

K3.1 The function and structure of the skin

The skin is the body's largest organ. It is part of the **integumentary system**, which also includes the hair and nails, and covers the body with a waterproof protective layer. Skin accounts for 15 per cent of a person's total body weight. It is composed of protein, lipids and minerals, and is kept hydrated with water. The skin regenerates and replenishes cells approximately every 28 days, with the outer layer shedding dead cells.

The main functions of skin

The skin has many functions, as described below.

Acts as a barrier for microbes

The skin acts as a **mechanical barrier** blocking pathogens from entering the body and acting as a seal against **microbes** with low permeability. If the skin is damaged, such as in the case of a paper cut, the opening provides a way for pathogens to enter the body. Under a microscope, the skin cells have the appearance of a brick wall, with a bricks and mortar formation. Cells called corneocytes look and act like the bricks, tightly bound, or stuck together, by glue-like fats (the mortar) such as ceramides, cholesterol and fatty acids.

Skin is also a biological barrier: it has trillions of harmless bacteria on it that act as a protective barrier against pathogens (harmful organisms). This is the body's first line of defence in immunity and demonstrates the importance of having good skin integrity.

Regulates the temperature of the body

The skin regulates the temperature of the body through the homeostasis mechanism, thermoregulation.

In vasodilation the blood vessels dilate (widen), causing blood to move towards the surface of the skin. This provides the body with a mechanism for heat loss, in addition to the production of sweat through the sweat glands/pores (see Figure 6.1a for an illustration of vasodilation).

A fall in body temperature stimulates muscle action, such as friction through shivering and raising surface hair to trap air. The hair-lifting arrector pili muscles can clearly be seen and are commonly known as goosebumps. In the dermis the muscles around the capillary circuit contract (vasoconstriction, see Figure 6.1b), allowing only minimal blood flow to the surface, to prevent heat radiating through the epidermis. The lumen of the arterioles decrease in circumference and blood is diverted to a shunt vessel in the hypodermis insulated with subcutaneous fat. The skin exposed to cold will appear lighter in colour when vasodilation takes place.

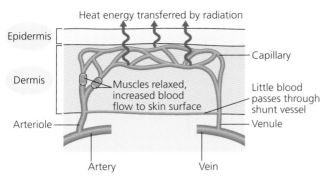

▲ Figure 6.1a Vasodilation in the skin

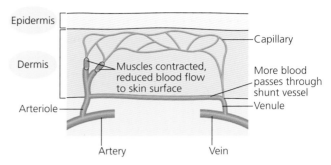

▲ Figure 6.1b Vasoconstriction in the skin

Prevents loss of essential body fluids

Transepidermal water loss is the term given to water that passes from inside the body through the epidermis to the surface via diffusion and evaporation processes. Skin has structures and mechanisms that control fluid loss, having their own role in osmoregulation (water balance).

Sudoriferous glands, also known as sweat glands, are located in the deeper layer of the skin, the dermis. Sweat glands occur all over the body but are most dense on the forehead, in the armpits, and on the palms and the soles of the feet. Eccrine sweat glands occur over most of the body and open directly onto the skin's surface. Apocrine glands are situated near hair follicles; they release sweat that follows the hair to the surface of the skin. Sweat is mainly water, but it also contains some salts. Its main function is to control body temperature. Nerve messages take information to sweat glands to tell them to secrete or retain fluids.

Provides protection against penetration of mechanical, physical and hazardous substances

Some hazardous substances can penetrate the skin due to its composition or the pre-existing skin integrity. The extent to which damage can occur depends on the health of the skin and any existing damage. Damage can be caused at any layer – to superficial or deep tissue. Skin can be damaged as a result of pressure across bony prominences, fractured bone tissue protruding through the skin layers, chemicals or heat causing burns, or friction caused by poor moving and handling techniques.

The stratum corneum (the top layer of the skin) is constructed of tough skin cells which provide the first layer of protection against the above causes of damage.

The ceruminous glands produce the wax that is found in the ear canal. This offers an element of physical protection from penetration with strength and elasticity, keeping friction minor and impact superficial, or preventing damage altogether.

Protection from harmful effects of the sun and radiation

The skin offers some protection from the harmful effects of the sun and radiation, as ultraviolet (UV) rays activate a chemical in the dermis layer called melanin. The radiation oxidises melanin, absorbing harmful rays, which darkens the skin. This is the first defence against the damage of skin cells and sunburn. UVA rays penetrate deeper than the less harmful UVB rays. Absorption of UVA radiation causes the formation of free radicals, which can damage proteins, DNA and RNA in cells.

Sunburn, caused by over exposure of skin to the UV rays of the sun, can range from a painful swelling and inflammation to the skin to blistering and peeling of the damaged layers. This exposure can damage the DNA of the skin cells and in some cases this can be instrumental in the development of some forms of skin cancer such as malignant melanomas.

Excretes toxic substances with sweat

Sweat includes an antibiotic agent called dermcidin. When sweat is excreted this natural antimicrobial peptide chemically protects the surface of the skin. Hairs help to disperse the liquid, so it does not merely sit on the top of the sweat gland exit.

During exercise, the body retains fluids which are usually excreted as urine. Urea and other toxic waste substances are not eliminated as efficiently and become more concentrated. Positive feedback instructs the sudoriferous glands to produce water and sodium salts to aid thermoregulation by evaporation from the skin's surface.

Uric acid is present in sweat. This is a toxin produced when the body breaks down purines which are natural substances found in every cell and in most foods. A patient with gout may overproduce uric acid.

The sudoriferous glands, the eccrine and apocrine glands, excrete some of these substances as a component of sweat. The quantity depends on a person's hydration status.

The sebaceous gland in the dermis produces oil (sebum), preventing the skin from drying out and cracking, offering a barrier with waterproofing to protect the skin in this situation.

Sensory organ for touch, heat and cold

The skin has some areas that are more **sensitive to touch and temperature** than others.

▶ The nerve endings are more dense and closer to the surface in the lips and fingertips.

▶ On the palms of the hands and the soles of the feet the epidermis layer is thicker and the nerve endings are more concentrated. For those areas without body hair, there is usually more subcutaneous fat present for warmth.

▶ The sensation of touch is increased in areas with multiple hair follicles as receptors can detect touch in the hair follicles before the skin is touched.

The skin's nerve receptors and locations differ in terms of receiving and interpreting sensations.

Scar tissue has impaired or no nerve endings, depending on the level and type of injury that caused the scar. Deterioration in nerve receptors and speed of sensory messages is part of the natural ageing process.

▶ An older person may not feel a light touch and good communication is essential to prevent them from becoming surprised by actions they are not expecting.

▶ Fragile skin has a tendency to tear rather than stretch when under pressure, and **care must be taken with moving and handling techniques to prevent damage**.

▶ Pain messages **may be reduced in the older adult and they may not recognise that their skin is becoming damaged by pressure until the injury has occurred**.

Vitamin D synthesis

In the presence of sunlight, a form of **vitamin D3** called cholecalciferol is **synthesised** from a derivative of the steroid cholesterol in the skin. The liver converts cholecalciferol to calciol (the active chemical form of the vitamin) in the kidneys.

Calcitriol is a man-made active form of vitamin D, which influences renal reabsorption of calcium, increasing intestinal absorption of calcium and phosphorus, and increasing the movement of calcium and phosphorus from bone (where it has been stored) to plasma.

Calcium stored in the bones is then released when foods in the intestines do not supply it in sufficient amounts.

Structure of the skin

The structure of the skin is made up of three layers, which provide different functions, as shown in Figure 6.2 and described in Table 6.1.

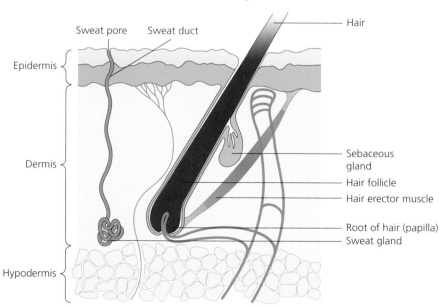

▲ Figure 6.2 Cross-section of human skin

▼ Table 6.1 The three layers of the skin

Skin layer	Explanation
Top layer: the epidermis	The outer layer of the skin is the thinnest; it has five layers of its own. Its role is to protect the body, producing skin cells, keeping the skin hydrated and keeping water in. Squamous cells are continuously shed and are known as stratum corneum (the surface). The basal layer is below, made up of basal cells, and the colour of the skin is produced by melanin, made by the melanocytes. A protein called keratin is produced by keratinocytes and forms a tight, **waterproof** barrier, which protects and strengthens the skin. Langerhans cells stop foreign substances penetrating the skin and are the skin's T-cell response, providing an immune barrier.
Middle layer: the dermis	Collagen is a protein that provides structural support; this gives the skin a plump, toned look and prevents sagging. Elastic tissues are fibres that allow the skin to stretch and recoil. The dermis is where **hair follicles**, **glands** and **nerve endings** sit, each with their own role. The capillaries play a key role in thermoregulation.
Bottom layer: the hypodermis	Sometimes known as the subcutaneous tissue layer, the hypodermis is made up of adipose cells that store fat (subcutaneous fat) for energy and **insulation**, and provide a varied amount of **cushioning** for protection. It also connects the dermis to muscle.

Test yourself

Describe the functions of the glands listed below:
1 eccrine
2 apocrine
3 sebaceous
4 ceruminous

K3.2 The pathophysiology of the skin ageing process and the factors affecting skin integrity

Pathophysiology of the skin ageing process

As we are unique, the **pathophysiology of the skin ageing process** differs between individuals. External factors such as sun and environmental pollution exposure, and internal factors such as poor nutrition and lifestyle choice, all have an impact.

Loss of elasticity

Elastin is a protein that combines with microfibrils to form elastic fibres, which allow the skin to stretch and retract. Collagen, also a protein, supports the structure of cells, and oestrogen stimulates oil production to keep skin supple, smooth and with a plump appearance. Part of the ageing process is that **skin loses its elasticity**. This is caused by hormone changes, a reduction in the production of collagen and external factors.

Thinning

Skin becomes thinner with age, in particular the epidermis layer, with the melanocytes increasing in size. Depending on an individual's skin tone, their skin may appear visually paler (pallor), become more translucent (transparent) and age spots (sometimes called liver spots) may be visible.

Thinner skin is fragile and vulnerable to friction damage, tears and pressure injuries as the level of protection it provides has weakened.

Slower regeneration

Skin cells are continuously **regenerating**; however, the **cycle slows** from around 30 days to replenish to between 60 and 90 days when a person is in their fifties. Increasing numbers of dead skin cells accumulate on the surface of the skin and the healing process may be up to four times slower.

Loss of fat

The insulating, cushioning layer of subcutaneous **fat also decreases**. At around the age of 70, an underweight patient will have less cover over the bony parts of their body, for example the pelvis and elbows. The nerves decrease in sensitivity, leaving an older person more likely to miss pain signals and the first signs of skin irritation, such as friction.

Reduced absorption of nutrients

With ageing, other body systems slow down and functioning is less effective, which impacts on skin health. The digestive system has a **reduced absorption of nutrients**; the cardiovascular capillaries have less muscle strength to co-ordinate vasodilation and vasoconstriction, and they may further be disrupted by the build-up of fatty plaque in the lumen of the veins and arteries. All these factors can affect the older person and make them more susceptible to the extremes of hot and cold resulting in hypothermia, sunstroke, skin infections and accidental skin damage.

Factors affecting skin integrity

Lifestyle factors

Smoking causes nicotine to enter the bloodstream; this is responsible for damage to blood capillaries, reducing the flow of oxygenated blood to the skin cells.

- ▶ Nicotine changes the structure of skin fibroblast, the main cells containing collagen, meaning skin ages prematurely, with more wrinkles developing at an earlier age.
- ▶ Identical twin research into facial skin ageing in Japan (Ichibori *et al.*, 2014) found a higher incidence of facial texture and wrinkles in the twin who smoked.
- ▶ Research conducted by the World Health Organization (WHO) in 2020 highlighted that smoking increases the risk of a wound opening and slows down healing, decreasing the body's inflammatory response and immune function.

Sources: Ichibori, R., Fujiwara, T., Tanigawa, T., Kanazawa, S., Shingaki, K., Torii, K., Tomita, K., Yano, K.; Osaka Twin Research Group; Sakai, Y. and Hosokawa, K. (2014), 'Objective assessment of facial skin aging and the associated environmental factors in Japanese monozygotic twins', *Journal of Cosmetic Dermatology*, 13(2): 158–63. **doi: 10.1111/jocd.12081.**

WHO (2020), 'Smoking greatly increases risk of complications after surgery', www.who.int/news/item/20-01-2020-smoking-greatly-increases-risk-of-complications-after-surgery

Alcohol is a diuretic, which causes water to be lost from the body. As a result, the skin can become very dehydrated which is damaging to the skin's composition. Alcohol can cause skin conditions such as psoriasis to worsen and the skin may become yellow as a result of liver damage caused by too much alcohol.

Diet can also affect the skin. Dietary planning has been covered in previous chapters, but needless to say if skin is made up of fat and protein, it requires the right amount of macronutrients and micronutrients. A number of factors may lead to reduced dietary intake of these nutrients; for example an older person may have less of an appetite than they used to, an individual may feel stressed by being admitted to hospital or pain may negatively impact on the enjoyment of eating. In this case a small amount of fresh orange juice can be more appealing than water and contains vitamin C, facilitating iron absorption. Smaller portions of highly nutritious foods and or protein-rich snacks in between meals such as yoghurt, rice pudding, custard pots, soya yoghurts or cheese and crackers can be considered to increase the consumption of protein and zinc to promote healing.

Environment

An external factor affecting skin integrity is **pollution** such as smoke and car exhaust. Air pollutants contain complex chemical compounds, and analysing these individually and then the combined effects of sun rays, pollution and ageing needs further research. It is thought that pollution reduces the skin's barrier effect, allowing chemicals in a work environment, say, to be absorbed through the skin and to act as irritants.

Particles in the air, such as **pollen**, can trigger dermatitis when they land on exposed skin. In some individuals, the skin's immune defence views pollen, a harmless substance, as a pathogen and reacts by flooding the bloodstream with inflammatory chemicals such as histamine. Skin may develop hives or rashes that are itchy or warm to the touch. For some people the blood vessels in the conjunctiva become swollen, giving the appearance of puffy eyes.

Skin reactions are more commonly a secondary symptom; the pollen is inhaled through the membrane of the nose and the effect of this is histamines, which can cause an outbreak of swelling and rashes in areas not directly exposed to pollen.

People who work outside, such as farmers, are exposed to the sun. UK research carried out in 2023 identified that 32 per cent of adults do not use sunscreen despite most burning at least once per year; 11 per cent say they always use sunscreen in the UK, dropping to 8 per cent for males alone. Application of sunscreen protects the skin from ultraviolet radiation from the sun, which damages skin cells. UVA rays penetrate deeper than UVB rays into the skin layer and mediate damage to both the epidermis and dermis.

Source: Cancer Research UK (2023), 'Melanoma skin cancer statistics', www.cancerresearchuk.org/health-professional/cancer-statistics/statistics-by-cancer-type/melanoma-skin-cancer#heading-Zero

Medical factors

Medication, such as blood thinners prescribed to address a clotting concern in middle-aged and older adults, compounds issues with a diminishing dermis layer. In this situation an impact injury causing bruising leaves the person more vulnerable to damage caused by bleeding for longer under the skin. Statins are given to patients to lower cholesterol levels in the blood and can also impact on lipids needed for a healthy layer of subcutaneous fat, another component of healthy skin. Anticoagulant medications are used to prevent clot formation and subsequently lead the individual to develop a hard-to-heal wound.

Certain **medical health conditions** can impact on skin integrity. An example of this is diabetes. A high concentration of glucose in the bloodstream can cause a condition called diabetic peripheral neuropathy which reduces the sensation felt by the skin on the feet. It also adds to the risk of tissue death and the loss of limbs as a result.

Polycystic ovary syndrome (PCOS) and lupus are other examples of health conditions that can impact skin integrity. PCOS symptoms include increased facial hair activity and acne due to hormonal imbalances in females. Lupus is an autoimmune condition which causes the body's immune system to attack the body. Cutaneous lupus causes a chronic skin condition in which rashes or sores typically appear on sun-exposed areas of the body, such as the face, scalp, chest, arms and legs.

K3.3 Common skin conditions seen in individuals and the possible causes of skin conditions

An understanding of the physiology of the skin, including its layers and structure, enables you to assess and grade skin injuries, according to the depth and level of damage you observe.

The skin's physiology, including the location of nerves as pain receptors, thermoregulation through sweat and shivering, and the skin's role in providing immunity to the body link this, the largest organ, to other body systems and functions.

Common skin conditions

Most common skin conditions are more visible in individuals with a lighter complexion compared to people with darker skin tones.

Pallor describes a pale appearance due to reduced oxyhaemoglobin levels in the blood, for instance when someone is in shock. In a patient who has a darker skin tone, looking at the palm of their hand – in particular the natural skin creases across the palm and finger joints – might show a paler colour than expected. A judgement on pallor for all skin complexions can be assessed by examining the blood flow status of the lower eyelid. When gently pulled down, the conjunctival colour should appear a healthy pink, confirming the presence of the red-coloured oxyhaemoglobin.

According to the British Skin Foundation, 60 per cent of people in the UK have a skin disorder currently or have had one in the past. The UK National Eczema Society states that 1 in 10 adults have eczema, which can make skin itchy. Further details of eczema are covered in hyperkeratosis on page 178.

Hives, also called urticaria, are a raised, itchy rash or welts usually caused by a reaction to things like food, pollen or insect bites. Antihistamines may resolve the outbreak.

Cellulitis is caused by bacteria. It usually affects the arms and legs since these are more likely to have minor injuries, which cause damage to the epidermis and a point of entry. It can also develop around the eyes, mouth and anus. Staphylococcus and streptococcus bacteria are common causes of cellulitis. Treatment is oral antibiotics or intravenous antibiotics for more serious infections.

Irritant reactions

Figure 6.3 lists some substances that are considered common skin irritants.

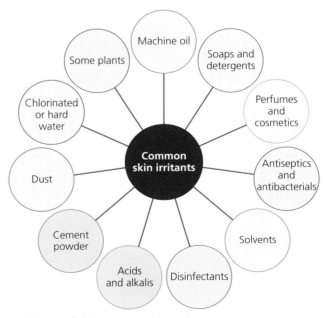

▲ Figure 6.3 Common skin irritants

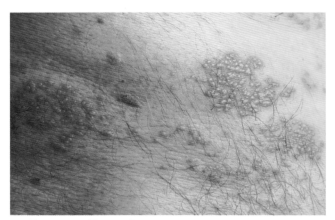 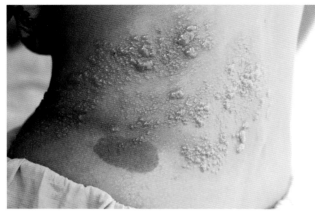

▲ Figure 6.4 Examples of skin eruptions caused by shingles (herpes zoster)

A non-allergic skin **irritant reaction** causes damage to the protective layer of the epidermis, either with a single contact or repeated exposure. The affected contact area may be raised, itchy, develop blisters and have a red appearance; this is called erythema.

Rashes

A rash is where the skin becomes red, inflamed and uneven.

▶ Some rashes become dry and itchy; others, such as shingles, are accompanied by pain.

▶ A heat rash is not caused by sun exposure; it happens when blocked pores trap sweat under the skin in warm, humid weather and during physical activity, causing itching and discomfort.

▶ A contact allergy differs; it involves the immune system, and the skin reaction can appear anywhere as welts (large raised patches of skin) or itchiness.

The most common causes of rashes are viral or chemical in nature such as contact dermatitis, hand, foot and mouth disease, or shingles. The first symptom of shingles (also known as herpes zoster) is pain; this is followed by raised, burning red skin and fluid-filled blisters (Figure 6.4).

Blisters

A blister usually takes the form of an oval-shaped bubble in between skin layers, filled with a clear fluid called serum.

▶ Blisters are usually caused by friction (repetitive movement across the skin's surface) or a burn, or they are a symptom of an allergic reaction.

▶ A new skin layer grows under the blister, the body reabsorbs the fluid, and eventually the top layer dries and flakes off.

▶ Once this happens the skin underneath is harder-wearing and usually a darker colour, thicker and more resistant to blistering again.

Hyperkeratosis

Hyperkeratosis occurs when a person's skin becomes thicker than usual in different places depending on the cause.

▶ In the case of a friction blister caused by shoes rubbing on a toe, continued rubbing will lead to a callus. Keratin is tough (it's a protein also found in fingernails) and the body produces extra keratin as an inflammatory response to protect the affected area. A callus is even in tone compared to a similar hyperkeratosis called a corn, which is cone-shaped.

▶ The surface of a corn is slightly raised and the cone grows inwards, for example into a toe that is under pressure, from, for example, tight-fitting shoes. The cone is made up of dead skin cells and, unlike calluses, a corn is painful. Corns can be removed by a qualified professional; hard skin can be removed by gently filing the skin.

Atopic dermatitis, also known as eczema, is also a hyperkeratosis condition, caused mainly by genetics or a skin irritant. Most people with eczema will have an environmental or biological trigger that makes the condition flare up, such as having a cold or eating/drinking dairy products.

Eczema takes the form of inflamed, itchy and cracked rough skin in patches across the body; common sites are the crease of the elbow, the backs of the knees, and around the eyes and mouth. In eczema, an opening appears between layers of skin, which prevents moisture reaching the skin's surface. This dries in the lower layers and forms an opening for bacteria to enter, causing infections. Topical corticosteroids (steroid creams) can be used to treat eczema. They come in different strengths; they will reduce inflammation, encourage vasoconstriction and supress the immune system, which speeds up healing.

Dehydration

The impact of dehydration on skin is temporary, causing a problem with the epidermis when the stratum corneum lipids are rearranged into deeper skin layers, and the lipid-to-water ratio is altered. The skin becomes stiffer and if the back of the hand is pinched the skin does not snap back as it should – its return is slower.

Possible causes

Common skin conditions can have a range of possible causes. Taking a detailed history from the patient or relative will provide a good indication of the cause of the condition. Some conditions are more common in babies (infantile eczema) or older adults (shingles).

Healthcare acquired skin conditions

Pressure injuries caused by excessive pressure to a specific part of the body are a common cause of patients staying in hospital for longer. People with reduced mobility or health conditions that prevent them from moving independently are at greater risk of developing pressure injuries. Continuous pressure applied to the layers of the skin causes blood supply to the skin to be reduced – resulting in the death of the surrounding tissues.

Pseudomonas aeruginosa is a type of germ that can cause skin infections and is a common hospital pathogen. Standard infection control precautions (SICPs) inform of the basic infection prevention control measures that reduce the transmission such as frequent handwashing, hand sanitiser and latex gloves to prevent transference.

Allergies

General allergies, such as a food allergy or insect bite, can be seen as a rash or **hives**. Areas of the skin that are in contact with an irritant such as jewellery or alcohol gel may show inflammation and, in some cases, small blisters or skin cracks and open sores.

Clinical conditions

Psoriasis is a clinical condition that is similar to eczema in appearance but has different causes and presents in some different locations. Eczema is more

> **Key terms**
>
> **Hives:** allergic reaction producing histamines, causing an area of skin swelling.
>
> **Psoriasis:** an abnormal immune response seen as areas of raised patches on the skin's surface.

> **Test yourself**
>
> Where are common sites for the conditions listed below? Give an example of a potential cause for each.
>
> 1 Hyperkeratosis   3 Pressure injury
>
> 2 Eczema   4 Contact dermatitis

common in children and psoriasis in individuals between the ages of 15 and 25 years.

▶ A person who is susceptible to psoriasis may experience a flare-up when they are stressed.

▶ Common sites for this itchy skin condition are the knees, elbow creases and lower back or scalp.

▶ Psoriasis causes a stinging, burning sensation and is less itchy compared to eczema; itchiness causes scratching and subsequent bleeding.

Trauma

Burns and scalds are damage to the skin usually caused by heat but can be caused by radiation, radioactivity, electricity, friction or contact with chemicals. Blisters and burns caused by heat are referred to as skin **trauma** injuries and vary in their severity.

Burns are measured in degrees, and these relate to how many layers of skin have been damaged. A first-degree burn, such as a steam thermal burn, affects only the epidermis. A second-degree burn, such as scalding from hot water, has damage to the epidermis and part of the dermis layer of skin. A third-degree burn, also known as a full-thickness burn, for example a hot object in contact with the skin for some time, destroys the epidermis and the dermis.

First- and second-degree burns are painful as there is damage to the nerves. A third degree burn burns through the layers where nerves are located meaning these may not hurt or may create less pain.

Friction, such as rubbing, generates heat that damages the skin's surface, and the damage becomes deeper the longer the friction continues. Similarly, the agent that causes a burn will affect the depth of burn depending on the type of agent (for example acid) and the length of time it is in contact with the skin.

A laceration is a cut to the skin and unlike an abrasion (graze), none of the skin is missing. A cut is typically caused by a sharp object, like a shard of glass, and is a split caused by a significant blunt force. A penetrating wound is caused when a foreign object pierces the skin and enters the body, creating a wound such as a thorn or stab wound.

An insect bite or sting can penetrate the skin's surface and introduce saliva or venom that causes the skin to swell, become red and, in some cases, itch. As the skin surface's protective layer has been penetrated the body is exposed, providing an opening for an infection to enter the bloodstream, particularly if the bite is scratched and any scab removed.

Practice points

S3.7 Assist with skin integrity assessments, treatment and care of skin conditions, working within scope of role, knowledge and responsibilities

You are a trainee nurse and have been tasked with producing a tri-folding leaflet to go in the GP waiting room's information area. The pamphlet will be in a leaflet rack, so the title needs to be eye-catching. For example, 'Common skin conditions'.

The aim of the leaflet is to educate patients and carers about different skin conditions. You will need to include informative images and text descriptions to illustrate the skin conditions listed below, with details of their transmission/cause, period of time they are likely to last (if appropriate) and an outline of treatments. Your images should include pale and darker skin tones and cover the following skin conditions:
- psoriasis
- eczema
- cuts and abrasions
- first- and second-degree burns
- dermatitis
- shingles
- allergy hives.

K3.4 How pressure injuries develop, the common sites, early symptoms and the preventative measures to avoid the development of a pressure injury

How pressure injuries develop

Pressure injuries develop when continuous pressure or friction is applied to an area of the body, causing damage to the surface of the skin and the underlying structures. This pressure has the effect of compressing the tissues and preventing oxygenated blood flow to pass through the skin layers, causing the tissue to die.

This area then develops into a pressure injury which can be graded from one to four in terms of its severity. Preventing pressure injuries is a safeguarding issue, and allowing them to develop is viewed as a form of neglect of duty of care.

Common sites of pressure injuries

Pressure damage can occur through lack of mobility or poor moving and handling techniques causing friction and shear to the skin layers. The most commonly affected sites across the body are bony prominences (see Figure 6.5). These are areas of the body that are exposed to additional pressure such as the heels, elbows, sacrum and shoulders (Figure 6.6).

The tips of ears and bridges of noses can also be affected by the presence of oxygen masks that are tightly applied to the face. Care must be taken to offload this pressure to prevent damage occurring.

Early symptoms of pressure injuries

Early signs of pressure injuries include:
- changes to the **colour** of the skin, for example redness in paler skin tones and blue/purple in darker skin tones
- depending on the depth of the damage and the presence of nerve endings at the site, the level of **pain** experienced may differ; some people will have a burning feeling, while others describe it as constant or **transient pain**; for some individuals the area affected can feel increasingly itchy. Older adults often have a higher pain threshold and may not notice that their skin is becoming damaged.
- the **area of damage may feel warmer or cooler than other areas** and will not blanch when additional pressure is briefly applied to it. This happens when there is no returning blood flow to the area as a result of the pressure damage caused.

The National Institute of Care Excellence (NICE) clinical guide, 'Pressure ulcers: prevention and management' (2014), suggests using the NPUAP/EPUAP Pressure Ulcer Classification System as a

---

Key term

Transient pain: pain that lasts for a short time.

Placements Of Pressure Ulcers

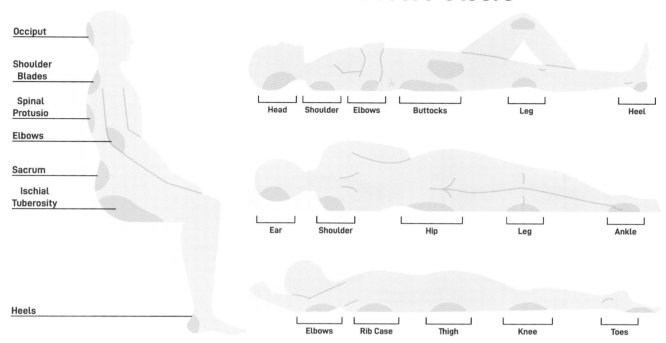

▲ Figure 6.5 Bony prominences

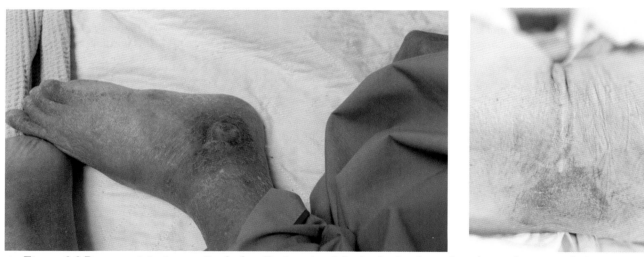

▲ Figure 6.6 Pressure injuries particularly affect parts of the body that have less fat and are weight-bearing

uniform guide when measuring the stage and level of damage of a pressure injury (Figure 6.7).

▶ Stage 1: injury has not caused the skin to be broken; it is a red/dusky coloured area.

▶ Stage 2: injury has caused a break in the epidermis and sometimes the top of the dermis.

▶ Stage 3: injury completely affects the epidermis, dermis and the fatty tissue. The skin may appear sloughy or infected.

▶ Stage 4: injury is a deep penetrating wound. Muscle, tendons, ligaments and bone may be visible.

Preventative measures

An estimated 700,000 patients are affected by pressure injuries each year in the UK, costing the NHS more than £3.8 million per day (Wood *et al.* 2019). Preventative measures must be in place for all patients, particularly those who are most at risk.

Source: Wood, J., Brown, B., Bartley, A., Margarida Batista Custódio Cavaco, A., Roberts, A. P., Santon, K. and Cook, S. (2019), 'Reducing pressure ulcers across multiple care settings using a collaborative approach', *BMJ Open Quality*, 8(3): e000409. **doi: 10.1136/bmjoq-2018-000409.**

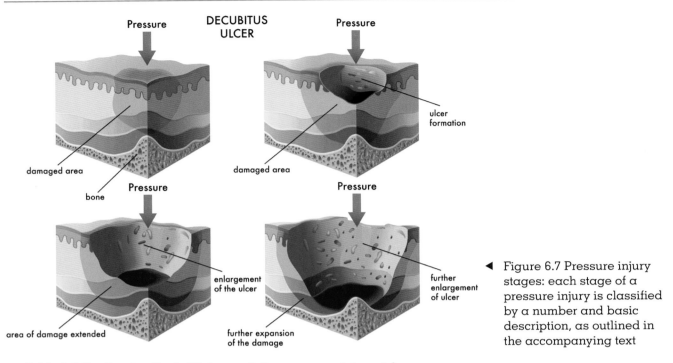

DECUBITUS ULCER

◀ Figure 6.7 Pressure injury stages: each stage of a pressure injury is classified by a number and basic description, as outlined in the accompanying text

▼ Table 6.2 The Braden Scale II© for predicting pressure injury risk

Sensory perception: ability to respond meaningfully to pressure-related discomfort	1. Completely Limited Is unresponsive (does not moan, flinch or grasp) to painful stimuli, due to diminished level of consciousness or sedation. OR Has limited ability to feel pain over most of the body.	2. Very Limited Responds only to painful stimuli. Cannot communicate discomfort except by moaning or restlessness. OR Has a sensory impairment that limits the ability to feel pain or discomfort over half of the body.	3. Slightly Limited Responds to verbal commands but cannot always communicate discomfort or need to be turned. OR Has some sensory impairment that limits ability to feel pain or discomfort in one or two extremities.	4. No Impairment Responds to verbal commands. Has no sensory deficit that would limit ability to feel or voice pain or discomfort.
Moisture: degree to which skin is exposed to moisture	1. Constantly Moist Skin is kept moist almost constantly by perspiration, urine, or other body fluids. Dampness is detected every time patient is moved or turned.	2. Often Moist Skin is often, but not constantly, moist. Linen must be changed at least three times a day.	3. Occasionally Moist Skin is occasionally moist. Linen must be changed at least twice a day.	4. Rarely Moist Skin is usually dry. Linen only requires changing at routine intervals.
Out of bed activity: degree of physical activity out of bed	1. Bedfast Confined to bed.	2. Chairfast Ability to walk severely limited or non-existent. Cannot bear own weight and/or must be assisted into chair or wheelchair.	3. Walks Occasionally Walks occasionally each shift, but for very short distances, with or without assistance.	4. Walks Frequently Walks outside the room at least twice a day and inside the room every two hours during waking hours.
In bed mobility: ability to change and control body position while in the bed or chair	1. Completely Immobile Does not make even slight changes in body or extremity position without assistance.	2. Very Limited Makes occasional slight changes in body or extremity position but unable to make frequent or significant changes independently.	3. Slightly Limited Makes frequent though slight changes in body or extremity position independently.	4. No Limitations Makes major and frequent changes in position without assistance.

Nutrition: food intake pattern	1. Very Poor	2. Probably Inadequate	3. Adequate	4. Excellent
	Never eats a complete meal. Rarely eats more than a third of any food offered. Eats two servings or less of protein per day. Takes fluids poorly. Does not take a liquid dietary supplement. OR Is NPO and/or maintained on clear liquids or IVs for more than five days.	Rarely eats a complete meal and generally eats only about half of any food offered. Protein intake includes only three servings per day. Occasionally will take a dietary supplement. OR Receives less than optimum amount of liquid diet or tube feeding.	Eats over half of most meals. Eats a total of four servings of protein per day. Occasionally will refuse a meal, but will usually take a supplement when offered. OR Is on a tube feeding or TPN regimen which meets nutrition needs.	Eats most of every meal. Never refuses a meal. Usually eats a total of four or more servings of protein per day. Occasionally eats between meals. Does not require supplementation.
Friction and shear	**1. Problem**	**2. Potential Problem**	**3. No Apparent Problem**	
	Requires moderate to maximum assistance in moving. Frequently slides down in bed or chair, requiring frequent repositioning with maximum assistance. Spasticity, contractures, or agitation leads to almost constant friction.	Moves feebly or requires minimum assistance. During a move, skin probably slides to some extent against sheets, chair, restraints, or other devices. Maintains relatively good position in chair or bed most of the time, but occasionally slides down.	Moves in bed and in chair independently and has sufficient muscle strength to lift up completely during move.	

A patient may have limited movement due to surgery, paralysis or an illness such as long COVID.

Adequate nutrition and hydration

Undertaking an appropriate nutritional risk assessment such as the Malnutrition Screening Tool (MST) on admission, and the monitoring of **adequate nutrition and hydration** during admission is one of the most important methods of preventing skin damage. Malnourishment will negatively impact wound healing and reduce the ability of the immune system to fight infection. Where a patient is identified as being at risk of malnourishment, they should be referred to a dietician and given dietary supplements as appropriate.

Malnutrition is a common complication in wound healing and has been cited as a key factor in the development of pressure injuries (NICE, 2014). Raising awareness of the importance of a balanced diet, and **advising individuals on nutritional** issues can be beneficial to those experiencing malnourishment as a result of illness or injury.

The average length of a hospital stay for a patient with a pressure injury is around 25 days (NHS Improvement, 2018). While an individual is in hospital, there is the opportunity to educate them and encourage **healthy eating habits** that can be continued after discharge.

Additional preventative measures include ensuring the skin is clean and protected from the damage caused by urine or faeces, applying barrier creams where continence management is required and monitoring any damage identified to the skin during repositioning. Furthermore, regularly inspecting the patients' skin over the bony prominences will enable action to be taken where damage is identified early.

Sources: NICE (2014), 'Pressure ulcers: prevention and management', www.nice.org.uk/guidance/cg179

NHS Improvement (2018), 'Pressure ulcer core curriculum', www.england.nhs.uk/wp-content/uploads/2021/09/Pressure-ulcer-core-curriculum.pdf

Comprehensive skin assessment

The Braden Scale is one example of a tissue viability risk assessment. It uses a scoring system to predict the likelihood of a patient developing a pressure injury and should be completed within six hours of an admission and then at regular planned intervals. You have already learned about this in ANPO1 K1.9. The document has six sub-categories, which are described and evidenced based on three studies that analysed its reliability as a written document to add to a care plan. NICE recommends the use of a tissue viability risk assessment such as Braden or Waterlow scales for the prevention and management of the risk of skin damage.

Sensory perception of skin damage must be considered, as pain is not always experienced during the development of skin damage. The ageing process can impact on the level of pain experienced by the older adult; therefore, using clinical judgement is also recommended when using any risk assessment tool. If communication or cognition are a barrier to understanding, other assessment tools can be used to aid understanding such as the Abbey Pain Scale. In the Abbey Pain Scale, the lower the score, the higher the risk: a score of 23 means no risk at all, while a score of 6 is severe risk.

The Waterlow assessment tool considers factors like nutrition, mobility, continence, age, pre-existing skin damage and current medication when assessing the risk of developing skin damage. It also takes into consideration a person's congitive ability and whether there has been a recent history of surgery. Like the Braden Scale, it uses a scoring system where a score of less than 10 means a low risk of developing skin damage, 10+ indicates someone is 'At Risk', 15+ is 'High Risk' and 20+ 'Very High Risk'.

As a result of these scores, additional pressure relieving equipment may be introduced, along with a strict repositioning regime and nutritional support. Body maps are also part of this risk assessment whereby the presence of damage is easily identified along with the grade of the damage and the subsequent healing.

Careful positioning

Careful and frequent repositioning, changing the points that are weight bearing to allow blood to the skin surface, will keep oxygenated blood going to the skin cells.

Attention must be paid to areas of skin that are already damaged and frail; it is of paramount importance that reposition should avoid these areas when shifting weight while positioning. A common site for minor skin friction is the heels; this may be an area that feels warm and on pale skin appears reddened. Being aware of potential areas which have been experiencing friction may mean that attention is paid to methods that reduce or prevent further friction.

A care plan will identify the regularity at which repositioning should take place, and two members of staff will be required to move the individual gently,

using the correct moving, handling and lifting techniques.

Use of equipment

Equipment used to relieve pressure when a patient is seated or lying down includes:

▶ Low-grade specialist mattresses: these are made of memory foam, or contain gel or water, and offer support-redistributing technology.

▶ Higher-grade mattresses: these are electrically powered, and use air inflation and deflation to constantly redistribute points of pressure.

▶ Pressure relief cushions can be used to off-set the pressure to areas such as heels and the sacral area.

▶ Healthcare professionals working in the community with patients in their own homes who have no specialist mattress can allocate air mattresses and pressure-relieving cushions to reduce the risk of skin damage.

Continence management

Incontinence can result in the skin coming into contact with urine and or faeces, causing damage to the outer layers and contributing to the risk of pressure injury.

▶ Continence-associated dermatitis starts as an inflamed rash caused by an increase in skin surface pH from urine and digestive enzymes from faeces.

▶ A patient with diarrhoea may have a skin burn as bile and stomach acid may be present in their loose stool.

▶ In extreme cases, a urinary catheter may be used to reduce the risk of urine being in contact with the skin. In the case of faecal continence issues, regular hygiene support, close monitoring and the use of barrier creams where prescribed are an important part of reducing the development of pressure injury.

Skin integrity assessments

Skin integrity means the overall health of the skin before any injury or burn. Impaired skin integrity can be caused by contact with an irritant or an inflammatory response due to contact with an allergen such as latex. Poor skin integrity refers to skin that has less blood flow to the surface due to age and pressure, is sensitive, susceptible to damage and has a slow healing rate. Damage to the skin is calculated in terms of depth of injury and extent, for example the size and depth of a pressure injury or burn.

Practice points

S3.9 Demonstrate the ability to provide the appropriate care to reduce the risk of pressure ulcers developing or deteriorating and record interventions

S3.10 Undertake and record interventions to treat and prevent skin conditions (for example repositioning of the individual) in line with your roles and responsibilities

Watch the video 'Prone positioning in severe acute respiratory distress syndrome' (NEJM Group, 2013), which you will find at this link: **www.youtube.com/watch?v=E_6jT9R7WJs**

You will need a manikin and a partner for this demonstration. Your task is to produce a training video where you narrate what you are doing and the purpose of each action.

Your patient is 82 years old. She has limited mobility and is confused. She is not ventilated but is having IV fluids. She has some areas of pressure concern when inspected, so she needs repositioning. You will need to make a sideways roll move with a partner.

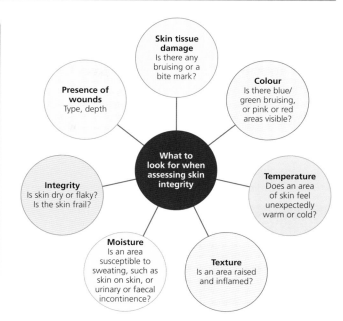

▲ Figure 6.8 What to look for when assessing skin integrity

K3.5 How to carry out assessments of skin integrity and why it is important to do so

Recognising those at risk of compromised skin integrity

A new patient admitted to a hospital or care setting should have a thorough examination of their skin and associated risk. This will **identify those most at risk of compromised skin integrity**, for example **someone with poor nutrition or someone who is immunocompromised**.

How to carry out assessments of skin integrity

Examine the skin

Figure 6.8 shows the aspects to look for when carrying out a detailed examination to assess skin integrity.

Document the outcome of the assessment

Using tools such as the Braden and Waterlow scales, along with a MST assessment, will ascertain those patients at risk. Swift preventative measures can then be put in place. Documentation should be completed and decisions made about the level and type of care needed

should be recorded in the patient's care plan. Patients admitted with existing pressure injuries will immediately be started with treatments and preventative methods to stop further deterioration. If a score identifies an individual is at high risk, escalation of concerns will be a requirement and an ongoing duty of care to stop further damage and begin the healing process.

Actions to be taken as a result of the assessment

Information relating to the actions to be taken as a result of the assessment is documented in the care plan:

▶ **Guidance** about the planned **dietary** needs and **fluid** intake will be given.

▶ A **positioning regime** will be established, and details of who is involved in this will be recorded; specific equipment may be needed, such as a slide sheet, repose boots or an air mattress.

▶ The care plan will state what **dressings are required as a result of existing skin damage**; those with clinical duties within their scope of practice for wound care will take responsibility.

Why it is important to carry out assessments of skin integrity

Reviewing measures put in place for monitoring purposes and assessing the effectiveness of a treatment plan are daily clinical requirements.

- **Early detection of risk and assessment of damaged skin** are important to maintaining skin integrity while an individual is hospitalised and after discharge.
- Any pre-existing pressure injuries will require accurate classifying using current guidelines, such as **EPUAP grading**, so that the **severity of existing damage** is known. This must be accurately recorded.
- The skin integrity assessment will **alert others** who are involved with the patient, including informal carers and relatives.

- **Frequent undertaking of skin integrity assessments reduces the risk of pressure injuries developing or deteriorating**. This is vital in reducing discomfort, length of hospitalisation and the likelihood of secondary infections such as sepsis.
- **Body mapping** highlights areas for concern in a visual document, **providing evidence** and information in a form that is easily understood.

Research

S3.8 Check skin integrity using appropriate assessment documentation and inform others

S3.9 Demonstrate the ability to provide the appropriate care to reduce the risk of pressure ulcers developing or deteriorating and record interventions

1 Visit the webpage at **www.torbayandsouthdevon.nhs.uk/services/care-of-the-elderly/support-videos/prevention-of-pressure-ulcers** to watch the following videos, which aim to educate patients and carers in different aspects of preventing pressure injuries:
   - Preventing pressure ulcers: top 10 tips
   - What to look for (identifying EPUAP grade 1 pressure injuries)
   - The power of food and drink
   - The importance of skin care
   - Using the right equipment.

   These informative videos are developed using language that is easy to understand, not medical terms.
   - Why do you think involving the patient, community carers and relatives is good practice for preventing and early detection of this type of skin wound?

2 Watch the video 'Pressure ulcer prevention: a guide for patients, carers and healthcare professionals' at **www.youtube.com/watch?v=0HRilRPjlY0**

   Reducing the risk of pressure injuries covers a multitude of aspects and can involve a multidisciplinary team (MDT), where all members have a role to play. The SSKIN care bundle (see page 187) is a resource pack that covers specific areas to assess risk, and this video presents discussions about preventative care from the perspective of different professionals working in the community.
   - How many professionals are involved in the community as part of the MDT?
   - Why is accurate recording of assessment and outcomes using uniform documentation good practice?

3 Watch the training video 'NHS Lothian induction: repositioning a patient in bed with minimal assistance', which you will find at **https://vimeo.com/402207032**
   - Would you be able to describe how you would carry out a solo move?

Case study

S3.8 Check skin integrity using appropriate assessment documentation and inform others

S3.9 Demonstrate the ability to provide the appropriate care to reduce the risk of pressure ulcers developing or deteriorating and record interventions

S3.11 Demonstrate the ability to advise and discuss with both individuals and carers about how to prevent pressure injuries

Carys is 82 and has been admitted to the ward at the start of your shift. She has a BMI of 17 and has fallen and hit her face on a table. Her nose is broken and face bruised so she cannot open her eyes. Doctors decided she needs monitoring as the head trauma is a concern and the cause of the fall was dizziness. She is responsive, a bit confused and does not want to stay in hospital as no one is home to take care of her cat.

You have been asked to check Braden and Waterlow scores, complete a body map and carry out a MST assessment, reporting any concerns to a line manager.

Carys responds to verbal commands but does not seem able to communicate discomfort or need to be turned. She has some urine incontinence, which may be temporary, and currently her skin is occasionally moist. Her pads are changed when she has leaked urine when moving, and she will require an extra linen change once a day and timely pad changes. She will be lying in bed with the side rails up as she is confused. Carys can reposition herself, but she is frail and makes only slight changes: she is mostly lying flat on her back, moving her legs and with some arm movements. Her heels and ankles glide along the sheet, but she tires easily. She has not eaten anything and had a cup of tea in A&E.

Although muddled, Carys is able to say she does not really have an appetite and that she misses meals since she no longer has her husband to cook for. She has lost at least a stone over the past six months. You have accessed previous blood tests, which show she is anaemic, and discovered she takes pain and anti-inflammatory (NSAID) medication for her osteoarthritis. Carys agrees for you to inspect her skin and you involve another staff member for a sideways roll so you can see her back. There is a pressure injury that has tissue damage in the dermis tissue on her lower back; it is uncovered and appears to be infected. Carys is unable to say how long she has felt uncomfortable as the pain medication she takes has masked this.

▶ Calculate scores and grade the pressure injury.
▶ Give any other relevant information referring to documents and images.
▶ Report your findings to your tutor, using appropriate technical language.

Your tutor will ask you to describe how you would reposition Carys and how frequently you would do this.

Treatment of skin conditions

Treatments for skin conditions vary greatly: a condition that causes inflammation, such as eczema, should improve with steroid cream; parasites found in the skin, such as scabies, are treated with an anti-parasitic cream; and dry skin conditions are treated with highly moisturising creams that do not have a perfume base. Other skin conditions can be improved with oral medication such as low-dose antibiotics for acne. Wounds that penetrate the skin are open to infection, as the barrier against microbes has been crossed; in such cases treatment of deeper wounds will focus on sealing the opening, if possible, and infection prevention measures. Pressure injuries, which are more common in older people, will require covering with gauze as a barrier following removal of any infected or dead skin. Good nutrition is an essential part of healing and will therefore form part of a care plan to support the wound healing process.

K3.6 The types of treatment that can be used to care for skin and prevent or treat skin conditions

The SSKIN care bundle is a framework for the management of skin integrity across all healthcare services. The bundle supports multidisciplinary team working with both care professionals and informal carers (or relatives) who may be offered training and education where appropriate.

Reflect

S3.11 Demonstrate the ability to advise and discuss with both individuals and carers about how to prevent pressure injuries

Communication can be in several formats. Care plan documents are continually updated – they can be handwritten or electronic, and patient history is available electronically. Training in the accurate and correct use of communication formats is needed before a trainee can enter clinical practice. Effective verbal and non-verbal communication is the number one tool in successful nursing. Medical professionals and nursing colleagues use medical terminology and acronyms, but understanding and using these are only half the story. Patients, informal carers and relatives require communications in a language they understand, with opportunities to ask questions of approachable staff. There is a level of translating one language to another, conveying empathy and providing information that overcomes communication barriers.

A patient may not understand information that is given to them but not ask for clarification, leading to fears, anxieties and stress.
▶ What might be the root cause of this?

Recognising this is a problem, observing and looking for signs of stress are important skills in effective communication.

Health and safety

Dead skin tissue around and in the pressure injury can slow healing. Removing the dead cells is a clinical process called **debridement**. A registered nurse may be able to remove the dead tissue as they clean a sore wound, and some dressings help with the clearing of dead tissue when removed. Not removing skin **necrosis** leads to infections and a further risk of sepsis.

▶ Gauze dressing is a less expensive form of dressing than some others but needs to be changed frequently. Surface dead tissue may come away from the wound when gauze is being replaced, which is a benefit.

▶ Alginate dressings absorb fluids produced by an infected pressure injury and will remove some dead tissue when changed but less frequently than gauze. This dressing is best for grade 3 and 4 pressure injuries.

▶ **Hydrocolloid dressings** are most suited to grade 2 and 3 pressure injuries. They are made of foam and contain a gel that absorbs some discharge. A **minimal adhesive covering**, for example **Melolin**, is placed over the dressing.

▶ Hydrogel dressings are gel based, 90 per cent water, and are ideal for dry and dehydrated wounds. They come as a thin fibre sheet, which is then sealed with **adhesive dressing**. Removal requires care and soaking the adhesive to prevent further skin damage.

▶ Transparent film dressings are for treating grade 1 pressure injuries. They offer a barrier against body excretions; the wound healing process can be seen and indicates when the dressing needs to be changed. Care in removing the dressing is needed so the adhesive does not rip the skin.

▶ Negative pressure wound therapy (NPWT) is for a deep wound. The necrosis tissue is removed and a foam dressing that is tailored to the patient's wound size and positioning is then used. A transparent covering is applied using a suction device, which creates a vacuum over the wound. Research has shown that this method of dressing speeds up the healing process.

The acronym SSKIN stands for:

S – Skin inspection: the use of Braden and Waterlow documentation

S – Surface: the patient's positioning (for example sitting or lying down) and current prevention methods

K – Keep moving: the patient's mobility and ability to reposition themselves

I – Incontinence: status of urine and faeces control/ retention

N – Nutrition: MST assessment, and nutrition and fluids monitoring.

In more recent years there have been improvements to the SSKIN bundle, with some additions: aSSKINg adds two letters to the acronym, the 'a' represents 'assess risk', while the 'g' highlights the need for 'giving information' to the patient and carers.

Topical treatments

Topical treatment refers to preventative or current treatment on a particular area of the body. A **barrier cream** is used to protect an area that is in contact with moisture such as urine. The cream creates a physical moisture-repellent barrier between the skin and urine or faeces while soothing any irritation.

Oral treatments

Oral treatments for skin may be given where there is an infection present. These medications are taken by mouth.

Dressings

Grade 3 and 4 pressure injuries may need necrosic tissue to be removed. Cleaning and wound care, such as dressing, speed up the healing process or slow further deterioration. In cases where an abscess has formed, this will need draining first before covering or packing to prevent it re-forming.

Other therapeutic interventions

Another pressure injury therapeutic intervention comes in the form of massaging the skin around the injury to increase blood flow; this will increase oxygen and hydration which will improve the speed of wound healing.

Phototherapy uses ultraviolet (UV) light directed onto an area of exposed skin and is used in the treatment of a wide range of inflammatory skin conditions. The

Key term

Necrosis: relating to the death of body tissue.

artificial intense light triggers a biological response, and a process that reduces inflammation and slows down skin cell renewal. Research into light therapy as treatment for psoriasis found that 50–90 per cent of people showed a noticeable improvement or complete remission.

Source: Institute for Quality and Efficiency in Health Care (IQWiG) (2021), 'Psoriasis: Learn More – Does light therapy (phototherapy) help reduce psoriasis symptoms?', www.ncbi.nlm.nih.gov/books/NBK435696/

Specialist equipment

Mattresses and cushions

In ANPO1 K1.13 you learned about pressure-relieving mattresses and their purpose: redistributing weight to change areas of pressure.

There are different types of specialist mattress that use this method, using an alternating flow of pressure relief to the body. For example:

▶ Hybrid mattresses use both foam and air in one support surface. Inflation of air bag 'cells' moves the body, working with gravity, onto foam in a different position depending on the location and intensity of inflation. This is often done manually but can be set up to be automated.

▶ Lateral rotation mattresses rotate the patient from side to side in order to cyclically change pressure points. It is a gentle continuous motion set electronically and provides pressure relief without disturbing the patient.

▶ Alternating or dynamic mattresses are made from air cells that inflate and deflate continuously. One cell will inflate and the next one deflate on a cycle, shifting weight distribution onto different points of the body.

In addition to a pressure-relieving mattress, it may be appropriate to use specialist cushions to put between a patient's knees or to temporarily have the weight of the head on the neck and lower head instead of the back of the head.

For seated areas, equipment other than mattresses and cushions directly addresses a need in a particular susceptible area.

Heel pads

A common location for pressure injuries is the heels of patients who spend a lot of time lying on their back. A ventilated patient, or an immobile individual, will have partial weight of the leg and foot on the surface of the back of the heel. Specialist foam or gel heel caps can be worn by the patient as cushioning, or an

inflatable foot protector can redistribute the weight, for example onto the calf, so the heel is not touching the bed. Similarly, foot elevation cushions that encircle the lower leg prevent the heel from surface contact. Fleece heel protectors allow air to circulate around the foot while cushioning and spreading the site of pressure.

Figure 6.9 depicts several methods of heel pressure injury prevention.

Repose boot

A repose boot is inflatable and can change pressure points with timely inflation and deflation without disturbing the patient. There are the same options to protect elbows as a bony prominence area.

Pressure ring

A foam seating cushion can relieve pressure from the tailbone area by simply having a hole cut out, so that pressure is on the top of the thighs instead. Pressure while seated is on the sitting bones at the bottom of the pelvis; relieving pressure from this bony prominence can be achieved by shape and design. Some pressure rings are inflatable and work using the same principle. However, the pressure ring is no longer used in practice after research questioned its suitability, as they cause additional pressure to build up at the sacral point.

Blanket cradle

A blanket cradle is a wire support that takes the weight of hospital bedding off an area of damage or potential damage.

Test yourself

S3.10 Undertake and record interventions to treat and prevent skin conditions in line with your roles and responsibilities

1   Describe the type of wound you would use the following dressings on and how you would apply and remove them safely:
    ▶ hydrocolloid
    ▶ non-adhesive dressing (such as Melolin)
    ▶ adhesive dressing.
2   Explain the purpose of steroid cream for treating eczema and psoriasis.
3   Explain the purpose of barrier creams.

You may want to use images to support your descriptions/explanations.

(a)   (b)   (c)

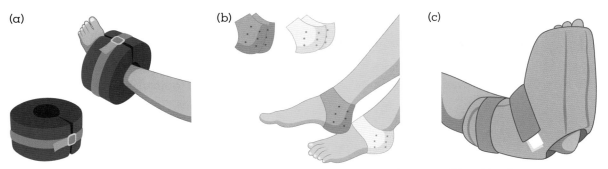

▲ Figure 6.9 Heel pressure injury prevention: (a) foot elevation cushioning; (b) gel heel cap protection; (c) inflatable heel protector

Assessment practice

Your task is to demonstrate the correct procedures when assisting with skin integrity assessments: maintain standards and health and safety and report any concerns you may have. You will need a manikin and a partner for moving and handling tasks.

You are to demonstrate your understanding of the Adult Nursing Performance Outcome 3 knowledge and skills, completing a number of tasks.

During your demonstration, you must narrate what you are doing using the correct terminology and explain why you are taking each action. You will need to describe skin conditions, expected patient pain and the expected response to skin treatments.

It would be an enhanced learning experience if you have your demonstration recorded, so you can evaluate your practical demonstration using Gibbs' reflective cycle to identify any areas for improvement.

You may refer to your notes related to:
▶ skin condition images (page 178)
▶ dressings (page 188)
▶ treatments (page 187)
▶ Braden Scale table (Table 6.2, page 182)
▶ Waterlow assessment tool (page 184)
▶ EPUAP pressure injury image grading stage (Figure 6.7, page 182).

You are working alongside a dermatologist. In the morning you are visiting patients on wards and in the afternoon you are working in outpatients. The dermatologist is using Peyton's four steps:
1 demonstrating assessment, diagnosing care and treatments, without commentary
2 breaking down steps, explaining and discussing these, deconstruction
3 demonstrating again, with explanation of different stages
4 observing your performance, which is video-recorded to enable you to self-reflect following feedback.

Tasks you will demonstrate:
1 a Carry out a Braden Scale assessment on a 70-year-old male patient who is sedated, ventilated and in the intensive care unit (ICU). He is malnourished and has open wounds on the tailbone area, elbow and the back of the head.
  b Dress the three areas of open pressure injury wound. Describe interventions to protect heels and further pressure injuries, and describe the importance of good nutrition and continence care.
2 Carry out a Waterlow assessment for a 42-year-old female patient with an estimated BMI of 34. Her diet is high in fats and sugars, and she tends to overeat. She has been diagnosed with type 2 diabetes, has stress incontinence when getting up, and has restricted movement due to her weight and oedema in the lower leg, wrists and hands. Inform the dermatologist of risk rating and make suggestions of how to support the patient to improve her situation.
3 Describe how the following skin conditions present in the different parts of the body listed, and explain the potential causes of these conditions:
  a psoriasis observed on the torso and scalp
  b eczema in elbow creases and on the back of knees
  c contact dermatitis around the neck and wrist
  d hives on the throat, upper arms and legs.
4 Describe the purpose of steroid creams, moisturisers and barrier creams.

Assessment

Assessment overview

The Occupational Specialism Assessment is a combination of three types of assignment:
- Case Study Assessment (CSA)
- Practical Activity Assessment (PAA) – split into parts A and B
- Professional Discussion Assessment (PDA)

These three assignments take place over a two-week window. There is an assessment task once a month from March until June.

These assignments are designed for you to incorporate learning from first year Core, second year Specialist Core and Supporting Adult Nursing component. You will demonstrate the foundation knowledge and specialist skills you have gained through industry placements and classroom-based simulations.

Assignment 1: Case Study Assessment (CSA)

You will be given an assignment brief and a case study, and you will be allocated 4 hours and 30 minutes to complete four tasks. This assessment focuses on appropriate care, accuracy, decision-making strategies, recommendations, principles and maintaining a professional standard.

The four tasks relate to one case study person. The assignment brief will contain several materials, for example a NEWS2 chart, which you will need to refer to as you work through each task.
- Task 1: Assessment of the patient and situation. [20 marks]
- Task 2: Goals/patient outcomes/planned outcomes [20 marks]
- Task 3: Care/treatment/support plan [20 marks]
- Task 4: Evaluation/monitoring effectiveness/clinical effectiveness [20 marks]

You are expected to produce a written analysis of each task. Drawing on your learning during the course; you will need to create a treatment plan using a person-centred approach and an evaluation of the evidence-based clinical actions to monitor effectiveness. Your completed work will be sent for external marking as one document.

The CSA is marked out of 80 and is 30 per cent of your end grade for the second year of this Health T Level qualification.

You will have internet access but only for specific web addresses indicated in the assignment brief.

Tips on how to prepare for the CSA

To prepare for the CSA, you could:
- Use the Practice points throughout this book as practice.
- Complete the Research and the Test yourself tasks throughout this book to broaden your understanding.
- Create your own glossary, noting down specialist terminology you could use in your four tasks.
- Refer to your Employer Set Project learning from your first year, as this assignment has similar content.
- Refer to past Assignment 1 tasks and compare the difference between mark band 1 and mark band 4 in the mark scheme for each of the four tasks.
- Refer to the reports from the Chief Examiner and Chief Moderator, which is commentary on what students across the country did well and where they could have improved their grade.
- Ensure you are using a person-centred approach when practising tasks.

Assignment 2 (Part A): Practical Activity Assessment (PAA) – Core

In the Core PAA, you will need to complete **three** practical activity scenarios that will assess your skills and knowledge in the Supporting Healthcare Core content.

The three practical assignment tasks will take place in three different assessment areas called 'stations'. The total time allowance is 1 hour 15 minutes, and you will have 5 minutes to familiarise yourself with the forms, equipment or manikin positions at each station.

Your teacher will give you an assessment booklet, the 'assignment brief', which contains the practical activity scenarios, and the timings for each. If you overrun on a task, your teacher will ask you to move onto the next.

Part A of the PAA is assessed against two mark schemes:

▶ A scenario-specific skills mark scheme
▶ An underpinning skills mark scheme

Your overall mark is for demonstrating the underpinning skills (duty of care, candour and person-centred care) and effective communication and health and safety actions.

At the end of this assignment, you will have three recorded demonstrations of you, focussed on specific healthcare competencies.

The assessment is marked out of 60, with 16 marks per task and an additional 12 marks for the underpinning skills. You will be awarded an underpinning skills mark for your performance across all three of the practical activity scenarios you demonstrate. The Core PAA is worth 20 per cent of your end grade for the second year of the Health T Level qualification.

The three practical activity scenarios are based on grouped healthcare Core Practical Assessments (CPAs), including CPA2 and two others from the list below.

Category heading	CPA	Skills/Knowledge	Description
Professional standards	1	S1.27, K1.4	Undertake a general or individual risk assessment in the healthcare environment: ▶ A general health and safety risk assessment ▶ A specific risk assessment for infection prevention ▶ An individual risk assessment relevant to the role in supporting healthcare.
	2	S1.34, S3.16, S3.17, S3.18, S3.19, S3.20, K3.1, K3.4, K3.5, K3.7, K3.8, K3.11, K3.14	Undertake and record a range of physiological measurements, recognising deteriorations in physical health and escalating as appropriate: ▶ Physiological measurements: — blood pressure, body temperature, respiration rate, heart rate, weight, height, urinary output, oxygen saturation and peak flow. ▶ Documentation: — blood pressure chart, body temperature chart, peak flow chart, weight/height chart, urine output chart and National Early Warning Scores 2 chart (NEWS2).
Health and safety, including infection prevention and control	3	S1.28, K1.5	Respond to an incident or emergency: ▶ Slip, trip or fall, an unresponsive patient, incidents of choking, bleeding wounds, a seizure and challenging behaviour (also referred to as 'behaviours that challenge').
	4	S1.29, K1.5	Demonstrate a range of techniques for infection prevention and control: ▶ Waste management, spillages and effective handwashing.
	5	S1.32, K1.9	Move and handle individuals safely when assisting them with their care needs, using moving and handling aids: ▶ Wheelchairs, a hoist, walking aids/frames, slide sheets, transfer belt, transfer board.
Clinical effectiveness	6	S1.31, S2.20	Assist in audit processes: ▶ Sharps boxes, clinical waste bins, manual and electronic information.

Category heading	CPA	Skills/Knowledge	Description
Comfort and wellbeing	7	S1.33, S1.34, S1.35, S1.39, K1.9, K1.12	Assist in the overall comfort and wellbeing of an individual, contributing, recording and following care plans and responding as appropriate: ▶ Pain management: medication ▶ Bed comfort and use of specialist mattress ▶ Environmental factors, considering heat and noise ▶ Social interaction, such as contact staff and visitors ▶ Access to media, including a mobile phone and TV ▶ Provide fluids and nutrition in terms of a balanced food and appropriate fluid intake ▶ Exercise or appropriate mobilisations.
Handling, recording, reporting and storing of information	8	S1.34, S1.39, S2.18, K1.10, K1.11, K1.15, K1.18	Assist in obtaining an individual's history and offer brief advice on health and wellbeing, recognising and responding as appropriate: ▶ Establish an individual's history, including physical, mental and social. ▶ Offer brief advice on physical activity, healthy lifestyle, smoking cessation, healthy eating and use of substances, including alcohol, legal and prescription drugs, illegal drugs, legal highs and solvent misuse.

Source: T Level Technical Qualification in Health, Occupational Specialism Assessment (OSA) Supporting Healthcare Tutor guidance, pages 13–16

Tips on how to prepare for the PAA – Core

To prepare for part A of the PAA, you could:

▶ Complete the healthcare Practice point demonstration tasks in this book: try to record yourself doing them and then carry out a thorough reflection afterwards. Use the recording to observe and note areas where you could improve. The more you practise, the more confident you will be in your demonstration and reflective practice.

▶ Refer to the 8 CPAs that group together knowledge and skills points that could be covered in a scenario station (see the table above).

▶ Refer to previous mark schemes for scenario-based competencies. Compare mark band 1 with mark band 4 and identify the areas to consider when carrying out Practice point scenario tasks.

▶ Refer to the mark scheme for underpinning skills. Compare mark band 1 with mark band 4 and identify the areas to focus on when carrying out Practice point scenario tasks; for example demonstrating duty of care, candour, and person-centred care, demonstrating your knowledge of health and safety and demonstrating effective communication.

▶ Work with peers, observing each other's demonstrations, marking them using the mark schemes and discussing the outcomes.

Assignment 2 (Part B): Practical Activity Assessment (PAA) – Option

For the Option PAA, you will need to complete four practical activity scenarios assessing skills and knowledge taken from the Adult Nursing Core content. The activities are grouped as separate Occupational Practical Assessments (OPAs).

The four practical assignment tasks take place in four different stations, and the time allowed is 1 hour and 15 minutes. You will have 5 minutes to familiarise yourself with the station at the start of each task.

The assessment is marked out of 76, with 16 marks per task and an additional 12 marks for the holistic underpinning Optional Core knowledge and skills. There are two mark schemes, which assess:

▶ Case study scenario specific skills
▶ General underpinning skills

At the end of the assignment, you will have four recorded demonstrations focussed on specific Supporting Adult Nursing competencies.

The grouped Supporting Adult Nursing Option Practical Assessment (OPAs) will include OPA6, OPA9 and two others from the list below. The Option PAA is worth 20 per cent of your end grade for the second year of the Health T Level qualification.

Theme	OPA	Skills/Knowledge	Description
Moving and positioning	1	S1.20, S2.12, S2.11, S2.13, S2.17	Move and/or position the individual for treatment or complete clinical skills, using moving and handling aids: ▶ Treatment: includes wound dressings, injections, catheterisation and administration of medication ▶ Clinical skills: include bathing of the body and hair, toileting, dressing and undressing, assisting with personal care needs and assisting with eating and drinking ▶ Aids: include wheelchairs, a hoist, sling, walking aids/frames, slide sheets and transfer board and belt.
Monitor and maintain clinical equipment	2	S1.22, K1.13	Perform first line calibration on clinical equipment: ▶ Automatic blood pressure monitor, manual blood pressure monitor, tympanic thermometer, pulse oximeter, weighing scales and glucometer.
Application of clinical skills	3	S1.17, K1.2	Perform the sequence to steps for basic life support (BLS).
	4	S1.18, K1.3, K1.4, K1.7	Demonstrate the ability to carry out clinical skills for individuals, including clinical assessments and reporting findings: ▶ Undertake and record physiological measurements including weight, height, temperature, blood pressure, BMI, respiration rate, heart rate, oxygen saturation, collection of urine and faecal specimens. ▶ Monitor fluid intake and output. ▶ Assess the need for a simple wound dressing.
	5	S2.19, K1.3, K1.4, K1.5, K1.7, K1.9	Support risk assessments for adults and escalate findings: ▶ Malnutrition Screening Tool (MST), wound, oral health assessment, continence, Bristol stool scale, fluid balance, nutrition assessment, pain assessment and mobility.

Theme	OPA	Skills/Knowledge	Description
Maintaining skin integrity and caring and treating skin conditions	6	S3.8, K3.5	Check skin integrity using appropriate assessment documentation and inform others: ▶ Body map, Waterlow or Braden risk assessment.
	7	S3.9, K3.5	Provide the appropriate care to reduce the risk of pressure ulcers developing or deteriorating and record interventions: ▶ Regular turning and positioning, support comfort and mobility by using bed type, seats and cushions.
	8	S3.7, S3.10, K3.6	Undertake and record interventions to treat and prevent skin conditions: ▶ Skin conditions, including psoriasis and eczema, cuts and abrasions, burns, and dermatitis ▶ Interventions, including apply non-prescription topical treatments (such as steroid creams, moisturisers and water-based creams) and apply and/or remove simple dressings, including cooling pads, hydrocolloid, adhesive dressing and non-adhesive dressing (such as Melolin).
	9	S3.11, K3.3, K3.4, K3.5	Advise and discuss with both individuals and carers about how to prevent pressure injuries: ▶ Areas of the individual's body that a carer should be assessing ▶ The signs of a pressure injury ▶ Simple techniques to prevent pressure injuries ▶ Signposting to appropriate services.
Promotion of health and wellbeing and independence	10	S1.18, S2.10, S2.17, S2.18, S2.19, K1.3, K2.1, K2.3, K2.6	Support or enable individuals to maintain good nutrition by promoting current healthy nutrition and hydration initiatives: ▶ Support individuals to make healthy choices, recording details using food and drink charts and nutritional plans and involving carers where appropriate.
	11	S2.12, S2.17, S2.18, S2.19, K2.1, K2.3, K2.6	Support or enable individuals to maintain good personal hygiene, involving carers where appropriate: ▶ Washing, bathing of the body and hair ▶ Promoting oral hygiene.
	12	S2.13, S2.17, S2.18, S2.19, K2.1, K2.3, K2.6	Support or enable individuals to dress and undress, involving carers where appropriate.
	13	S2.14, S2.19, K2.1	Support or enable individuals to be mobile in accordance with their individual needs: ▶ Walking frames, walking stick and crutches.

Source: T Level Technical Qualification in Health, Occupational specialism assessment (OSA) Supporting Healthcare Tutor guidance, pages 17–21

Tips on how to prepare for the PAA – Option

To prepare for Part B of the PAA, you could:

▶ Complete the Adult Nursing Practice point demonstration tasks, preferably recording yourself and thoroughly reflecting afterwards, using the recording to observe and note areas where you could improve. As with Part A, the more you practise the more confident you will be in your demonstration and reflective practice.

▶ Refer to the specification content for Adult Nursing Performance Outcomes 1, 2 and 3 for both knowledge and skills. Tick off what you feel competent in as this will highlight areas where you need to work on.

▶ Refer to the 13 OPAs that group together knowledge and skills points which could be covered in a scenario.

▶ Refer to previous mark schemes for scenario-based competencies: look at what is required for mark band 4 and identify the areas that you should consider when carrying out Practice point scenario tasks.

▶ Refer to the mark scheme for underpinning skills: compare mark band 1 with mark band 4 and identify the areas to consider when carrying out Practice point scenario tasks, for example person-centred care and service frameworks, demonstrating effective communication and demonstrating health and safety knowledge.

Assignment 3: Professional Discussion Assessment (PDA)

This assignment requires you to demonstrate your skills, knowledge and competencies in the context of an interview about your reflective practice. You will need to refer to your reflective practice portfolio that you should have compiled during the course. Identify where you have reflected on a demonstration of a specific healthcare Core skill (the CPAs) or an Adult Nursing skill (the OPAs). This can be knowledge and skills you have used in your industry placement or in a classroom practical demonstration, then reflected upon and recorded in your portfolio.

You will have 45 minutes preparation time for the discussion under exam conditions. This preparation time is your opportunity to refer to your reflection portfolio and make notes. The time allowed for the professional discussion is 1 hour.

You will be given an assignment with three themes. A theme relates to a topic area (for example assisting with a skin integrity assessment) and the knowledge, skills and professional behaviours and values that were required when supporting the Adult Nursing team. The theme will be integrated in tasks you have completed yourself or have observed a professional demonstrating.

For each theme, you will be asked two questions, which have a Part A and B. Each theme is worth 32 marks, made up of one 12-mark question and one 20-mark question. You will need to answer Part A first, followed by Part B when prompted. In total, the PDA is marked out of 96 and is 30 per cent of your end grade for the second year of the Health T Level qualification.

Tips on preparing for the PDA

To prepare for your Assignment 3, you could:

▶ Ensure you are building a reflective portfolio that is organised and clear throughout your course (you have only 45 minutes to refer to this when preparing for your professional discussion). Your answers will be based on your own learning and experience.

▶ Use the reflective model you prefer and practise applying this to your classroom and work placement demonstrations, for example Kolb's or Gibbs' reflective cycles.

▶ Prepare terminology used when discussing emotions relating to professional challenges that have contributed to your self-development and limitations you discovered.

▶ When receiving feedback from your placement mentor or tutor, evaluate the purpose and principles to enable you to develop actions to help you improve.

▶ Be aware of your personal behaviours during demonstrations that positively contribute to your performance and professional competencies, such as a person-centred approach.

▶ Be prepared to identify and describe areas for your short- and long-term future personal development when evaluating the last stage of your reflective model, for example professional shadowing for a particular purpose.

Glossary

5 Manual Handling Principles The 5Ps guidance on good practice – Plan, Position, Pick, Proceed, Place.

Adipose tissue A type of connective tissue that specialises in the storage of fat.

Angina Chest pain caused by reduced blood flow to the heart muscles.

Appendectomy Surgery under general anaesthetic to remove the appendix.

Arrhythmia A problem with the rate or rhythm of the heartbeat.

Aseptic technique The technique that healthcare professionals use to prevent cross-infection during procedures such as dressing changes, wound management, surgery etc.

Asperger's syndrome A developmental disorder that is a form of autism spectrum disorder. Symptoms include difficulties in socialising, misunderstanding sarcasm and social cues, and having behaviours and thinking patterns that can be rigid and repetitive.

Bariatric patient An individual who has a BMI greater than 30 and is classified as obese.

Barium swallow A medical examination of the oesophagus and stomach. The patient drinks a liquid called barium while having an X-ray which records the position of the barium and identifies any blockages along the gastrointestinal (GI) tract.

Biomedical scientists Scientists who conduct laboratory testing on fluids and tissue to support diagnosis and treatment of disease.

Biopsychosocial Involving the interaction of biological, psychological and social factors.

Calibration A procedure for detecting and fixing uncertainties in equipment used to take measurements.

Cellulitis Painful bacterial infection of the dermis layer of the skin.

Clostridium Difficile A bacterial infection of the colon, transmitted by poor hygiene when toileting, spread in faeces.

Coercion The practice of persuading someone to do something by using force or threatening them.

Colonoscopy A procedure similar to an endoscopy, in which the flexible tube camera is used to inspect the colon and rectum.

Colostomy surgery An operation to divert the end of the colon through an opening, usually in the mid- to lower abdomen, called a stoma.

Communicable disease Illness spread from one person to another caused by bacteria and viruses.

Consolability The rate/level to which an individual can be consoled, for instance feel less uncomfortable or respond to reassurance over a period of time, as a measurement.

Cytoplasm The material or protoplasm within a living cell.

Defecation Discharging faeces from the digestive system.

Delirium A decline in mental state characterised by disorientation, paranoia, hallucinations and agitation.

Deviations from the norm Readings that are higher or lower than the healthy norm of the physiological measurement.

Digital rectal examination An examination where a healthcare professional uses their finger (digit) to check for any problems inside a patient's bottom (rectum).

Dispensing A process where a qualified pharmacist prepares an order of medication(s) prescribed by a doctor, confirms a patient's details and checks they have understood the instructions.

Dorsum The back of a structure, in this case the hand.

Dosette box A tablet organiser with separate compartments for days of the week and time of day, for example morning, lunchtime and evening.

Duty of candour The legal obligation to be open and honest with individuals and/or their families about incidents as promptly as possible.

Duty of care The legal obligation to always act in the best interest of individuals and others to prevent negligence causing harm. It means you should act within your level of competence and not take on anything you do not believe you can safely do.

Emotional intelligence An individual's ability to manage their own emotions and to understand the emotions of the people they come into contact with.

Endoscopy A procedure where a tube camera, controlled by a doctor, is inserted in the anus for a lower bowel inspection. A tissue biopsy can be taken at the same time if necessary.

Enteral Passing through the intestine, either naturally via the mouth and oesophagus, or through an artificial means such as a nasogastric tube.

Epidermis Outer layer of skin, which acts as a protective barrier.

Family The people identified by an individual as significant and important to them.

Fluctuating readings The rise and fall of a numerical amount, such as blood glucose levels.

Gait The way a person walks, or their pattern of walking.

Gram-negative bacteria (GNB) Bacteria such as E. coli. that are highly resistant to antibiotics and therefore represent one of the world's most significant public health challenges.

Guthrie test A heel-prick capillary test to detect the presence of phenylketonuria markers.

Hives Allergic reaction producing histamines, causing an area of skin swelling.

Holistic A way of approaching the delivery of healthcare that considers the whole person, not just the part that requires physical treatment. It also takes into account an individual's intellectual, emotional and social needs.

Hydraulic stretchers Stretchers used in medical emergencies that are powered to lift and drop their height, are on wheels for smooth movement, and have side rails and straps to keep a patient safely in position.

Hyperthermia A core body temperature of above 38°C.

Hypothermia A core body temperature of below 35°C.

Ileostomy surgery An operation to divert the end of the small intestine, the ilium, through an opening in the mid-abdomen.

Immunocompromised It refers to individuals who have a weakened immune system, making them vulnerable to infections. The cause can be a medical condition, such as cancer, or immunosuppressive medication treatment, such as that for lupus.

Individual A person who may require care, assessment, investigation, support or treatment.

Informed consent Before making a final decision, a person receiving care or treatment has the right to be given all the relevant information about it.

Insomnia Changes in sleep patterns making it difficult to fall asleep, have quality sleep and stay asleep.

Integrated service Various health services collaborating as a multidisciplinary team, enabling them to offer responsive, easily accessible services that meet the population's health needs.

Least restrictive It refers to practice decisions that support a person's basic rights to freedom, with care actions that interfere with these rights at the lowest level necessary to provide safety.

Microscopical Using a microscope.

Multidisciplinary team (MDT) A group of professionals from one or more clinical disciplines collaborating to provide the appropriate medical treatment for an individual.

National Patient Safety Agency Body responsible for identifying and reducing risks to patients receiving NHS care. The organisation leads national initiatives to improve patient safety.

Necrosis Relating to the death of body tissue.

Neurodegenerative disease A group of health conditions where nerve cells do not transmit neural messages as they should and an individual loses normal functioning over time.

Octogenarian A person aged from 80 to 89.

Oedema A fluid build-up, often in ankles and hands, causing swelling and puffiness.

Palliative care Care that aims to achieve the best quality of life possible, as actively as possible, until the individual's death from a terminal illness. It is a holistic approach and supports the individual and their family.

Partner The person considered by an individual to be their life partner.

Patient A person receiving care, support or treatment.

Penile sheath Silicone tube condom attached to a urine collection bag.

Perineal care A cleaning method for genital hygiene to prevent infection; there are different methods for patients of different genders.

Person-centred care Focusing care on the needs, values and preferences of the individual, and ensuring any clinical decisions are guided by these needs, values and preferences.

Postnatal depression A type of depression experienced by parents that impacts on functioning; symptoms are low mood, anxiety and crying, causing concerns for the baby's welfare.

Postpartum depression Similar to postnatal depression, but in this case care for the baby is not considered a concern.

Practitioner A person appropriately qualified in the practice of an occupation, for example a maternity support worker or a midwife. Practitioners may be registered or unregistered.

Pre-op clinic An outpatients department that specialises in carrying out tests in advance of a surgical procedure, to measure a person's health and suitability.

Proctoscopy An examination where a medical professional looks directly at the anal canal using a rigid inflexible proctoscope.

Psoriasis An abnormal immune response seen as areas of raised patches on the skin's surface.

Reflux When stomach acid repeatedly backflows through the oesophagus sphincter.

Revalidation a process that all nurses and midwives in the UK must complete to check their competence and maintain their registration with the NMC.

Roper–Logan–Tierney Model It defines what living means and the daily tasks a person needs to perform. It provides a framework to assess a patient's ability to carry out these tasks independently.

Scope of practice Sets out the limits of responsibility and ensures individuals do not undertake work outside their level of training or competence.

Scope of role Range of activities, duties or responsibilities that an employee is reasonably expected to carry out or fulfil within the remit of their job or position.

Service user A person receiving or using healthcare services.

Skin turgor The skin's elasticity and its ability to change shape and return to normal.

Sluice room A specialist infection prevention room for storing bed/bedside toileting equipment, and for the safe and effective disposal of human waste.

Sphygmomanometer An instrument with a rubber cuff, gauge and inflation bulb, used for measuring blood pressure manually.

Spirometer Assessment equipment to assist with diagnosing and monitoring of certain lung conditions by measuring how much air is inhaled and exhaled in one forced breath.

Standard infection control precautions (SICPs) Basic infection prevention and control measures as part of good practice to reduce the risk of infection transmission.

Stigma Negative perception associated with a particular person or circumstance.

Talking therapies Treatments that involve talking to a trained professional, such as a counsellor, about thoughts, feelings and behaviour.

Therapeutic intervention A course of action with the intention of managing a patient's physical or mental wellbeing to achieve a positive outcome, with the aim of avoiding the need for further treatment.

Transient pain Pain that lasts for a short time.

Tympanic membrane sensors Infrared sensors used to measure body temperature, usually inside the ear.

Index